Evidence-based Clinical Chinese Medicine

Volume 18

Cancer Pain

Evidence-based Clinical Chinese Medicine

Print ISSN: 2529-7562
Online ISSN: 2529-7554

Published

Vol. 1 *Chronic Obstructive Pulmonary Disease*
by Charlie Changli Xue and Chuanjian Lu

Vol. 2 *Psoriasis Vulgaris*
Lead Authors: Claire Shuiqing Zhang and Jingjie Yu

Vol. 3 *Chronic Urticaria*
Lead Authors: Meaghan Coyle and Jingjie Yu

Vol. 4 *Adult Asthma*
Lead Authors: Johannah Shergis and Lei Wu

Vol. 5 *Allergic Rhinitis*
Lead Authors: Claire Shuiqing Zhang and Qiulan Luo

Vol. 6 *Herpes Zoster and Post-herpetic Neuralgia*
Lead Authors: Meaghan Coyle and Haiying Liang

Vol. 7 *Insomnia*
Lead Authors: Johannah Shergis and Xiaojia Ni

Vol. 8 *Alzheimer's Disease*
Lead Authors: Brian H May and Mei Feng

Vol. 9 *Vascular Dementia*
Lead Authors: Brian H May and Mei Feng

Vol. 10 *Diabetic Kidney Disease*
Lead Authors: Johannah Shergis and Lihong Yang

Vol. 11 *Acne Vulgaris*
Lead Authors: Meaghan Coyle and Haiying Liang

More information on this series can also be found at https://www.worldscientific.com/series/ebccm

(*Continued at end of book*)

Evidence-based Clinical Chinese Medicine

Co Editors-in-Chief

Charlie Changli Xue
RMIT University, Australia

Chuanjian Lu
Guangdong Provincial Hospital of Chinese Medicine, China

Volume 18

Cancer Pain

Lead Authors

Brian H May
RMIT University, Australia

Yihong Liu
Guangdong Provincial Hospital of Chinese Medicine, China

World Scientific

NEW JERSEY • LONDON • SINGAPORE • BEIJING • SHANGHAI • HONG KONG • TAIPEI • CHENNAI • TOKYO

Published by

World Scientific Publishing Co. Pte. Ltd.
5 Toh Tuck Link, Singapore 596224
USA office: 27 Warren Street, Suite 401-402, Hackensack, NJ 07601
UK office: 57 Shelton Street, Covent Garden, London WC2H 9HE

Library of Congress Cataloging-in-Publication Data
Names: Xue, Charlie Changli, author. | Lu, Chuan-jian, 1964– author.
Title: Evidence-based clinical Chinese medicine / Charlie Changli Xue, Chuanjian Lu.
Description: New Jersey : World Scientific, 2016. | Includes bibliographical references and index.
Identifiers: LCCN 2015030389| ISBN 9789814723084 (v. 1 : hardcover : alk. paper) |
ISBN 9789814723091 (v. 1 : paperback : alk. paper) |
ISBN 9789814723121 (v. 2 : hardcover : alk. paper) |
ISBN 9789814723138 (v. 2 : paperback : alk. paper) |
ISBN 9789814759045 (v. 3 : hardcover : alk. paper) |
ISBN 9789814759052 (v. 3 : paperback : alk. paper)
Subjects: | MESH: Medicine, Chinese Traditional--methods. | Clinical Medicine--methods. |
Evidence-Based Medicine--methods. | Psoriasis. | Pulmonary Disease, Chronic Obstructive.
Classification: LCC RC81 | NLM WB 55.C4 | DDC 616--dc23
LC record available at http://lccn.loc.gov/2015030389

Volume 18: Cancer Pain
ISBN 978-981-123-793-5 (hardcover)
ISBN 978-981-123-928-1 (paperback)
ISBN 978-981-123-794-2 (ebook for institutions)
ISBN 978-981-123-795-9 (ebook for individuals)

British Library Cataloguing-in-Publication Data
A catalogue record for this book is available from the British Library.

For any available supplementary material, please visit
https://www.worldscientific.com/worldscibooks/10.1142/12306#t=suppl

Disclaimer

The information in this book is based on systematic analyses of the best available evidence for Chinese medicine interventions both historical and contemporary. Every effort has been made to ensure accuracy and completeness of the data herein. This book is intended for clinicians, researchers and educators. The practice of evidence-based medicine consists of consideration of the best available evidence, practitioners' clinical experience and judgment, and patients' preference. Not all interventions are acceptable in all countries. It is important to note that some of the substances mentioned in this book may no longer be in use, may be toxic, may be prohibited in some jurisdictions, or may be restricted under the provisions of the Convention on International Trade in Endangered Species of Wild Fauna and Flora (CITES). Practitioners, researchers and educators are advised to comply with the relevant regulations in their country and with the restrictions on the trade in species included in CITES appendices I, II and III. This book is not intended as a guide for self-medication. Patients should seek professional advice from qualified Chinese medicine practitioners.

Foreword

Since the late 20th century, Chinese medicine, including acupuncture and herbal medicine, has been increasingly used throughout the world. The parallel development and spread of evidence-based medicine have provided challenges and opportunities for Chinese medicine.

The opportunities have been evidence-based medicine's emphasis on the effective use of the best available clinical evidence, incorporating the clinicians' clinical experience, subject to patients' preference. Such practices have a patient focus which reflects the historical nature of Chinese medicine practice. However, the challenges are also significant due to the fact that, despite the long-term development and very rich literature accumulated over 2,000 years, there is an overall lack of high-level clinical evidence for many of the interventions used in Chinese medicine.

To address this knowledge gap, we need to generate clinical evidence through high-quality clinical studies, evaluate evidence to enable effective use of the available evidence, and promote evidence-based Chinese medicine practice.

Modern Chinese medicine is rooted in its classical literature and the legacies of ancient doctors, grounded in the practice of expert clinicians and increasingly informed by clinical and experimental research efforts. In recognition of the unique features of Chinese medicine, for each of the conditions in this series a 'whole-evidence' approach is used to provide a synthesis of different types and levels of evidence to enable practitioners to make clinical decisions informed by the current best evidence.

There are four main components of this 'whole-evidence' approach. In the first component, we present the current approaches to the diagnosis, differentiation and treatment of each condition based on expert consensus, as published in textbooks and clinical guidelines. This provides an overview of how the condition is currently managed. The second component provides an analysis of the condition in historical context based on systematic searches of the *Zhong Hua Yi Dian* 中华医典 which includes the full texts of more than 1,000 classical medical books. These analyses provide objective views on how the condition has been treated over two millennia, reveal continuities and discontinuities between traditional and modern practice, and suggest avenues for future research.

The third component is the assessment of evidence derived from modern clinical studies of Chinese medicine interventions. The methods established by the *Cochrane Collaboration* are used for conducting systematic reviews and undertaking meta-analyses of outcome data for randomised controlled trials (RCTs). In addition, the clinical relevance of meta-analysis data is enhanced by examining the herbal formulas, individual herbs and acupuncture treatments that were assessed in the RCTs and the evidence base is broadened by the inclusion of data from controlled clinical trials and non-controlled studies. The fourth component is to determine how the herbal medicine interventions may achieve the effects indicated by the clinical trials. Thus for each of the most frequently used herbs we provide reviews of their effects in pre-clinical models and their likely mechanisms of action.

For each condition, this 'whole-evidence' approach links clinical expertise, historical precedent, clinical research data and experimental research to provide the reader with assessments of the current state of the evidence of efficacy and safety for Chinese medicine interventions using herbal medicines, acupuncture and moxibustion and other health care practices such as *tai chi* 太赤.

Since these books are available in Chinese and English, they can benefit patients, practitioners and educators internationally and enable practitioners to make clinical decisions informed by the current best evidence.

These publications represent a major milestone in Chinese medicine development and make a significant contribution to the progess of evidence-based Chinese medicine globally.

Co-editors-in-Chief

Distinguished Professor Charlie Changli Xue,
RMIT University, Australia

Professor Chuanjian Lu, Guangdong Provincial Hospital of
Chinese Medicine, China

Purpose of This Book

This book is intended for clinicians, researchers and educators. It can be used to inform tertiary education and clinical practice by providing systematic, multi-dimensional assessments of the best available evidence for using Chinese medicine to manage each common clinical condition.

How to Use This Book

Some Definitions

A glossary is included, containing terms and definitions which frequently appear in the book. It also describes the definitions of statistical tests, methodological terms, evaluation tools and interventions. For example, in this book, *integrative medicine* refers to the combined use of a Chinese medicine treatment with conventional medical management, and *combination therapies* refer to two or more Chinese medicines from different therapy groups (Chinese herbal medicine, acupuncture or other Chinese medicine therapies) administered together. Terminology used throughout the book is based on the World Health Organisation's *Standard Terminologies on Traditional Medicine in the Western Pacific Region* (2007) where possible or from the cited reference.

Data Analysis and Interpretation of Results

In order to synthesise the clinical evidence, a range of statistical analysis approaches is used. In general, the effect size for dichotomous data is reported as a risk ratio (RR) with 95% confidence interval (CI), and for continuous data, effect size is reported as mean difference (MD) with 95% CI. Statistically significant effects are indicated with an asterisk*. Readers should note that statistically significant does not necessarily correspond with a clinically important effect. Interpretation of results should take into consideration the clinical significance, quality of studies (expressed as high, low or unclear risk of bias in this book) and heterogeneity amongst the studies. Tests for heterogeneity are conducted using the I^2 statistic. An I^2 score greater than 50% was considered to indicate substantial or considerable heterogeneity.

Use of Evidence in Practice

The Grading of Recommendations Assessment, Development and Evaluation (GRADE) approach was used to summarise the quality of evidence and results of the strength of evidence for critical and important comparisons and outcomes. Due to the diverse nature of Chinese medicine practice, treatment recommendations are not included with the summary-of-findings tables. Therefore readers will need to interpret the evidence with reference to the local practice environment.

Limitations

Readers should note some of the methodological limitations on classical literature and clinical evidence.

- Search terms used to search the *Zhong Hua Yi Dian* 中华医典 database may not include all terms that have been used for the condition. Inclusion of additional terms may alter the findings.
- Chinese language has changed over time. Citations have been interpreted for analysis, and such interpretations may be subject to disagreement.
- Chinese medicine theory has evolved over time. As such, concepts described in classical Chinese medical literature may no longer be found in contemporary works.

- Symptoms described in classical citations may be common to many conditions, and a judgement was required to determine the likelihood of the citation being related to the condition. This may have introduced some bias due to the subjective nature of the judgement.
- The vast majority of the clinical evidence for Chinese medicine treatments has come from China. The applicability of the findings to other populations and other countries requires further assessment.
- Many studies included participants with varying disease severity. Where possible, subgroup analyses were undertaken to examine the effects in different subpopulations. As this was not always possible, the findings may be limited to the population included, and not to subpopulations.
- The potential risk of bias found in many included studies suggested methodological limitations. The findings for GRADE assessments based on studies of very low to moderate quality evidence should be interpreted accordingly.
- Nine major English- and Chinese-language databases plus clinical trial registeries were searched to identify clinical studies. Other studies may exist which were not identified through searches, and which may alter the findings.
- The calculation of frequency of herbal formula use was based on formula names. It is possible that studies evaluated herbal treatments with the same or similar herb ingredients, but the herbal treatments were unamed or were given different formula names. Due to the complexity of herbal formulas, it was considered not appropriate to make a judgement as to the similarity of formulas for analysis. As such, the frequency of formulas reported in Chapter 5 may be underestimated.
- The most frequently utilised herbs which may have contributed to the treatment effect have been described in Chapter 5. These herbs may provide leads for further exploration. Calculation of the herbs with potential effect is based on frequency of formulas reported in the studies, and does not take into consideration the clinical implications and functions of every herb in a formula.

Authors and Contributors

CO-EDITORS-IN-CHIEF

Dist. Prof. Charlie Changli Xue (*RMIT University, Australia*)
Prof. Chuanjian Lu (*Guangdong Provincial Hospital of Chinese Medicine, China*)

CO-DEPUTY EDITORS-IN-CHIEF

Assoc. Prof. Anthony Lin Zhang (*RMIT University, Australia*)
Dr. Brian H May (*RMIT University, Australia*)
Prof. Xinfeng Guo (*Guangdong Provincial Hospital of Chinese Medicine, China*)
Prof. Zehuai Wen (*Guangdong Provincial Hospital of Chinese Medicine, China*)

LEAD AUTHORS

Dr. Brian H May (*RMIT University, Australia*)
Dr. Yihong Liu (*Guangdong Provincial Hospital of Chinese Medicine, China*)

CO-AUTHORS

RMIT University (*Australia*):
Assoc. Prof. Anthony Lin Zhang
Prof. Charlie Changli Xue

Guangdong Provincial Hospital of Chinese Medicine (*China*):
Dr. Yihan He
Dr. Haibo Zhang
Prof. Xinfeng Guo
Prof. Chuanjian Lu

Members of Advisory Committee and Panel

Co-chairs of Project Planning Committee

Prof. Peter J Coloe (*RMIT University, Australia*)
Prof. Yubo Lyu (*Guangdong Provincial Hospital of Chinese Medicine, China*)
Prof. Dacan Chen (*Guangdong Provincial Hospital of Chinese Medicine, China*)

Centre Advisory Committee (in Alphabetical order)

Prof. Keji Chen (*The Chinese Academy of Sciences, China*)
Prof. Aiping Lu (*Hong Kong Baptist University, China*)
Prof. Caroline Smith (*University of Western Sydney, Australia*)
Prof. David F Story (*RMIT University, Australia*)

Methodology Expert Advisory Panel (in Alphabetical order)

Prof. Zhaoxiang Bian (*Hong Kong Baptist University, China*)
The late Prof. George Lewith (*University of Southampton, United Kingdom*)
Prof. Jianping Liu (*Beijing University of Chinese Medicine, China*)
Prof. Frank Thien (*Monash University, Australia*)
Prof. Jialiang Wang (*Sichuan University, China*)

Content Expert Advisory Panel (in Alphabetical order)

Assoc. Prof. Depei Li (*Department of Critical Care, University of Texas MD Anderson Cancer Center, United States*)
Prof. Pingping Li (*Beijing Cancer Hospital, China*)
Prof. Zhongjun Xia (*Sun Yat-Sen University Cancer Hospital, China*)

Distinguished Professor Charlie Changli Xue

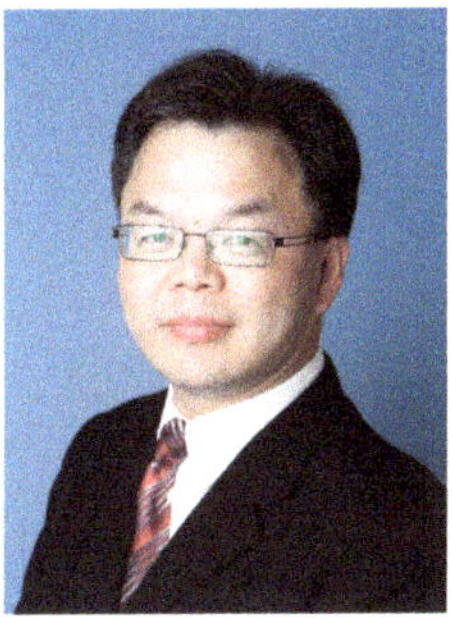

Distinguished Professor Charlie Changli Xue holds a Bachelor of Medicine (majoring in Chinese Medicine) from Guangzhou University of Chinese Medicine, China (1987) and a PhD from RMIT University, Australia (2000). He has been an academic, researcher, regulator and practitioner for almost three decades. Professor Xue has made significant contributions to evidence-based educational development, clinical research, regulatory framework and policy development and provision of high-quality clinical care to the community. Distinguished Professor Xue is recognised internationally as an expert in evidence-based traditional medicine and integrative health care.

Distinguished Professor Xue was the Inaugural National Chair of the Chinese Medicine Board of Australia appointed by the Australian Health Workforce Ministerial Council (in 2011). He was reappointed for a second term in 2014 and a third term in 2017. Since 2007, he has been a Member of the World Health Organisation (WHO) Expert Advisory Panel for Traditional and Complementary Medicine, Geneva. Distinguished Professor Xue is also Honorary Senior Principal Research Fellow at the Guangdong Provincial Academy of Chinese Medical Sciences, China.

At RMIT, Distinguished Professor Xue is Executive Dean, School of Health and Biomedical Sciences. He is also Director, WHO Collaborating Centre for Traditional Medicine.

Between 1995 and 2010, Distinguished Professor Xue was Discipline Head of Chinese Medicine at RMIT University. He led the development of five successful undergraduate and postgraduate degree programmes in Chinese Medicine at RMIT University which is now a global leader in Chinese medicine education and research.

Distinguished Professor Xue's research has been supported by research grants of over AUD 15 million, including six project grants from the Australian Government's National Health and Medical Research Council (NHMRC) and two Australian Research Council (ARC) grants. He has contributed over 200 publications and has been frequently invited as keynote speaker for numerous national and international conferences. Distinguished Professor Xue has contributed to over 300 media interviews on issues related to complementary medicine education, research, regulation and practice.

Professor Chuanjian Lu

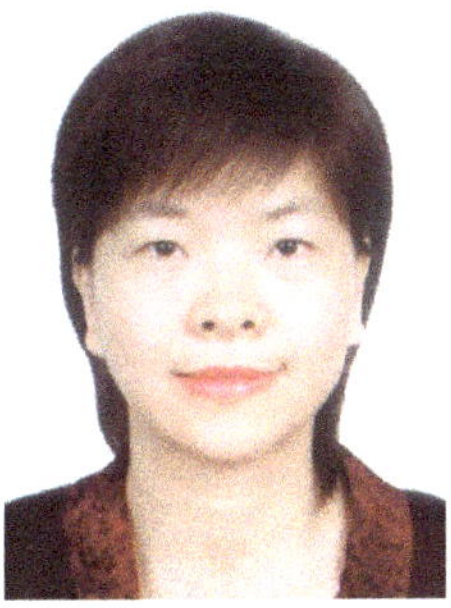

Professor Chuanjian Lu is Vice-president of Guangdong Provincial Hospital of Chinese Medicine (Guangdong Provincial Academy of Chinese Medical Sciences, Second Clinical Medical College of Guangzhou University of Chinese Medicine). She also is Chair of the Guangdong Traditional Chinese Medicine (TCM) Standardisation Technical Committee, and the Vice-chair of the Immunity Specialty Committee of the World Federation of Chinese Medicine Societies (WFCMS).

Professor Lu has engaged in scientific research into TCM, clinical practice and teaching for some 25 years. Her research has been devoted to integrating traditional and Western medicine. She has edited and published 12 monographs and 120 academic research articles as first author and corresponding author with over 30 articles being included in SCI journals.

She has received widespread recognition for her achievements with awards for Excellent Teacher of South China, National Outstanding Women TCM Doctor and National Outstanding Young Doctor of TCM. She also received the Science and Technology Star of the Association of Chinese Medicine, the National Excellent Science and Technology Workers of China Award and the Five-continent Women's Scientific Award of China Medical Women's Association.

Professor Lu has won the Award of Science and Technology Progress over ten times from Guangdong Provincial Government, China Association of Chinese Medicine and Chinese Hospital Association.

Acknowledgements

The authors and contributors would like to acknowledge the valuable contributions of the following people who assisted with database searches, data extraction, data screening, data assessment, translation of documents, editing and/or administrative tasks: Su-yueh Chang, Dr. Menghua Chen, Dr. Meaghan Coyle, Dr. Jhodie Duncan, Jiaming Fan, Shaonan Liu, Lihong Yang, Jing Chen, Dr. Claire Zhang and Dr. Iris Zhou.

Contents

List of Figures

List of Tables

1

Introduction to Cancer Pain

OVERVIEW

This chapter introduces cancer pain from the perspective of modern medicine. It outlines the features of cancer pain, its prevalence and risk factors, how cancer pain is diagnosed and the intensity determined, and it provides a summary of cancer pain syndromes. The management of cancer pain in conventional medicine is described, including the application of the analgesic ladder, the management of breakthrough pain and the alleviation of the adverse effects of opioids. In addition, interventional approaches, radiotherapy, and topical pharmacotherapy and non-pharmacotherapy approaches are outlined, and rehabilitation and palliative care are briefly discussed.

Definition of Cancer Pain

The clinical guideline in adult cancer pain issued by the National Comprehensive Cancer Network (NCCN) adopted the definition of pain from the International Association for the Study of Pain (IASP) as follows: 'An unpleasant sensory and emotional experience associated with actual or potential tissue damage, or described in relation to such damage'.[1] In the *International Statistical Classification of Diseases* (ICD10), the term 'neoplasm-related pain (acute) (chronic)' (Diagnosis Code G89.3) refers to cancer-associated pain, pain due to malignancy (primary) (secondary), and/or tumour-associated pain.[2,3]

In this book, we include pain in adults relating to the presence of neoplasms and pain associated with cancer treatments, but we exclude pain associated with surgery for cancer (time ≤ three months) since such pain is classified under the various ICD10 codes for postoperative and postprocedural pain (G89.18, G89.28) which are not specific to cancer.[3]

Clinical Presentation and Subtypes

Pain in cancer may be directly due to the tumour, may be related to the various therapies the patient has received, may be due to issues not directly related to the cancer such as immobility, atrophy and degeneration, or may be due to a combination of these and other factors. Usually pain is part of a cluster of symptoms and signs that include social and psychological aspects.[4] Cancer-related pain may be acute or chronic. It can be described according to its apparent causes, such as nociceptive pain due to stimulation of pain receptors by tumour growth; neuropathic pain due to pressure on nerves or injury of nerve tissues by chemotherapy; and by its presentation and/or location, such as bone pain, soft tissue pain, visceral pain and referred pain. Other types include pain following radiotherapy, pain associated with adverse reactions to chemotherapy and phantom pain in the part of the body removed by surgery.[5,6] Currently, the types of cancer pain are categorised into syndromes which are outlined below.[1,4,7,8]

Epidemiology

A review of 64 studies found only a few reports of pain prevalence at the time of cancer diagnosis (range 35–38%).[9] In cancer patients, considerably more data were available. The weighted mean pain prevalence was 45.6% (range 21.4–84.1%), but in advanced cancer the weighted mean prevalence was 76.1% (range 53–100%) and in the last year of life it was 73.9% (range 53–100%). However, rates varied considerably by cancer type. In breast cancer, prevalence ranged from 23% to 92% based on 18 studies; in lung/respiratory cancers the range was 17–86% (13 studies); in head and neck cancers it was 25–91% (ten studies); whereas in pancreatic cancer it was 72–100% (5 studies). All estimates showed wide ranges, which was likely reflective of disease severity. For example, 40% of patients with non-metastatic breast cancer reported pain versus 64% in patients with metastatic disease.[9] Another systematic review found that rates varied with the stage of treatment with an overall pain prevalence of 39.3% after curative treatment, and in breast cancer survivors this was 45.1%. During anticancer treatment pain prevalence was 55.0% and there was a prevalence of 66.4% in advanced or metastatic cancers, or terminal disease. In terms of pain severity, the prevalence of moderate to severe pain (NRS≥5) was 38.0%. Age was not associated with overall pain prevalence but patients with poor Eastern Cooperative Oncology Group (ECOG) performance status (ECOG 2–3) had a higher prevalence of pain than those with better performance status (ECOG 1).[10]

Burden of Disease

An American study of patients reported outcomes in cancers at a median of nine months after diagnosis. It found the highest burden was for 'pain interference' at 52.4% (49.1% prostate cancer, 55.5% lung cancer) which increased with disease stage.[11]

In advanced cancers, metastasis to the bone can lead to skeletal-related events (SREs) including pathological fracture, the need for radiotherapy to the bone (to relieve pain), the need for surgery to the bone (to relieve pain), spinal cord compression and hypercalcaemia. The incidence of SREs was highest in breast cancer and was also high in prostate and lung cancer.[12] Of the features of SREs, those with the greatest negative impact on survival were presence of hypercalcemia, spinal cord compression, and then radiation to the bone.[13] A multivariate analysis of the independent predictive effect of pain on overall survival (OS) in various cancers, found mixed results for breast, colorectal and lung cancer, but pain showed a significant negative impact on OS in prostate cancer.[14] In terms of economic burden based on 20 studies mainly from Europe and the United States, the highest costs of SREs were those related to spinal cord compression; the cost was estimated at a mean of USD 20,434 per event, with a mean of USD 17,734 for bone surgery and a mean of USD 3,546 for bone radiation, with higher costs in the United States compared to European countries.[13]

Taking advanced prostate cancer as an example, up to 65–75% of patients will develop SREs, which can be associated with severe bone pain that requires treatment with radiotherapy or surgery. These treatments can relieve pain in about 70% of patients, but up to 24% continue to have pain with pain worsening in 18%. Such bone pain is associated with poorer quality of life and survival outcomes.[15] In an economic analysis, the cost of bone surgery was USD 88,838 per episode and the cost of radiotherapy was USD 7,553 per episode.[16] In a longitudinal study (median 19 months), men with one or more SREs were twice as likely to die, compared to men with no SREs, with the greatest increase in risk being due to pathological fracture. Emergency department visits were twice as frequent in men who had an SRE and hospitalisations increased almost four-fold. The increase in health care resource utilisation was a mean of USD 21,191 for one or more SREs, based on all Medicare claim reimbursement amounts between diagnosis of prostate cancer with bone metastasis and death or the end of the study.[17] In another longitudinal study of 1,071 US patients who had been newly diagnosed with an SRE, after the SRE diagnosis the number of long-term opioid users increased by about 50%, and the proportion of time on opioid therapy doubled, but a substantial percentage of patients (42.0%) did not receive opioids or radiotherapy post-diagnosis.[18]

A review of the burden of cancer pain in developing countries found a wide range in prevalence (31.9–87.5%) based on ten studies, with a median prevalence of 42.1% (Brazil), 51.9% (East Asia), 61.6% (Africa) and 70% (Middle East) based on location. In many countries pain management was not adequately provided, often due to regulatory and other barriers against opioid use, leading to poorer quality of life outcomes and increased burden on caregivers. The author noted that the economic burden of cancer pain in developing countries was difficult to quantify, but due to the lack of adequate insurance the costs tended to be out-of-pocket and borne by the patient and family.[19]

Risk Factors

The prevalence and severity of cancer pain vary with the site of the cancer, the stage of the disease, the type of therapy and the type of pain control. For pain directly associated with the tumour, pain has a higher prevalence in advanced disease. Age does not appear to be a predictor.[9]

Greater levels of psychological distress appear to be associated with more frequent, or more intense, pain.[9] Conversely, suboptimal pain management is associated with psychological distress and impaired quality of life. It has been reported that pain was poorly controlled in almost half of cancer patients and two thirds reported that their pain interfered with their activities of daily living (ADL).[5]

Pathological Processes and Mechanisms

The pathological processes that led to the stimulation of pain receptors (nociceptors) vary considerably with the type and stage of the cancer. Pressure on nerves can produce nociceptive pain which is described as deep, dull, aching and constant, and can get worse over time. Distension of a hollow organ can produce visceral pain, which is described as cramping and bloating that is intermittent and can be associated with obstruction. Direct damage to the nerves produces neuropathic pain, which can be due to the cancer and to chemotherapy. The pain tends to be localised, sharp and shooting, burning or stabbing, and can be associated with allodynia or hyperalgesia. Neuropathic pain due to chemotherapy can produce numbness, tingling and pain of the hands and feet and is described as 'stocking-glove' neuropathy. Damage to bone and pathological fractures can produce incidents of movement pain, which is triggered by movement and relieved by rest, and can be very severe and hard to control. Also, pain perception can be influenced by depression, anxiety and distraction.[5]

The mechanisms of pain are complex and multi-dimensional.[20] Cancer pain can be viewed as a distinctive pain syndrome that involves a mixed mechanism that combines the mechanisms of other types of pain[21] including nociceptive transduction,[22] peripheral and neuropathic sensitisation,[23–25] spinal sensitisation and disinhibition,[26,27] spinal cord disinhibition[28,29] and immune modulation,[30–33] as well as supraspinal changes.[34–36] At the central level, the perception of chronic pain involves a complex mix of nociception, emotional processing, behaviour, learning and memory that induces a range of neuroplastic changes in the somatosensory-limbic pathway.[37] Such changes are evident on imaging studies which suggest different patterns of brain activation between acute and chronic pain.[34] A diagnosis of cancer and its associated tests and procedures can lead to increased psychological distress, especially fear and anxiety, and heightened central nervous system activity even prior to the experience of physical pain. In addition, stressful states can increase nociception and emotional pain can sensitise perception of nociceptive pain.[37] In addition, there is a complex relationship between chronic pain and depression, with pain causing depression and depression being associated with worse pain and poorer treatment response.[38]

Diagnosis

Pain is a psychosomatic experience reported by the pain sufferer. When acute, it is normally associated with an acute injury or illness, recent treatment or procedure, or by movement, physical position or pressure. Appearance of acute pain in a cancer patient may indicate an oncological emergency such as spinal cord compression or internal bleeding.[4,39] Chronic pain is more complex and is usually associated with multiple symptoms and with psychological, social and existential challenges.[4,7] Breakthrough pain is a transitory increase in pain to greater than moderate intensity, which may be spontaneous or due to an identifiable event such as movement in patients with metastatic bone pain.[40]

The assessment of pain requires a detailed history from the patient and their family members or carers. This should include the following: the specific pain(s) experienced, since many patients will suffer pain in multiple locations, not all of which are cancer-related; the intensity of the pain (right now, at its worst, on average); its location and radiation; the quality of the pain (aching, sharp, burning); any associated symptoms (redness, numbness, tingling, hypersensitivity); aggravating and relieving factors; previous treatments and their effects; its temporal pattern (onset, course, daily fluctuation, breakthrough pain); its effects on quality of life (physical functioning, mood, sleep, social and psychological well-being); comorbidities (physical and psychiatric); burden on caregivers and difficulties in managing or coordinating care.[4,7,39]

In the assessment of pain intensity, patients need to be taught the use of a pain scale such as the Numerical Rating Scale (NRS), the Verbal Rating Scale (VRS), or the Visual Analogue Scale (VAS). Multidimensional instruments, such as the McGill Pain Questionnaire and the Brief Pain Inventory, provide a broader assessment. Each pain should be assessed separately and its features recorded.[1,4]

The physical examination involves the following: observation of any deformation in limbs or joints, muscle wasting, posture, gait and changes in skin; palpation for any pain, tenderness or masses; auscultation to help distinguish functional from organic obstruction; percussion of bone to determine tenderness; and movement (active and passive) to assess pain in the musculoskeletal system. In neuropathic pain, a neurological examination is needed.[4,7,39]

Additional investigations can include biological markers of the severity, or progress, of the particular cancer; serum calcium since increased levels are associated with bone pain; radiological examination to identify skeletal lesions; and computerised tomography (CT), magnetic resonance imaging (MRI) and/or bone scintigraphy to identify bone metastases. These methods are important to identify the type and location of lesions and the guide treatment.[4]

Patients must be screened at each contact to assess their pain intensity and quality, any changes, any experience of breakthrough pain, the patient's level of comfort and satisfaction with the pain relief currently provided, and whether there is a risk of opiate abuse or misuse.[1]

Cancer Pain Syndromes

Based on an international survey, in the majority of cancer patients (>92%) pain was directly due to the tumour, while in more than 20% of patients pain was attributable to anticancer therapies and almost 25% of patients had two or more forms of pain.[4,7] Pain due to tumours was mainly associated with tumours of the bones and joints (42%), visceral organs (28%), soft tissue infiltration (28%) and peripheral nerve injury (28%). Of patients treated for cancer pain with opioids, the main pain mechanisms were nociceptive somatic pain (72%), nociceptive visceral pain (35%) and neuropathic (mostly mixed neuropathic nociceptive) pain (40%).[4,7,41]

In general, nociceptive visceral pain tends to be diffuse. Cramping or gnawing pain is associated with hollow organ obstruction while sharp, aching or throbbing pain suggests involvement of organ capsules or mesentery. Superficial pain of the skin or mucosa tends to be localised, sharp, hot or stinging. Deep well-localised throbbing, aching or dull pain is associated with somatic pain of the muscles, joints and bones. Neuropathic pain can be burning, stabbing, shooting, hot, searing or shock-like, and be associated with tingling, numbness or allodynia and hyperesthesia. It may be located along nerves or dermatomes.[4]

In recent years the diversity of pain in cancer has been classified into acute and chronic syndromes that reflect the sources or causes of the pain. The following list is a brief (not comprehensive) outline of the classification of chronic cancer pain syndromes, with some examples.

Related to tumour:

- Neuropathic syndromes;
- Visceral nociceptive syndromes;
  - Hepatic distension syndrome;
  - Midline retroperitoneal syndrome;
  - Chronic intestinal obstruction;
  - Malignant perineal pain;
- Somatic nociceptive syndromes;
  - Tumour-related bone pain;
  - Tumour-related soft tissue pain;
  - Paraneoplastic pain syndromes.

Related to treatment:

- Chemotherapy;
  - Painful peripheral neuropathy;
  - Mucositis;
  - Taxol-induced arthralgia and myalgia;
- Radiation;
  - Radiation-induced brachial plexopathy;
  - Chronic radiation myelopathy;

- Surgery
  - Postmastectomy pain syndrome;
  - Post-radical neck dissection pain;
  - Stump pain and phantom pain;
- Other antitumour treatments;
  - Aromatase inhibitor-induced arthralgia (breast cancer).

Due to cancer-related complications:

- Paraneoplastic sensory neuropathy;
- Paraneoplastic nociceptive pain syndromes;
- Myofascial pain syndrome;
- Constipation;
- and others.

Note: This list is not comprehensive.[4,7]

Of these, the most common causes of chronic pain in cancer patients are bone metastases. These can cause focal or referred pain and impede movement. In diagnosis it is essential to rule out pain due to non-cancer causes such as osteoporotic fracture, osteoarthritis, focal osteonecrosis, osteomalacia and nerve compression. Bone invasion is most common in the thoracic spine, followed by the lumbosacral and cervical vertebrae. Other sites include the ischiopubic, iliosacral or periacetabular regions of the pelvis, hip joint, proximal femur and base of the skull. Of the visceral nociceptive syndromes, the most common are hepatic distension syndrome (liver cancer), midline retroperitoneal syndrome (pancreatic cancer), chronic intestinal obstruction (gastrointestinal cancers) and malignant perineal pain (colon, rectal, female reproductive, genitourinary cancers).[4]

Principles of Cancer Pain Management

The overarching goals of pain management are to:

- Optimise analgesia;
- Optimise activities of daily living;

- Minimise adverse effects;
- Avoid aberrant drug taking.

The management of cancer pain is optimally done by a multidisciplinary team and involves psychosocial support and education of the patient, family members and other carers. Pain is managed in conjunction with other symptoms and symptom clusters within the overall management of the disease.[1]

The importance of the multidisciplinary team is illustrated in a study that compared the pain management approaches of oncologists, pain management specialists and palliative medicine specialists, and found that prescriptions by oncologists were less than adequate.[5]

Pharmacological Management

The 'pain ladder' or 'analgesic ladder' introduced by the World Health Organization (WHO) in 1986 has been the basis for care in cancer pain. The basic principle is that non-opioid analgesics should be used as the first step. If the pain persists, treatment should move to Step 2, then Step 3 to provide continuous pain relief (Table 1.1).

Table 1.1 World Health Organization's Analgesic Ladder for Cancer Pain Management

Step on Ladder	Pain Severity	Analgesic Approach	Actions
Step 1	Mild pain	Non-opioid (aspirin[1] or NSAID) ± optional adjuvant.	If pain persists or increases, go to Step 2.
Step 2	Moderate pain	Weak opioid (codeine[2]) ± non-opioid (as above) ± optional adjuvant.	If pain persists or increases, go to Step 3.
Step 3	Severe pain	Strong opioid (morphine[3]) ± non-opioid (as above) ± optional adjuvant.	Aim is freedom from pain.

[1]Alternative was acetaminophen/paracetamol.
[2]Alternative was oxycodone.
[3]Alternative was methadone or others.[39,42]
Abbreviations: NSAID, non-steroidal anti-inflammatory drug.

Analgesics should be administered orally, at regular intervals based on the duration of efficacy of the particular medication, and the dose should be sufficient to control the pain. Two products from the same drug class should not be used simultaneously. Prescription should be based on the patient's perception of pain level; dosage should be adapted to individual response and monitored to balance analgesic effect and side effects. Patient response should be monitored regularly and in detail. Patients should be provided with a personalised programme which is written and also available to staff and family. At each step, adjuvant treatments can be included to manage neuropathic pain or other symptoms.[43]

Since that time, additional opioid drugs have become available such as tramadol, fentanyl, hydromorphone and buprenorphine, as well as transdermal patches. Tramadol has been added to Step 2 and the others have been added to Step 3. Also, in patients presenting with severe pain requiring urgent relief, parenteral opioids (subcutaneous or intravenous) with dose titration are used. For neuropathic pain, gabapentin or gabapentin plus opioids can be used. A modified version of the ladder includes a fourth step when pain is not well managed by Step 3 which involves the use of interventions such as nerve block epidurals, neurolytic block therapy, spinal stimulators and patient-controlled analgesia.[5,43–45]

A wide range of adjuvant drugs can be used for certain presentations. Corticosteroids reduce inflammation and oedema, and are used for bone pain, neuropathic pain, lymphoedema pain, headache and bowel obstruction. Antidepressants (notably tricyclics) or anticonvulsants (notably gabapentin) are used for opioid-refractory neuropathic pain, and there is good evidence for intravenous lidocaine. Bone strengtheners, such as bisphosphonates, are routinely used for lytic bone metastases.[5,7,44]

Contemporary clinical guidelines are considerably more complex than the WHO ladder, although they preserve many of the same features. This chapter can only provide an overview of current cancer pain management (Table 1.2). The main clinical guidelines used internationally are produced by the European Society for Medical Oncology (ESMO)[45,46] and the NCCN.[1] Readers should consult the

Table 1.2 Treatment Algorithm

Opioid-naïve Patient[1]			
Pain Intensity	**Treatment***		
Mild pain (NRS 1–3)	• See general principles; • First consider non-opioids and adjuvant therapies, then short-acting opioids for patients who require further intervention.		
Moderate to severe pain (NRS ≥4)	• For acute, severe pain or pain crisis, consider hospital or in-patient hospice admission to achieve patient-specific goals for comfort and function; • See general principles; • Start and rapidly titrate short-acting opioids.		
Pain ≥4 (moderate to severe) or as indicated for uncontrolled pain (patient goals not met)	Initial dose: • Oral or intravenous[2] short-acting morphine sulfate or equivalent; • Reassess efficacy and adverse effects.	Subsequent dose: • Pain unchanged or increased: Increase dose by 50–100%; • Pain decreased but inadequately controlled: Repeat same dose; • Pain improved and adequately controlled: Continue at current effective dose as needed over initial 24 hours.	After 2–3 cycles, consider rotating oral to IV titration and/or consider subsequent management and treatment (see below).
Opioid-tolerant Patient[3]			
Pain Intensity	**Treatment***		
Pain ≥4 (moderate to severe); or as indicated for uncontrolled pain (patient goals not met)	Initial dose: • Administer oral or IV[2] opioid dose equivalent to 10–20% of total opioid taken in the previous 24 hours; • Reassess efficacy and adverse effects.	Subsequent dose: • Pain unchanged or increased: Increase dose by 50–100%; • Pain decreased but inadequately controlled: Repeat same dose; • Pain improved and adequately controlled: Continue at current effective dose as needed over initial 24 hours.	After 2–3 cycles, consider rotating oral to IV titration and/or consider subsequent management and treatment (see below).

Table 1.2 (*Continued*)

Subsequent Pain Management

Pain Intensity	Treatment*	Goals*
Mild pain (NRS 0–3)	• See general principles; • Reassess and modify regimen to minimise adverse effects; taper opioids and other treatments when no longer needed.	Routinely re-evaluate pain at each contact and as needed to meet patient-specific goals for comfort, function and safety.
Moderate to severe pain (NRS ≥4)	• See general principles; • If pain is inadequately controlled re-evaluate opioid titration; • If pain is inadequately controlled re-evaluate working diagnosis with a comprehensive pain assessment; • Consider specific pain syndrome problems; • Consider pain specialty consultation; • Consider opioid rotation if dose-limiting adverse effects are noted.	

*See National Comprehensive Cancer Network (NCCN) Guidelines Version 1, 2018 for more detail.

[1]Opioid-naïve patients are those not chronically receiving opioid analgesic on a daily basis and therefore have not developed significant tolerance.

[2]Subcutaneous can be substituted for intravenous.

[3]Opioid-tolerant patients include those who are chronically receiving opioid analgesic on a daily basis.

latest versions of these guidelines and other country-specific guidelines for more detailed information.

Interventional Techniques

With morphine, about 63% of patients have successful pain relief and the other opioids can provide alternatives for most of the remaining patients. However, in about 15% of patients analgesics will not provide effective pain relief and/or produce severe adverse effects.[5] When pharmacological therapies titrated to maximum doses cannot deliver the required level of analgesia, or the side effects of these therapies limit further dose escalation, interventional therapies can be considered. In refractory cancer pain a number of surgical neuroablative techniques are used to irreversibly interrupt the transmission of painful stimuli. These methods include celiac neurolytic plexus block which is used in pancreatic carcinoma, hypogastric neurolytic plexus block which is used for visceral cancer pain originating from advanced cancers of the pelvic organs, and percutaneous cervical cordotomy for pain in head and neck cancer. Other interventions include neuraxial infusions of drugs (mainly opioids) to the spinal cord; epidural administration of anaesthetics, and vertebroplasty for painful pathological fractures of vertebra.[47]

Radiotherapy

In patients whose pain originates from compression of nerve structures, from bone metastases or from cerebral metastases, and has proven difficult to control using analgesic therapies, external beam radiotherapy (EBRT) or radioisotope treatment can be considered.[46,48] Reviews have concluded that single fraction radiation therapy (SFRT) was as effective in pain relief as multiple fraction radiation therapy (MFRT) and SFRT has been recommended for uncomplicated bone metastases.[5,49–51]

Topical Pharmacological Methods

A number of topical medications are used as adjuvant treatments. Topical administration of local anaesthetic creams can produce a reversible nerve block. Baclofen-amitriptylineketamine gel has been used for peripheral neuropathy caused by chemotherapy. Lidocaine patch (5%) has been used for neuropathic pain and myofascial pain. Menthol creams (1%) twice daily may provide pain relief but higher-dose creams should not be used. Capsaicin patch (8%) and 0.25%, 0.75% creams have shown effects in postherpetic neuralgia and may be effective for peripheral neuropathic pain.[5,7,52]

Non-pharmacological Methods

Transcutaneous electrical nerve stimulation (TENS) is used for local pain relief, such as for lumbar pain.[52] Although the few randomised controlled trials of TENS in cancer pain and neuropathic pain suggest a benefit, the evidence remains inconclusive.[53,54] Acupuncture is also in frequent use and has been suggested as an option due to its relatively low risk,[5] but a systematic review concluded there was insufficient evidence to judge its efficacy for cancer pain.[55] A clinical guideline for supportive care in breast cancer graded the evidence for acupuncture as grade C for anxiety/stress reduction, depression/mood disturbances, quality of life/physical functioning, and pain associated with aromatase inhibitors.[56] In addition, a recent comprehensive report from the United States on non-pharmacologic therapies for pain management, including cancer pain, called for increased awareness and application of evidence-based therapies including acupuncture therapy, massage therapy, mind–body interventions and TENS.[57]

Various mind–body approaches aimed at managing pain, reducing anxiety, improving sleep and enhancing coping skills play a supportive role in cancer care, and there is some clinical evidence supporting their use.[7,58,59] For pain relief, one systematic review found low-quality evidence for massage and aromatherapy massage based on small studies.[60] The clinical guideline for breast cancer recommended meditation for anxiety and stress reduction (grade A), followed by music therapy (grade B), stress management (grade B) and yoga (grade B). For depression/mood disturbances meditation was again assessed as grade A, relaxation was grade A, followed by massage (grade B). For quality of life/physical functioning meditation was grade A followed by yoga (grade B).[56]

Prevention and Management of Adverse Effects of Analgesics

Adverse effects of opiates typically include constipation, nausea, sedation, itching and opioid-induced hyperalgesia (OIH).[5,61] Constipation is a predictable adverse effect that can be proactively managed with stimulant laxatives (such as senna), stool softeners (such as docusate), polyethylene glycol, adequate fluid intake, adequate dietary fibre and exercise. In people with a history of opioid-induced nausea, antiemetics can be used prophylactically and opioid rotation can be used when nausea persists. Pruritus is treated symptomatically but when accompanied by a rash may indicate an allergy. When severe or persistent, opioid rotation can be used. Adverse effects of higher opioid doses include excessive sedation, respiratory depression and delirium.[1]

Opioid-induced hyperalgesia is a nociceptive sensitisation that mainly occurs after longer-term opioid use. It manifests as heightened sensitivity to the pre-existing pain and/or the appearance of more generalised diffuse hyperalgesia/allodynia, which can resemble neuropathic pain and may be accompanied by myoclonus. It needs to be distinguished from opioid tolerance and withdrawal-associated hyperalgesia. Treatment is based on anecdotal reports and can involve opioid rotation or switching and dose reduction.[61]

Rehabilitation

Following a cancer diagnosis, people may reduce their normal daily living activities and this is particularly the case when they experience pain. This decline in activity can lead to progressive motor deconditioning with the onset of fatigue, and muscle, bone and joint pains not associated with the cancer. In people who exercise regularly, studies have found less fatigue, and exercise can improve mood and reduce the consumption of antidepressants. Rehabilitation is of particular importance during remission, when fatigue, pain and depressed mood may limit participation in activities of daily living. At these times, a rehabilitation programme tailored to the individual patient that involves education of the family and other caregivers can empower the person to participate in daily life, undertake physical activities and manage their pain and body weight. In longer-term survivors rehabilitation also involves improving positive self-image, overcoming the stigma of cancer and the adverse effects of its treatment, and gaining maximum independence.[62] It is notable that 33% of cancer survivors report pain five years after treatment.[63]

Palliative Care

Palliative care focuses on the effective management of pain and suffering and supports the best possible quality of life for patients and their family. Collaboration between the multidisciplinary oncology team and the palliative care team enables development of a care plan that integrates physical and psychosocial aspects of care. The benefits and burdens of anticancer treatment relative to estimated life expectancy should be assessed and discussed with the patient. When the assessment indicates months to weeks, discontinuation of cancer treatment should be considered in favour of treatment of specific symptom complexes. Besides pain, these can include constipation, diarrhea, bleeding, bowel obstruction, dyspnea, anorexia and cachexia, nausea and vomiting, insomnia, sedation and delirium. Pain from obstructive tumours and metastases can be relieved with radiotherapy or surgery depending on the case.[64] Early involvement of the rehabilitation unit may enable the person to return to home-based care. Management of bed posture and physiotherapies to maintain joint movement and muscle tone are important in all patients and massage therapies can induce feelings of well-being.[62]

Prognosis

Cancer pain can be successfully managed in most patients with appropriate techniques and the available drugs. The NCCN guideline advises that clinicians should base management on routine pain assessments, utilise both pharmacologic and non-pharmacologic interventions, and carefully monitor and re-evaluate the patient. If the algorithms presented are systematically applied, cancer pain can be well managed in the majority of patients.[1]

However, pain response in the individual patient is variable and related to interactions between patient characteristics, the pain syndrome and the nature of the pain treatment.[65] A longitudinal study of advanced cancer patients who were receiving opioids identified the following predictors of pain outcomes at two weeks following initial assessment (in descending order): initial pain intensity, initial pain relief, pain localisation, cancer diagnosis (lung), incident pain and age.[66] Initial pain intensity was a negative predictor since this was associated with more complex or difficult-to-treat conditions. Incident pain also predicted poorer pain control. A likely reason is, this is often associated with bone metastases and triggered by movement. This makes it difficult to optimise opioid dosage because the background pain intensity is much lower than the peak intensity.[66,67] Conversely, initial pain relief and pain localisation in the thorax/abdomen were positive predictors of pain relief. Of the cancer diagnoses, lung cancer predicted the poorest outcome. Younger age was also associated with less pain relief but the reason for this difference may be complex. Poor sleep was another negative predictor. This may have been due to poorly controlled pain leading to poor sleep or poor sleep itself contributing to worse pain outcomes.[66] Another longitudinal study of patients with advanced cancer undergoing palliative care found that younger age, neuropathic pain, incident pain, psychological distress and pain intensity were all negatively associated with the number of days required to achieve stable pain control.[68] A number of studies have found associations between depressive mood and anxiety and poorer treatment outcomes but the reasons for the association may be complex.[67]

Genetic variation is another important factor in response to pain management. Polymorphisms of the gene for the mu 1 opioid receptor (OPRM1) affect the pharmacodynamics of opioids. Approximately 20% of the population carries at least one copy of the G allele while about 4% are homozygous for the G allele (i.e. GG). These patients appear to be less sensitive to the effects of morphine and have higher incidence of adverse effects. From the perspective of pharmacokinetics, opioids are metabolized via the cytochrome P450 family member CTP2D6 which has multiple alleles, some of which are functionally null while others result in ultra-rapid opioid metabolism. In the case of opioid pro-drugs (codeine, oxycodone, hydrocodone, tramadol) which require metabolism via CTP2D6 to form their active metabolites, subnormal metabolisers (approximately 20%) will receive reduced pain relief but ultra-rapid metabolisers (approximately 3%)

may suffer acute opioid toxicity while failing to obtain the steady concentration of the drug required for effective pain relief. Furthermore, these polymorphisms can interact with each other and with environmental inhibitors of CTP2D6, such as some drugs, foods and herbs, to reduce or increase a person's responses to opioids.[69] Another gene associated with variation in response to opioids is the catechol-O-methyltransferase (COMT) gene, which is associated with the metabolism of dopamine, epinephrine and norepinephrine. People with a certain polymorphism (Val) require higher morphine doses.[70] As pharmacogenetic testing progresses, clinicians will be able to identify those at risk of opioid intolerance and increased toxicity risk to improve pain management.

References

1. National Comprehensive Cancer Network. (2018) Clinical practice guidelines in oncology: Adult cancer pain, version 1. Available from: www.nccn.org.
2. World Health Organisation. (2004) ICD-10 international statistical classification of diseases and related health problems. Geneva, World Health Organisation.
3. National Center for Health Statistics, Centers for Disease Control and Prevention. (2018) ICD-10-cm guidelines for coding and reporting. Available from: www.cdc.gov/nchs/icd/data/10cmguidelines-FY2019-final.pdf.
4. Krajnik M, Zylicz Z. (2013) Pain assessment, recognising clinical patterns, and cancer pain syndromes. In: Hanna M, Zylicz Z (eds), *Cancer Pain*. Springer London, London, pp. 95–108.
5. Smith TJ, Saiki CB. (2015) Cancer pain management. *Mayo Clin Proc* **90(10):** 1428–1439.
6. Hansen DMH, Kehlet H, Gartner R. (2011) Phantom breast sensations are frequent after mastectomy. *Dan Med Bull* **58(4):** A4259.
7. Portenoy RK. (2011) Treatment of cancer pain. *Lancet (London, England)* **377(9784):** 2236–2247.
8. Portenoy RK, Ahmed E. (2018) Cancer pain syndromes. *Hematol Oncol Clin North Am* **32(3):** 371–386.

9. Higginson IJ, Murtagh FEM, Osborne TR. (2013) Epidemiology of pain in cancer. In: Hanna M, Zylicz Z (eds). *Cancer Pain*, Springer London, London, pp. 5–24.
10. van den Beuken-van Everdingen MH, Hochstenbach LM, Joosten EA, *et al.* (2016) Update on prevalence of pain in patients with cancer: Systematic review and meta-analysis. *J Pain Symptom Manage* **51(6):** 1070–1090.
11. Jensen RE, Potosky AL, Moinpour CM, *et al.* (2017) United States population-based estimates of patient-reported outcomes measurement information system symptom and functional status reference values for individuals with cancer. *J Clin Oncol* **35(17):** 1913–1920.
12. Coleman R, Body JJ, Aapro M, *et al.* (2014) Bone health in cancer patients: ESMO Clinical Practice Guidelines. *Ann Oncol* **25 (Suppl 3):** iii124–iii137.
13. Carter JA, Ji X, Botteman MF. (2013) Clinical, economic and humanistic burdens of skeletal-related events associated with bone metastases. *Expert Rev Pharmacoecon Outcomes Res* **13(4):** 483–496.
14. Zylla D, Steele G, Gupta P. (2017) A systematic review of the impact of pain on overall survival in patients with cancer. *Support Care Cancer* **25(5):** 1687–1698.
15. Broder MS, Gutierrez B, Cherepanov D, Linhares Y. (2015) Burden of skeletal-related events in prostate cancer: Unmet need in pain improvement. *Support Care Cancer* **23(1):** 237–247.
16. Yong C, Onukwugha E, Mullins CD. (2014) Clinical and economic burden of bone metastasis and skeletal-related events in prostate cancer. *Curr Opin Oncol* **26(3):** 274–283.
17. McDougall JA, Bansal A, Goulart BHL, *et al.* (2016) The clinical and economic impacts of skeletal-related events among medicare enrollees with prostate cancer metastatic to bone. *Oncologist* **21(3):** 320–326.
18. Yaldo A, Wen L, Ogbonnaya A, *et al.* (2016) Opioid use among metastatic prostate cancer patients with skeletal-related events. *Clin Ther* **38(8):** 1880–1889.
19. Li Z, Aninditha T, Griene B, *et al.* (2018) Burden of cancer pain in developing countries: A narrative literature review. *Clinicoecon Outcomes Res* **10:** 675–691.
20. Vardeh D, Mannion RJ, Woolf CJ. (2016) Toward a mechanism-based approach to pain diagnosis. *J Pain* **17(Suppl 9):** T50–T69.
21. Urch CE, Suzuki R. (2008) Pathophysiology of somatic, visceral, and neuropathic cancer pain. In: Sykes N, Bennett MI, Yuan CS (eds).

Clinical Pain Management: Cancer Pain, 2nd ed. Hodder & Stoughton Limited, London, pp. 3–11.
22. Binshtok AM. (2011) Mechanisms of nociceptive transduction and transmission: A machinery for pain sensation and tools for selective analgesia. In: Kobayashi M, John LW (eds). *International Review Of Neurobiology Volume 97*. Academic Press, pp. 143–177.
23. Costigan M, Scholz J, Woolf CJ. (2009) Neuropathic pain: A maladaptive response of the nervous system to damage. *Annu Rev Neurosci* **32:** 1–32.
24. Woolf CJ. (2011) Central sensitization: Implications for the diagnosis and treatment of pain. *Pain* **152(Suppl 3):** S2–S15.
25. Djouhri L, Koutsikou S, Fang X, *et al.* (2006) Spontaneous pain, both neuropathic and inflammatory, is related to frequency of spontaneous firing in intact c-fiber nociceptors. *J Neurosci* **26(4):** 1281–1292.
26. Latremoliere A, Woolf CJ. (2009) Central sensitization: A generator of pain hypersensitivity by central neural plasticity. *J Pain* **10(9):** 895–926.
27. Duan B, Cheng L, Bourane S, *et al.* (2014) Identification of spinal circuits transmitting and gating mechanical pain. *Cell* **159(6):** 1417–1432.
28. Inquimbert P, Bartels K, Babaniyi OB, *et al.* (2012) Peripheral nerve injury produces a sustained shift in the balance between glutamate release and uptake in the dorsal horn of the spinal cord. *Pain* **153(12):** 2422–2431.
29. Zeilhofer HU, Ralvenius WT, Acuña MA. (2015) Chapter 4: Restoring the spinal pain gate: Gabaa receptors as targets for novel analgesics. In: Uwe R (ed), *Advances in Pharmacology Volume 73*. Academic Press, pp. 71–96.
30. Grace PM, Hutchinson MR, Maier SF, Watkins LR. (2014) Pathological pain and the neuroimmune interface. *Nat Rev Immunol* **14(4):** 217–231.
31. Milligan ED, Watkins LR. (2009) Pathological and protective roles of glia in chronic pain. *Nat Rev Neurosci* **10(1):** 23–36.
32. Xin WJ, Weng HR, Dougherty PM. (2009) Plasticity in expression of the glutamate transporters glt-1 and glast in spinal dorsal horn glial cells following partial sciatic nerve ligation. *Mol Pain* **5(1):** 15.
33. Harvey RJ, Depner UB, Wässle H, *et al.* (2004) Glyr α3: An essential target for spinal pge-2-mediated inflammatory pain sensitization. *Science* **304(5672):** 884–887.
34. Apkarian AV, Hashmi JA, Baliki MN. (2011) Pain and the brain: Specificity and plasticity of the brain in clinical chronic pain. *Pain* **152(Suppl 3):** S49–S64.

35. Gussew A, Rzanny R, Gullmar D, *et al.* (2011) 1h-mr spectroscopic detection of metabolic changes in pain processing brain regions in the presence of non-specific chronic low back pain. *Neuroimage* **54(2):** 1315–1323.
36. Geha PY, Baliki MN, Harden RN, *et al.* (2008) The brain in chronic crps pain: Abnormal gray-white matter interactions in emotional and autonomic regions. *Neuron* **60(4):** 570–581.
37. Prinsloo S, Gabel S, Lyle R, Cohen L. (2014) Neuromodulation of cancer pain. *Integr Cancer Ther* **13(1):** 30–37.
38. Doan L, Manders T, Wang J. (2015) Neuroplasticity underlying the comorbidity of pain and depression. *Neural Plast* **2015:** 504691.
39. Woodruff R. (1996) *Cancer Pain.* Asperula, Heideberg.
40. Mercadante S, Portenoy RK. (2016) Breakthrough cancer pain: Twenty-five years of study. *Pain* **157(12):** 2657–2663.
41. Caraceni A, Portenoy RK. (1999) An international survey of cancer pain characteristics and syndromes. *Pain* **82(3):** 263–274.
42. World Health Organisation. (1986) *Cancer Pain Relief.* World Health Organisation, Geneva.
43. Vargas-Schaffer G. (2010) Is the WHO analgesic ladder still valid? Twenty-four years of experience. *Can Fam Physician* **56(6):** 514–517.
44. Scarborough BM, Smith CB. (2018) Optimal pain management for patients with cancer in the modern era. *CA Cancer J Clin* **68(3):** 182–196.
45. Ripamonti CI, Santini D, Maranzano E, *et al.* (2012) Management of cancer pain: ESMO Clinical Practice Guidelines. *Ann Oncol* **23:** 139–154.
46. Fallon M, Giusti R, Aielli F, *et al.* (2018) Management of cancer pain in adult patients: ESMO Clinical Practice Guidelines. *Ann Oncol* **29(Suppl 4):** iv166–iv191.
47. Schweiger V, Polati E, Paladini A, Varrassi G. (2013) Interventional techniques in cancer pain: Critical appraisal. In: Hanna M, Zylicz Z (eds), *Cancer Pain.* Springer London, London, pp. 231–247.
48. Ripamonti CI, Bandieri E, Roila F, Grp EGW. (2011) Management of cancer pain: ESMO Clinical Practice Guidelines. *Ann Oncol* **22:** vi69–vi77.
49. Lutz S, Berk L, Chang E, *et al.* (2011) Palliative radiotherapy for bone metastases: An astro evidence-based guideline. *Int J Radiat Oncol Biol Phys* **79(4):** 965–976.
50. Chow R, Hoskin P, Hollenberg D, *et al.* (2017) Efficacy of single fraction conventional radiation therapy for painful uncomplicated bone metastases: A systematic review and meta-analysis. *Ann Palliat Med* **6(2):** 125–142.

51. Conway JL, Yurkowski E, Glazier J, *et al.* (2016) Comparison of patient-reported outcomes with single versus multiple fraction palliative radiotherapy for bone metastasis in a population-based cohort. *Radiother Oncol* **119(2):** 202–207.
52. Lecybyl R. (2013) The non-pharmacological and local pharmacological methods of pain control. In: Hanna M, Zylicz Z (eds). *Cancer Pain.* Springer London, London, pp. 143–151.
53. Hurlow A, Bennett MI, Robb KA, *et al.* (2012) Transcutaneous electric nerve stimulation (TENS) for cancer pain in adults. *The Cochrane Database of Systematic Reviews* **3:** CD006276.
54. Gibson W, Wand BM, O'Connell NE. (2017) Transcutaneous electrical nerve stimulation (TENS) for neuropathic pain in adults. *The Cochrane Database of Systematic Reviews* **9:** CD011976.
55. Paley CA, Johnson MI, Tashani OA, Bagnall AM. (2015) Acupuncture for cancer pain in adults. *Cochrane Database of Systematic* **2015(10)**: CD007753.
56. Greenlee H, DuPont-Reyes MJ, Balneaves LG, *et al.* (2017) Clinical practice guidelines on the evidence-based use of integrative therapies during and after breast cancer treatment. *CA Cancer J Clin* **67(3):** 195–232.
57. Tick H, Nielsen A, Pelletier KR, *et al.* (2018) Evidence-based nonpharmacologic strategies for comprehensive pain care: The consortium pain task force white paper. *Explore (NY)* **14(3):** 177–211.
58. Kwekkeboom KL, Cherwin CH, Lee JW, Wanta B. (2010) Mind-body treatments for the pain-fatigue-sleep disturbance symptom cluster in persons with cancer. *J Pain Symptom Manage* **39(1):** 126–138.
59. Cassileth BR, Keefe FJ. (2010) Integrative and behavioral approaches to the treatment of cancer-related neuropathic pain. *Oncologist* **15:** 19–23.
60. Shin ES, Seo KH, Lee SH, *et al.* (2016) Massage with or without aromatherapy for symptom relief in people with cancer. *The Cochrane Database of Systematic Reviews* **6:** CD009873.
61. Sørensen J, Sjøgren P. (2013) Opioid-induced hyperalgesia. In: Hanna M, Zylicz Z (eds), *Cancer Pain.* Springer London, London, pp. 131–142.
62. Casale R, Miotti D. (2013) Rehabilitation of cancer patients: A forgotten need? In: Hanna M, Zylicz Z (eds), *Cancer Pain.* Springer London, London, pp. 203–209.
63. Harrington CB, Hansen JA, Moskowitz M, *et al.* (2010) It's not over when it's over: Long-term symptoms in cancer survivors: A systematic review. *Int J Psychiatry Med* **40(2):** 163–181.

64. National Comprehensive Cancer Network. (2017) Clinical practice guidelines in oncology: Palliative care, version 2.2017. Available from: www.nccn.org.
65. Bruera E. (2012) The challenges of prognosis in cancer pain. *Pain* **153(3):** 513–514.
66. Knudsen AK, Brunelli C, Klepstad P, *et al.* (2012) Which domains should be included in a cancer pain classification system? Analyses of longitudinal data. *Pain* **153(3):** 696–703.
67. Mercadante S. (2019) The patient with difficult cancer pain. *Cancers (Basel)* **11(4):** 565.
68. Fainsinger RL, Nekolaichuk C, Lawlor P, *et al.* (2010) An international multicentre validation study of a pain classification system for cancer patients. *Eur J Cancer* **46(16):** 2896–2904.
69. Ruano G, Kost JA. (2018) Fundamental considerations for genetically-guided pain management with opioids based on cyp2d6 and oprm1 polymorphisms. *Pain Physician* **21(6):** E611–E621.
70. Reyes-Gibby CC, Shete S, Rakvag T, *et al.* (2007) Exploring joint effects of genes and the clinical efficacy of morphine for cancer pain: Oprm1 and comt gene. *Pain* **130(1–2):** 25–30.

2

Cancer Pain in Chinese Medicine

OVERVIEW

This chapter introduces the main aetiology, pathogenesis and syndromes of cancer pain in contemporary Chinese medicine based on guidelines and major textbooks. For each syndrome a guiding herbal formula is provided based on an authoritative clinical guideline and additional formulas from major textbooks are provided in a table. Treatments with external herbal preparations and acupuncture and related therapies, as well as management with other Chinese medicine therapies, prevention, nursing and care of the patient are included based on major textbooks.

Introduction

In modern Chinese medicine (CM) the term for 'cancer pain' is *ai tong* 癌痛. However, this term was not used in pre-modern and ancient times. Nevertheless, traditional terms for cancers included pain as one of the symptoms of the disorder (see Chapter 3).[1–9]

Aetiology and Pathogenesis

In CM, the aetiology and pathogenesis of cancer pain involves two categories: deficiency (*xu* 虚) and excess (*shi* 实). The excess is 'stagnation causing pain' (*bu tong ze tong* 不通则痛) and the deficiency is 'lack of nourishment causing pain' (*bu rong ze tong* 不荣则痛). Cold, heat, wind, dampness, *qi* stagnation, Blood stasis, phlegm accumulation and many other disorders can cause masses (*zheng jia* 癥/症瘕, *ji ju* 积聚), which can lead to stagnation in the movement of *qi* 气 within the internal organs (*zang fu* 脏腑), and/or the obstruction of movement in the meridians causing pain. This is the meaning of 'stagnation causing pain' (*bu tong ze tong* 不通则痛). Healthy *qi* deficiency, fluid and humour (*jin ye* 津液) drying up, loss of nourishment to the bones, vessels, sinews and muscles, or prolonged illness causing *yin* and *yang* dual deficiency (*yin yang liang xu* 阴阳两虚) and loss of nourishment to the internal organs (*zang fu* 脏腑), can all cause pain. This is the meaning of 'lack of nourishment causing pain' (*bu rong ze tong* 不荣则痛). In the early and middle stages of the disease, excess syndromes are the main reasons for pain, while in the late stages mixed deficiency-excess is the main cause.[1–9]

Syndrome Differentiation and Treatments

There was no national standard for syndrome differentiation in cancer pain at the time of writing. Syndromes can vary considerably from patient to patient and according to the different cancers, the clinical symptoms and the stage of the disease, so this is a complex area. We consulted textbooks and other books on cancer pain and obtained expert advice to select the Guideline of Diagnosis and Treatment of Tumours in Chinese Medicine 肿瘤中医诊疗指南 which was produced in 2008 by the China Association of Chinese Medicine 中华中医药学会 as the basis for syndrome differentiation and treatment.[1]

Treatment Based on Syndrome Differentiation

Six syndromes are described, each with typical symptoms and signs, a principle of treatment and oral herbal formulas.

1. Wind-cold blockage and obstruction (*feng han bi zu* 风寒闭阻)

Clinical manifestations: Cold pain, sudden pain and sharp pain. Aggravated by cold and the pain is fixed in location. There is a pale tongue body, with a thin white tongue coat and a string-like (*xian mai* 弦脉) or tight pulse (*jin mai* 紧脉).

Treatment principle: Dispelling wind and dissipating cold to relieve pain (*qu feng san han zhi tong* 祛风散寒止痛).

Oral formula: *Xiao huo luo dan* 小活络丹 or *Xiao feng san* with modifications 消风散加减.

Herbs: *Chuan wu* 川乌, *cao wu* 草乌, *xi xin* 细辛, *chuan xiong* 川芎, *bai zhi* 白芷, *sang ji sheng* 桑寄生, *lu feng fang* 露蜂房, *wu zhu yu* 吴茱萸, *jiang can* 僵蚕, *di long* 地龙 and *bai hua she* 白花蛇.

Main actions of herbs: *Chuan wu* 川乌, *cao wu* 草乌 and *xi xin* 细辛 dispel wind and dissipate cold (*qu feng san han* 祛风散寒) to relieve pain; *chuan xiong* 川芎, *bai zhi* 白芷, *lu feng fang* 露蜂房 and *jiang can* 僵蚕 dispel wind and relieve pain; *sang ji sheng* 桑寄生, *di long* 地龙 and *bai hua she* 白花蛇 dispel wind and free the collateral vessels (*tong luo* 通络) to relieve pain; *wu zhu yu* 吴茱萸 warms *yang* and dissipates cold (*wen yang san han* 温阳散寒) to relieve pain.

2. *Qi* movement depressed and bound (*qi ji yu jie* 气机郁结)

Clinical manifestations: Chest and abdomen bloated and painful (*zhang tong* 胀痛), pain that moves, often aggravated by gloomy mood. There is a pale tongue body with a white tongue coat, and a string-like pulse.

Treatment principle: Regulating *qi* and relieving pain (*li qi zhi tong* 理气止痛).

Oral formula: *Si ni san* 四逆散 or *Chai hu shu gan san* with modifications 柴胡疏肝散加减.

Herbs: *Chai hu* 柴胡, *qing pi* 青皮, *chen pi* 陈皮, *ba yue zha* 八月札, *wu yao* 乌药, *xiang fu* 香附, *chuan lian zi* 川楝子, *hou pu* 厚朴, *yan hu suo* 延胡索, *zhi shi* 枳实, *bai shao* 白芍 and *fo shou* 佛手. Of these herbs, *zhi shi* 枳实, *chai hu* 柴胡 and *bai shao* 白芍 are components of *Si ni san* 四逆散.

Main actions of herbs: *Chai hu* 柴胡 soothes the liver (*shu gan* 疏肝) and regulates *qi* (*li qi* 理气); *qing pi* 青皮, *ba yue zha* 八月札, *xiang fu* 香附 and *fo shou* 佛手 soothe the liver and regulate *qi* to relieve pain; *chen pi* 陈皮 and *hou pu* 厚朴 regulate *qi* and harmonise the middle (*he zhong* 和中); *wu yao* 乌药, *chuan lian zi* 川楝子 and *yan hu suo* 延胡索 move *qi* and relieve pain; *zhi shi* 枳实 breaks *qi* (*po qi* 破气), disperses nodules (*xiao ji* 消积) and dissipates stuffiness (*san pi* 散痞); *bai shao* 白芍 emolliates the liver (*rou gan* 柔肝) and relieves pain.

3. Phlegm-dampness congealing and binding (*tan shi ning jie* 痰湿凝结)

Clinical manifestations: When a phlegm-damp pathogen stays in chest and lungs, there is cough and rapid breathing, chest and costal pain, epigastric fullness and rigidity (*xin xia pi ying* 心下痞硬). When a pathogen stays in the chest and costal region, there is cough that causes pain, cough and dysnoea, and the person cannot lay supine. When a pathogen stays in the abdomen, there is abdominal distension like a drum, with a feeling of heaviness like being tightly wrapped (*zhong zhuo ru guo* 重浊如裹), and distending pain that is unbearable (*zhang tong nan ren* 胀痛难忍). The tongue body is pale red or pale white with a white slimy tongue coat, and there is a slippery pulse.

Treatment principle: Resolving phlegm and dispersing nodules to relieve pain (*hua tan san jie zhi tong* 化痰散结止痛).

Oral formula: *Ting li da zao xie fei tang* with modifications 葶苈大枣泻肺汤加减.

Herbs: *Ting li zi* 葶苈子, *bai jie zi* 白芥子, *ban xia* 半夏, *bei mu* 贝母, *nan xing* 南星, *kun bu* 昆布, *gua lou* 瓜蒌, *huang yao zi* 黄药子, *da zao* 大枣 and *chen pi* 陈皮.

Main actions of herbs: *Ting li zi* 葶苈子 purges the lung to calm panting (*xie fei ping chuan* 泻肺平喘) and induces diuresis to alleviate oedema (*li shui xiao zhong* 利水消肿); *bai jie zi* 白芥子 warms the middle and dissipates cold, resolves phlegm and frees the collateral vessels to relieve pain; *ban xia* 半夏, *nan xing* 南星 and *chen pi* 陈皮 dry dampness to resolve phlegm (*hua tan* 化痰); *bei mu* 贝母, *gua lou* 瓜蒌 and *huang yao zi* 黄药子 clear heat and resolve phlegm; *kun bu* 昆布 induces diuresis to alleviate oedema, eliminates phlegm (*xiao tan* 消痰) and disperses nodules (*san jie* 散结); *da zao* 大枣 tonifies the middle and replenishes *qi*, fortifies Spleen (*jian pi* 健脾) and harmonises Stomach (*he wei* 和胃).

4. Heat and toxins congealing and binding (*re du ning jie* 热毒凝结)

Clinical manifestations: Burning pain (*zhuo tong* 灼痛), distended pain or red swollen hot pain (*hong zhong re tong* 红肿热痛), accompanied by high fever, thirst for cold drinks, flushed face and red eyes, reddish urine and constipation; or low fever in the afternoon, feeling of heat in the chest, palms and soles (*wu xin fan re* 五心烦热), night sweats (*dao han* 盗汗) and dry throat. There is a red or purple tongue body, and a rapid pulse.

Treatment principle: Clearing heat and resolving toxins to relieve pain (*qing re jie du zhi tong* 清热解毒止痛).

Oral formula: *Ru yi jin huang san* 如意金黄散 or *Long dan xie gan tang* with modifications 龙胆泻肝汤加减.

Herbs: *Huang qin* 黄芩, *huang lian* 黄连, *zhi zi* 栀子, *jin yin hua* 金银花, *liao qiao* 连翘, *long dan cao* 龙胆草, *pu gong ying* 蒲公英, *dang gui* 当归, *mu xiang* 木香, *xia ku cao* 夏枯草, *chi shao* 赤芍, *tu bei mu* 土贝母 and *gan cao* 甘草.

Main actions of herbs: *Huang qin* 黄芩, *huang lian* 黄连, *jin yin hua* 金银花, *long dan cao* 龙胆草 and *tu bei mu* 土贝母 clear heat and resolve toxins (*qing re jie du* 清热解毒); *zhi zi* 栀子 clears heat and relieves pain; *lian qiao* 连翘, *pu gong ying* 蒲公英 and *xia ku cao* 夏枯草 clear heat and resolve toxins, disperse swelling and dissipate nodules (*xiao zhong san jie* 消肿散结); *dang gui* 当归 tonifies Blood and activates Blood (*huo xie* 活血), resolves stasis and relieves pain (*hua yu zhi tong* 化瘀止痛); *mu xiang* 木香 moves *qi* to relieve pain;

chi shao 赤芍 cools Blood and activates Blood to relieve pain; *gan cao* 甘草 clears heat and resolves toxins, relaxes tension (*huan ji* 缓急) and relieves pain, and harmonises each herb (*tiao he zhu yao* 调和诸药).

5. Static blood obstruction and stagnation (*yu xue zu zhi* 瘀血阻滞)

Clinical manifestations: Pain that is like needles piercing, fixed and does not move, especially at night. There is a dark purple (*zi an* 紫暗) tongue body, with ecchymosis (*yu ban* 瘀斑) and a white tongue coat, and a rough pulse.

Treatment principle: Activating Blood and relieving pain (*huo xue zhi tong* 活血止痛).

Oral formula: *Tao hong si wu tang* 桃红四物汤 or *Fu yuan huo xue tang* with modifications 复元活血汤加减.

Herbs: *Dang gui* 当归, *chi shao* 赤芍, *chuan xiong* 川芎, *dan shen* 丹参, *yan hu suo* 延胡索, *san qi* 三七, *ru xiang* 乳香 and *mo yao* 没药.

Main actions of herbs: *Dang gui* 当归, *chuang xiong* 川芎, *dan shen* 丹参 and *yan hu suo* 延胡索 activate the blood and resolve stasis to relieve pain; *chi shao* 赤芍 activates the blood and resolves stasis (*hua yu* 化瘀); *san qi* 三七, *ru xiang* 乳香 and *mo yao* 没药 dissipate stasis (*san yu* 散瘀) and disperse swelling (*xiao zhong* 消肿) to relieve pain.

6. Deficiency cold pain (*xu han tong* 虚寒痛)

Clinical manifestations: Fatigue, bright pale complexion (*mian se huang bai* 面色晄白), limbs are cold and there is mental fatigue, continuous abdominal pain, better with warmth and light pressure. There is a thin tongue body with a white tongue coat, and a sunken and fine pulse.

Treatment principle: Warming the meridian and dissipating cold to relieve pain (*wen jing san han zhi tong* 温经散寒止痛).

Oral formula: *Gui zhi jia shao yao tang* 桂枝加芍药汤 or *Ren shen jia shao yao gan cao tang* 人参加芍药甘草汤.

Herbs: *Gui zhi* 桂枝, *shao yao* 芍药, *da zao* 大枣, *sheng jiang* 生姜, *ren shen* 人参, *gan cao* 甘草, *bai zhu* 白术, *gan jiang* 干姜, *fu ling* 茯苓, *huang qi* 黄芪, *dang gui* 当归 and *du zhong* 杜仲.

Main actions of herbs: *Gui zhi* 桂枝 warms and smooths the meridians (*wen tong jing luo* 温通经脉); *shao yao* 芍药 nourishes blood and constrains the *yin* (*lian yin* 敛阴) to relieve pain; *da zao* 大枣 tonifies the middle and replenishes *qi*, fortifies Spleen and nourishes Blood; *sheng jiang* 生姜 warms the middle and dissipates cold; *ren shen* 人参 greatly tonifies the original *qi* (*da bu yuan qi* 大补元气), restores the pulse and relieves collapse syndrome (*fu mai gu tuo* 复脉固脱); *gan cao* 甘草 fortifies Spleen and replenishes *qi*, relaxes tension and relieves pain and harmonises each herb; *bai zhu* 白术 and *fu ling* 茯苓 fortify Spleen and replenish *qi*; *gan jiang* 干姜 warms the middle and dissipates cold, restores *yang* (*hui yang* 回阳) and promotes Blood circulation; *huang qi* 黄芪 tonifies *qi* and secures the exterior (*gu biao* 固表); *dang gui* 当归 tonifies Blood and relieves pain; *du zhong* 杜仲 tonifies Liver and Kidney 补肝肾, strengthens the waist (*qiang yao* 强腰) and relieves pain. Table 2.1 gives a summary of syndromes and treatments.

Additional Sources for Treatment Based on Syndrome Differentiation

Since there was no single national standard for the CM differential diagnosis and management of cancer pain, a summary is provided in Table 2.2 of the syndromes, principles of treatment and guiding oral formulas from five additional authoritative monographs and textbooks.[2–5] These books list between three and eight syndromes and their associated formulas.

Manufactured Medicines

A number of orally-administered manufactured medicines (*zhong cheng yao* 中成药) are available for use in cancer pain.[1–4,6–8]

Table 2.1 Summary of Chinese Herbal Medicine for Cancer Pain

Syndrome Differentiation	Treatment Principle	Oral Formula
Wind-cold blockage and obstruction 风寒闭阻	Dispelling wind and dissipating cold to relieve pain 祛风散寒止痛	*Xiao huo luo dan* 小活络丹 or *Xiao feng san* with modifications 消风散加减
Qi movement depressed and bound 气机郁结	Regulating *qi* and relieving pain 理气止痛	*Si ni san* 四逆散 or *Chai hu shu gan san* with modifications 柴胡疏肝散加减
Phlegm-dampness congealing and binding 痰湿凝结	Resolving phlegm and dispersing nodules to relieve pain 化痰散结止痛	*Ting li da zao xie fei tang* with modifications 葶苈大枣泻肺汤加减
Heat and toxins congealing and binding 热毒凝结	Clearing heat and resolving toxins to relieve pain 清热解毒止痛	*Ru yi jin huang san* 如意金黄散 or *Long dan xie gan tang* with modifications 龙胆泻肝汤加减
Static blood obstruction and stagnation 瘀血阻滞	Activating Blood and relieving pain 活血止痛	*Tao hong si wu tang* 桃红四物汤 or *Fu yuan huo xue tang* with modifications 复元活血汤加减
Deficiency cold pain 虚寒痛	Warming the meridian and dissipating cold to relieve pain 温经散寒止痛	*Gui zhi jia shao yao tang* 桂枝加芍药汤 or *Ren shen jia shao yao gan cao tang* 人参加芍药甘草汤

1. *Yuan hu zhi tong ke li* 元胡止痛颗粒

Actions: Regulates *qi* and activates Blood to relieve pain. Can be used by patients with *qi* stagnation pain (*qi zhi teng tong* 气滞疼痛).

Dose: 1 packet, three times per day.[1,6]

2. *Xin huang pian* 新癀片

Actions: Clears heat and resolves toxins, activates Blood and resolves stasis, disperses swelling to relieve pain. Used in the middle and later stages of cancer pain, and also has antipyretic actions.

Dose: 2–4 tablets, three times per day.[1–3,6,7]

Table 2.2 Summary of Chinese Herbal Medicine for Colorectal Cancer in Additional Monographs and Textbooks

Book Name	Syndrome Differentiation	Treatment Principle	Oral Formula
Shi Yong Zhong Yi Zhong Liu Shou Ce 实用中医肿瘤手册[2]	*Qi* movement stagnation 气机阻滞	Regulating *qi* and resolving stagnation 理气导滞, 调畅气机	*Mu xiang shun qi wan* with modifications 木香顺气丸加减
	Blood stasis blocking the interior 瘀血内阻证	Activating Blood and resolving stasis, dispersing swelling to relieve pain 活血化瘀, 消肿止痛	*Xue fu zhu yu tang* with modifications 血府逐瘀汤加减
	Dual deficiency of *qi* and blood 气血两亏	Tonifying *qi* and nourishing Blood 补气养血	*Ba zhen tang* with modifications 八珍汤加减
E Xing Zhong Liu Zhong Yi Zhen Liao Zhi Nan 恶性肿瘤中医诊疗指南[3]	Liver depression and *qi* stagnation 肝郁气滞	Moving *qi* to relieve pain 行气止痛	*Chai hu shu gan san* 柴胡疏肝散
	Static blood obstruction and stagnation 瘀血阻滞	Dispelling stasis and freeing the collateral vessels 祛瘀通络	*Shi xiao san* 失笑散, *Xue fu zhu yu tang* 血府逐瘀汤, etc.
	Phlegm-dampness stagnation 痰湿中阻	Resolving phlegm and excreting dampness 化痰渗湿	*Dao tan tang* 导痰汤, *Ping wei san* 平胃散, etc.
	Heat toxin obstruction 热毒壅盛	Clearing heat and resolving toxins 清热解毒	*Wu wei xiao du yin* 五味消毒饮
Shi Yong Zhong Xi Yi Jie He Zhong Liu Xue 实用中西医结合肿瘤学[4]	*Qi* movement stagnation 气机郁滞	Moving *qi* to relieve pain 行气止痛	*Chai hu shu gan san* 柴胡疏肝散 or *Si ni san* with modifications 四逆散加减
	Blood stasis and toxin agglomeration 血瘀毒结	Activating Blood and resolving stasis, dispersing nodules and relieving pain 活血化瘀, 散结止痛	*Tong qiao huo xue tang* 通窍活血汤, *Xue fu zhu yu tang* 血府逐瘀汤, *Shao fu zhu yu tang* 少腹逐瘀汤, *Shi xiao san* 失笑散, etc.

(*Continued*)

Table 2.2 (*Continued*)

Book Name	Syndrome Differentiation	Treatment Principle	Oral Formula
	Phlegm-dampness agglomeration 痰湿凝聚	Fortifying Spleen and dry dampness, resolving phlegm and relieving pain 健脾燥湿, 化痰止痛	*Chen xia liu jun zi tang* 陈夏六君子汤, *Dao tan tang* 导痰汤, *Ban xia tian ma bai zhu tang* 半夏天麻白术汤, etc.
	Heat toxin obstruction 热毒蕴结	Clearing heat and resolving toxins, dispersing nodules and relieving pain 清热解毒, 散结止痛	*Wu wei xiao du yin* 五味消毒饮, *Huang lian jie du tang* 黄连解毒汤, etc.
	Dual deficiency of *qi* and blood 气血亏虚	Tonifying *qi* and engendering Blood, nourishing Blood and relieving pain 补益气血, 养血止痛	*Ba zhen tang* 八珍汤, *Fu zi li zhong tang* 附子理中汤, etc.
Zhong Liu Nei Ke Zhong Xi Yi Jie He Zhi Liao 肿瘤内科中西医结合治疗[5]	Qi stagnation pain 气滞疼痛	Moving *qi* to relieve pain 行气止痛	*Chai hu shu gan san* with modifications 柴胡疏肝散加减
	Blood stasis pain 血瘀疼痛	Activating Blood and relieving pain 活血止痛	*Shi xiao san* 失笑散, *Xue fu zhu yu tang* 血府逐瘀汤, etc. with modifications
	Phlegm-dampness pain 痰湿疼痛	Resolving phlegm and draining dampness 化痰利湿	*Er chen tang* plus *Yi yi ren tang* 二陈汤合薏苡仁汤, etc. with modifications
	Heat pain 热邪疼痛	Clearing heat and resolving toxins 清热解毒	*Wu wei xiao du yin* with modifications 五味消毒饮加减
	Yang deficiency and cold pain 阳虚寒痛	Warming the meridian and dissipating cold 温经散寒	*Yang he tang* 阳和汤, *Da zhui feng wan* 大追风丸, *Gu sui bu wan* with modifications 骨碎补丸加减
	Qi deficiency pain 气虚疼痛	Replenishing *qi* and relieving pain 益气止痛	*Bu zhong yi qi tang*补中益气汤, *Shi quan da bu tang* with modifications 十全大补汤加减
	Blood deficiency pain 血虚疼痛	Nourishing Blood and relieving pain 养血止痛	*Gui pi tang* with modifications 归脾汤加减
	Yin deficiency pain 阴虚疼痛	Enriching *yin* and relieving pain 滋阴止痛	*Zuo gui wan* with modifications 左归丸加减

3. *Xiao jin dan* 小金丹

Actions: Resolves phlegm and dispels dampness (*hua tan qu shi* 化痰祛湿), dissipates nodules and disperses swelling, resolves stasis and relieves pain. For cancer pain patients who have the syndrome of binding of phlegm and Blood stasis (*tan yu hu jie* 痰瘀互结).

Dose: 0.6g, twice a day.[6,8]

4. *Mei hua dian she dan* 梅花点舌丹

Actions: Clears heat and resolves toxins, disperses swelling to relieve pain. Used for cancer pain.

Dose: 2 pills, three times per day.[6,8]

5. *Liu shen wan* 六神丸

Actions: Cools and resolves toxins (*qing liang jie du* 清凉解毒), disperses inflammation (*xiao yan* 消炎) and relieves pain. Used for cancer pain.

Dose: 10–15 pills, four times per day.[6,8]

6. *Fu fang tian xian jiao nang* 复方天仙胶囊

Actions: Clears heat and resolves toxins, activates Blood and resolves stasis, dissipates nodules and relieves pain. It can be used by esophageal cancer or gastric cancer patients who have the symptom of pain.

Dose: 2–3 pills, three times per day.[6,8]

External Chinese Herbal Medicine Treatment

External herbal medicine is an important component of traditional CM treatment. It can have effects that are similar to those of oral CHM and can be used in cases where oral CHM cannot be applied. External herbal medicine therapies used in cancer pain include topical applications (*wai fu* 外敷) and enemas (*guan chang* 灌肠).

Topical Applications

1. *Chan su gao* 蟾酥膏: 18 herbs including *chan su* 蟾酥, *sheng chuan wu* 生川乌, *liang mian zhen* 两面针, *gong ding xiang* 公丁香, *rou gui* 肉桂, *xi xin* 细辛, *qi ye yi zhi hua* 七叶一枝花 and *hong hua* 红花. Make into a paste, apply to the local pain area and change every six hours. Its actions are activating Blood and resolving stasis and dispersing swelling to relieve pain, and it can be used for cancer pain.[2,3,6,8]
2. *Xiao ji zhi tong fang* 消积止痛方: *Zhang nao* 樟脑, *a wei* 阿魏, *ding xiang* 丁香, *bai zao xiu* 白蚤休 and *teng huang* 藤黄, made into powders and combined in equal proportions. Sprinkle on adhesive plaster, use on the painful area, and then cover with a 50°–60°C wet towel for half an hour, three times per day. Continue for 5–7 days. Can be used for cancer pain.[1,2,8]
3. *Ru mo zhi tong ding* 乳没止痛酊: Includes *ru xiang* 乳香, *mo yao* 没药, *song xiang* 松香, *xue jie* 血竭 and *bing pian* 冰片. Make into a powder and add wine to form a liquid, use on the local pain area, 4–6 g per time. It can be used for upper limb pain caused by brachial plexus involvement.[1,8]
4. *Shen ai zhi tong san* 肾癌止痛散: Includes *bing pian* 冰片, *teng huang* 藤黄, *she xiang* 麝香 and *sheng nan xing* 生南星. Make into a power and add wine and vinegar to form a paste, apply to painful area in kidney cancer.[1,8]
5. *Xiang song san* 香松散: Includes *she xiang* 麝香, *wu gong* 蜈蚣, *ru xiang* 乳香, *mo yao* 没药, *sheng ban xia* 生半夏, *chen pi* 陈皮, *peng sha* 硼砂, *zao xiu* 蚤休, *quan xie* 全蝎, *zi hua ding ding* 紫花地丁 and *yin zhu* 银朱. Make into a powder and add buckwheat noodles to form a paste, and apply to the local painful area. It can be used to stop liver pain; change every 1–2 days.[1,6,8]
6. *Tian xian zi san* 天仙子散: *tian xian zi* 天仙子, *bing pian* 冰片. Make into a powder and add warm water to form a paste, put on a tissue and apply to the local painful area, change every 1–2 days.[1,6,8]

Herbal Enema

Shou nian san with modifications 手拈散加味 (*yan hu suo* 延胡索, *mo yao* 没药, *xiang fu* 香附, *wu ling zhi* 五灵脂). It can be used for gastric cancer patients with pain.[1,6]

Acupuncture and Related Therapies

Acupuncture and moxibustion therapy, as specific treatments in CM, have been documented since at least the era of the *Huang Di Nei Jing* 黄帝内经. Modern innovations include electro-acupuncture and ear acupuncture. These treatments are used to alleviate various symptoms including cancer pain. These are summarised in Table 2.3.

1. Lung cancer pain: TE6 *Zhigou* 支沟, LR14 *Qimen* 期门, LI4 *Hegu* 合谷, PC6 *Neiguan* 内关, BL12 *Fengmen* 风门, BL13 *Feishu* 肺俞, EX-B1 *Dingchuan* 定喘, ST40 *Fenglong* 丰隆.[2,3,6]
2. Liver cancer pain: LU5 *Chize* 尺泽, LR14 *Qimen* 期门, ST36 *Zusanli* 足三里, SP6 *Sanyinjiao* 三阴交, LI4 *Hegu* 合谷, PC6 *Neiguan* 内关, SP9 *Yinlingquan* 阴陵泉, GB34 *Yanglingquan* 阳陵泉, *Ashi* points 阿是穴, *Ganyandian* 肝炎点 which is located 2 cun 寸 below the lower edge of the rib arch on a line intersecting the midline of the clavicle (Fig. 2.1).[1–3,6,9]
3. Gastrointestinal cancer pain: ST36 *Zusanli* 足三里, ST37 *Shangjuxu* 上巨虚, LI4 *Hegu* 合谷, PC6 *Neiguan* 内关, SP9 *Yinlingquan* 阴陵泉, GB34 *Yanglingquan* 阳陵泉, *Ashi* points 阿是穴.[2,3,6]
4. Gynaecologic cancer pain: SP6 *Sanyinjiao* 三阴交, LR3 *Taichong* 太冲.[2]
5. Head and face pain: EX-HN5 *Taiyang* 太阳, *Yintang* 印堂, GV20 *Baihui* 百会, LI4 *Hegu* 合谷, TE5 *Waiguan* 外关, LU7 *Lieque* 列缺, GB15 *Toulinqi* 头临泣.[4]
6. Neck pain: GV21 *Qianding* 前顶, GV13 *Taodao* 陶道, TE5 *Waiguan* 外关, GB11 *Touqiaoyin* 头窍阴, SI7 *Zhizheng* 支正.[4]

Table 2.3 Summary of Acupuncture Therapies for Cancer Pain

Type	Acupuncture Points
Lung cancer pain[2,3,6]	TE6 *Zhigou* 支沟, LR14 *Qimen* 期门, LI4 *Hegu* 合谷, PC6 *Neiguan* 内关, BL12 *Fengmen* 风门, BL13 *Feishu* 肺俞, EX-B1 *Dingchuan* 定喘, ST40 *Fenglong* 丰隆
Liver cancer pain[1–3,6,9]	LU5 *Chize* 尺泽, LR14 *Qimen* 期门, ST36 *Zusanli* 足三里, SP6 *Sanyinjiao* 三阴交, LI4 *Hegu* 合谷, PC6 *Neiguan* 内关, SP9 *Yinlingquan* 阴陵泉, GB34 *Yanglingquan* 阳陵泉, *Ashi* points 阿是穴, *Ganyandian* 肝炎点
Gastrointestinal cancer pain[2,3,6]	ST36 *Zusanli* 足三里, ST37 *Shangjuxu* 上巨虚, LI4 *Hegu* 合谷, PC6 *Neiguan* 内关, SP9 *Yinlingquan* 阴陵泉, GB34 *Yanglingquan* 阳陵泉, *Ashi* points 阿是穴
Gynaecologic cancer pain[2]	SP6 *Sanyinjiao* 三阴交, LR3 *Taichong* 太冲
Head and face pain[4]	EX-HN5 *Taiyang* 太阳, *Yintang* 印堂, GV20 *Baihui* 百会, LI4 *Hegu* 合谷, TE5 *Waiguan* 外关, LU7 *Lieque* 列缺, GB15 *Toulinqi* 头临泣
Neck pain[4]	GV21 *Qianding* 前顶, GV13 *Taodao* 陶道, TE5 *Waiguan* 外关, GB11 *Touqiaoyin* 头窍阴, SI7 *Zhizheng* 支正
Chest pain[3,4]	LU2 *Yunmen* 云门, LU4 *Xiabai* 侠白, LU6 *Kongzui* 孔最, LU8 *Jingqu* 经渠, LU9 *Taiyuan* 天泉, PC7 *Daling* 大陵, PC6 *Neiguan* 内关, PC5 *Jianshi* 间使, HT1 *Jiquan* 极泉, TE6 *Zhigou* 支沟, LI4 *Hegu* 合谷, ST40 *Fenglong* 丰隆, HT8 *Shaofu* 少府
Hypochondriac pain[3]	LI4 *Hegu* 合谷, PC6 *Neiguan* 内关, LR3 *Taichong* 太冲, GB40 *Qiuxu* 丘墟
Shoulder and upper limb pain[4]	LI5 *Yangxi* 阳溪, LI10 *Shousanli* 手三里, LI11 *Quchi* 曲池, LI14 *Binao* 肩臑, LI15 *Jianyu* 肩髃, TE10 *Tianjing* 天井, TE13 *Naohui* 臑会, SP21 *Dabao* 大包
Abdominal pain[3,4]	PC6 *Neiguan* 内关, LI4 *Hegu* 合谷, ST36 *Zusanli* 足三里, CV12 *Zhongwan* 中脘, CV4 *Guanyuan* 关元, CV3 *Zhongji* 中极, ST29 *Guilai* 归来, SP6 *Sanyinjiao* 三阴交
Lower back pain[4]	BL23 *Shenshu* 肾俞, BL25 *Dachangshu* 大肠俞, EX-B2 *Jiaji* 夹脊, BL52 *Zhishi* 志室, GV4 *Mingmen* 命门, GV3 *Yaoyangguan* 腰阳关, *Ashi* points 阿是穴

Table 2.3 (*Continued*)

Type	Acupuncture Points
Buttock and lower limb pain[4]	Points painful on pressure *Ya tong dian* 压痛点, EX-B2 *Jiaji* 夹脊, GB30 *Huantiao* 环跳, BL25 *Dachangshu* 大肠俞, BL54 *Zhibian* 秩边, BL36 *Chengfu* 承扶, BL37 *Yinmen* 殷门, BL40 *Weizhong* 委中, GB36 *Yanglingquan* 阳陵泉, BL57 *Chengshan* 承山, BL58 *Feiyang* 飞扬, BL39 *Xuanzhong* 悬钟, BL60 *Kunlun* 昆仑
Various malignant tumour patients with pain, including lung cancer, liver cancer and brain tumour[1,6,9]	Ear acupuncture Main points: AT4 *Pizhixia* 皮质下, CO15 *Xin* 心, HX6,7i *Erjian* 耳尖 Auxiliary points: AH6a *Jiaogan* 交感, CO12 *Gan* 肝, TF4 *Shenmen* 神门

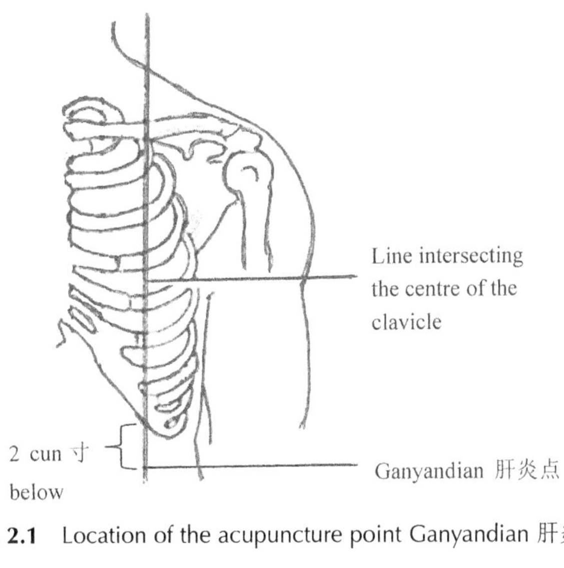

Fig. 2.1 Location of the acupuncture point Ganyandian 肝炎点

7. Chest pain: LU2 *Yunmen* 云门, LU4 *Xiabai* 侠白, LU6 *Kongzui* 孔最, LU8 *Jingqu* 经渠, LU9 *Taiyuan* 天泉, PC7 *Daling* 大陵, PC6 *Neiguan* 内关, PC5 *Jianshi* 间使, HT1 *Jiquan* 极泉, TE6 *Zhigou* 支沟, LI4 *Hegu* 合谷, ST40 *Fenglong* 丰隆, HT8 *Shaofu* 少府.[3,4]

8. Hypochondriac pain: LI4 *Hegu* 合谷, PC6 *Neiguan* 内关, LR3 *Taichong* 太冲, GB40 *Qiuxu* 丘墟.[3]
9. Shoulder and upper limb pain: LI5 *Yangxi* 阳溪, LI10 *Shousanli* 手三里, LI11 *Quchi* 曲池, LI14 *Binao* 肩臑, LI15 *Jianyu* 肩髃, TE10 *Tianjing* 天井, TE13 *Naohui* 臑会, SP21 *Dabao* 大包.[4]
10. Abdominal pain: PC6 *Neiguan* 内关, LI4 *Hegu* 合谷, ST36 *Zusanli* 足三里, CV12 *Zhongwan* 中脘, CV4 *Guanyuan* 关元, CV3 *Zhongji* 中极, ST29 *Guilai* 归来, SP6 *Sanyinjiao* 三阴交.[3,4]
11. Lower back pain: BL23 *Shenshu* 肾俞, BL25 *Dachangshu* 大肠俞, EX-B2 *Jiaji* 夹脊, BL52 *Zhishi* 志室, GV4 *Mingmen* 命门, GV3 *Yaoyangguan* 腰阳关, *Ashi* points 阿是穴.[4]
12. Buttock and lower limb pain: Points that are painful on pressure (*ya tong dian* 压痛点), EX-B2 *Jiaji* 夹脊, GB30 *Huantiao* 环跳, BL25 *Dachangshu* 大肠俞, BL54 *Zhibian* 秩边, BL34 *Chengfu* 承扶, BL37 *Yinmen* 殷门, BL40 *Weizhong* 委中, GB36 *Yanglingquan* 阳陵泉, BL57 *Chengshan* 承山, BL58 *Feiyang* 飞扬, BL39 *Xuanzhong* 悬钟, BL60 *Kunlun* 昆仑.[4]
13. Ear acupuncture: Main points include AT4 *Pizhixia* 皮质下, CO15 *Xin* 心, HX6,7i *Erjian* 耳尖; auxiliary points include AH6a *Jiaogan* 交感, CO12 *Gan* 肝, TF4 *Shenmen* 神门. Can be used for various malignant tumour patients with pain, including lung cancer, liver cancer and brain tumour.[1,6,9]

Other Chinese Medicine Therapies

In addition to Chinese herbal medicine and acupuncture therapies, CM includes a range of other therapies to treat cancer pain. Examples include appropriate exercise therapies, *qi gong* 气功,[8] music therapy[8,10] and others. In particular, music therapy is a non-pharmacological adjuvant therapy whose purpose is to alleviate the cancer pain of patients by reducing their physiological, psychological, social and spiritual distress, and improving their quality of life. It has the advantages of convenience, low price and low risk. The history of music therapy in China can be traced back to the Spring and Autumn periods and the Warring States period. In the *Huang Di Nei Jing* 黄帝内经, there were records of using the traditional musical notes *gong* 宫, *shang* 商, *jue* 角, *zhi* 徵 and *yu* 羽 to regulate the *qi* of the five internal organs (*wu zang* 五脏) and treat various diseases.[8,10,11,12]

Prevention

Cancer pain is the most common symptom in cancer patients, especially in patients with middle- and late-stage cancers. Therefore, the fundamental way to prevent cancer pain is effective and timely treatment of the cancer so that patients without pain do not develop pain, and those with moderate pain do not progress to severe pain. In addition, it is important to prevent and/or treat at an early stage any opioid-induced adverse reactions such as constipation.[3,8]

Lifestyle

Appropriate physical exercise not only helps patients to enhance immunity, it also has the effects of distracting the patient's attention from the pain, making people more energetic and emotionally stable, and increasing appetite. These all improve a person's quality of life. Patients with cancer pain can choose recreational activities suitable for their physical strength and physical condition, such as watching TV, listening to music, and reading books and newspapers, to distract them from the pain and make them feel more comfortable.[2,6]

Psychology

The psychological condition is closely related to a person's physiological functions and affects pathological changes. A stable mental and emotional state can smooth the *qi* and Blood (*qi xue liu tong* 气血流通), regulate the internal organs (*zang fu* 脏腑), increase resistance to disease, and promote physical and mental health. Patients can be provided with psychological support therapy, relaxation therapy and cognitive therapy to help them relieve the psychological burden of cancer, relieve their emotional distress, build up their confidence and enhance their initiative to take an active role in their pain management.[6,8]

Diet

Patients with cancer pain are recommended to choose food according to their physical condition, their constitution and the flavour and nature of the food. They should avoid excessively hot foods, fried food and roasted food. The effects of the five flavours can be used to regulate *zang-fu* 脏腑 disharmony, to counter cancer progression and prevent or alleviate pain.[6]

Prognosis

The prognosis of cancer pain depends on many factors including the person's condition and the effectiveness of the treatment of the cancer, whether the use of analgesics is standardised and sufficient, and whether a multidisciplinary comprehensive treatment is adopted for refractory cancer pain. Different painful areas have a different prognosis; individual differences and the different causes of cancer pain will also affect prognosis.[8]

References

1. 中华中医药学会. (2008) 肿瘤中医诊疗指南. 北京: 中国中医药出版社.
2. 刘嘉湘. (1996) 实用中医肿瘤手册. 上海: 上海科技教育出版社.
3. 林洪生. (2014) 恶性肿瘤中医诊疗指南. 北京: 人民卫生出版社.
4. 张蓓，周志伟. (2004) 实用中西医结合肿瘤学. 广州: 广东人民出版社.
5. 王居祥. (2009) 肿瘤内科中西医结合治疗. 北京: 人民卫生出版社.
6. 王洪武. (2010) 癌性疼痛的综合治疗. 北京: 科学普及出版社.
7. 何裕民. (2005) 现代中医肿瘤学 (普通高等教育"十五"国家级规划教材面向21世纪课程教材). 北京: 中国协和医科大学出版社.
8. 李佩文, 蔡光蓉. (2002) 癌症疼痛中西医汇通. 沈阳: 辽宁科学技术出版社.
9. 郑伟达. (1998) 肿瘤的中医防治. 北京: 中国中医药出版社.
10. 余怡，许青. (2016) 音乐疗法治疗癌痛应用进展概述. 现代肿瘤医学 **24(22):** 3667–3669.
11. Zhang H, Lai H. (2017) Five Phases Music Therapy (FPMT) in Chinese medicine: Fundamentals and application. *Open Access Library Journal* **4**: e4190, 1–11.
12. Wu Y. (2019) The development of music therapy in mainland China. *Music Therapy Perspectives* **37(1):** 84–92.

3

Classical Chinese Medicine Literature

OVERVIEW

References to conditions that may have been cancers are found throughout Chinese medicine classical literature. In addition, some of these conditions manifested pain and treatments were recorded. Hence this literature provides a valuable record of how cancer-like conditions were conceptualised and pain was managed using Chinese herbal medicine, acupuncture, moxibustion and other therapies. This chapter reports the results of searches of the collection of classical Chinese medicine texts *Zhong Hua Yi Dian* 中华医典. Terms relating to masses (*ji ju* 积聚, *zheng jia* 癥瘕/症瘕, *yan* 岩) and bone lesions (*gu ju* 骨疽) were combined with terms for pain (*tong* 痛, *teng* 疼) to identify 121 citations of conditions broadly consistent with cancer pain. The citations provided descriptions of the symptoms, and included treatments using orally and/or topically administered herbal medicines as well as treatments using acupuncture, moxibustion and a form of *qi gong* 气功.

Introduction

The earliest written records of medical practice in China were found in the Spring and Autumn (770–476 BC) and Warring States (474–221 BC) periods which showed that the practices of moxibustion, herbal decoction and acupuncture were in use.[1]

For this chapter, classical and pre-modern medical literature was searched electronically using the *Zhong Hua Yi Dian* 中华医典 (ZHYD) Fifth Edition, which is a database containing more than 1,150 classical and pre-modern Chinese medical books.[2] This is one of the largest collections of such books, and comparisons with other large collections found it to be broadly representative of the classical and pre-modern literature on Chinese medicine (CM).[3,4]

Search Terms

Searches were based on combinations of terms relevant to 'cancer' and terms relevant to 'pain'. To obtain candidate terms, books and guidelines were consulted[5–13] and lists of terms used in pre-modern and ancient times were compiled. Then, ten clinical experts and consultant physicians provided their rankings of these terms regarding their relevance to cancer pain. For the more relevant terms, test searches were conducted to determine combinations of terms that identified passages relevant to cancer pain in the literature. Terms which had high frequencies but low specificity for cancer pain were excluded, including *fei ji* 肺积, *e he* 恶核 and others. Finally, we selected the terms *ji ju* 积聚, *zheng jia* 癥瘕, *zheng jia* 症瘕, *fan hua* 翻花, *yan* 岩, *gu ju* 骨疽 and *ai* 癌 as potentially relevant to cancer. For pain we selected the terms *tong* 痛 and *teng* 疼 since they both have the meaning of pain and are used throughout the literature.

Procedures for Search, Data Coding and Data Analysis

Each of the seven search terms relevant to cancer was combined with each of the two terms for pain to produce 14 combinations. These were searched separately in the ZHYD database. The search results were downloaded to spreadsheets. Each distinct passage of text referring to one or more of the search terms was defined as a 'citation' and duplicate citations were identified and removed. Each distinct citation was allocated a number. Candidate citations were read in detail and those unrelated to cancer pain were excluded. Additional codes were added for the book in which the citation was located, the dynasty and year in which the book was written and the type of intervention used. Books written after 1949 were excluded.[14]

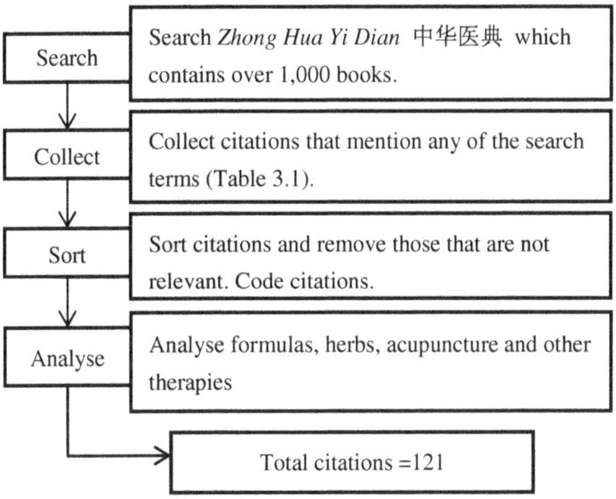

Fig. 3.1 Process for identifying classical literature citations

Further codes were allocated to identify citations that were more or less specific to cancer pain, including whether a mass was mentioned and the location of the mass, whether pain was an associated symptom and the location of the pain, and whether the symptoms suggested malignancy. Only citations that mentioned the presence of a mass and pain were included. Analyses were conducted in SPSS® to identify the herbal formulas, their constituent herbs, acupuncture points and any other CM therapies used for cancer pain (Fig. 3.1).

Search Results

The 14 pairs of search terms produced 9,186 'hits' in the ZHYD database. One 'hit' was the co-occurrence of the two terms within 100 characters of text, so many hits were not relevant. After the process of duplicate removal and exclusion of irrelevant and unclear passages of text, 121 citations were included. Some of these were located by multiple combinations of search terms.

Of the terms for pain, *tong* 痛 was used more frequently than *teng* 疼. The terms *ji ju* 积聚, *zheng jia* 癥瘕, *zheng jia* 症瘕, *yan* 岩, *fan hua* 翻花 and *ai* 癌 can all refer to a range of solid tumours. Of these, *ai* 癌 is the main modern term for cancer whereas *ji ju* 积聚 and the closely related terms *zheng jia* 癥瘕 and *zheng jia* 症瘕 are common in pre-modern literature. The term *gu ju* 骨疽 was selected due to its relation to possible bone cancer.

The most productive combination of terms was *ji ju* plus *tong* (积聚 + 痛) which identified 3,906 hits and 62 included citations. The combination *ji ju* plus *teng* (积聚 + 疼) was less productive with 21 citations, many of which were also found by *ji ju* plus *tong* (积聚 + 痛). The terms *zheng jia* plus *tong* (癥瘕 + 痛) located 1,186 hits and 17 citations and *zheng jia* plus *tong* (症瘕 + 痛) had 1,134 hits and 30 citations. The terms *yan* plus *tong* (岩 + 痛) were the next most productive with 15 citations while *fan hua* plus *tong* (翻花 + 痛) located one citation. The combination *ai* plus *tong* (癌 + 痛) only identified one citation which was in a relatively recent book (*Zhong Guo Nei Ke Yi Jian* 中国内科医鉴 c. 1933). *Gu ju* 骨疽 plus the two terms for pain did not locate any relevant citations (Table 3.1).

Table 3.1 Hit Frequency by Search Term

Pinyin	Chinese Characters	Hit Frequency (%)[1]	Included Citations *n* (%)[2]
Ji ju + tong	积聚 + 痛	3,906 (42.5)	62 (35)
Ji ju + teng	积聚 + 疼	703 (7.7)	21 (11.9)
Zheng jia + tong	癥瘕 + 痛	1,186 (12.9)	17 (9.6)
Zheng jia + teng	癥瘕 + 疼	202 (2.2)	12 (6.8)
Zheng jia + tong	症瘕 + 痛	1,134 (12.3)	30 (16.9)
Zheng jia + teng	症瘕 + 疼	226 (2.5)	16 (9)
Fan hua + tong	翻花 + 痛	92 (1)	1 (0.6)
Fan hua + teng	翻花 + 疼	25 (0.3)	0 (0)
Gu ju + tong	骨疽 + 痛	570 (6.2)	0 (0)
Gu ju + teng	骨疽 + 疼	73 (0.8)	0 (0)
Yan + tong	岩 + 痛	822 (8.9)	15 (8.5)
Yan + teng	岩 + 疼	112 (1.2)	1 (0.6)
Ai + tong	癌 + 痛	113 (1.2)	1 (0.6)
Ai + teng	癌 + 疼	22 (0.2)	1 (0.6)
Totals		9186	121*

*Some citations were located by two or more search terms.

[1]Before duplicate removal and screening.

[2]After duplicate removal and screening.

The included citations were derived from 48 different books written between c. 282 AD (*Zhen Jiu Jia Yi Jing* 针灸甲乙经) and c. 1937 (*Jin Zhen Mi Chuan* 金针秘传). The book that provided the most citations was *Pu Ji Fang* 普济方 with 24 citations, followed by *Tai Ping Sheng Hui Fang* 太平圣惠方 with 11 citations. The largest proportion of citations were from the *Ming* 明 dynasty (c. 1369–1644) with 49.6%, followed by the *Song* and *Jin* 宋金 dynasties (c. 961–1271) which provided 21.5% and the *Qing* 清 dynasty (c. 1645–1911) with 18.2%.

In the 121 citations, herbal interventions were used in 87 citations. Orally administered Chinese herbal medicine (CHM) was used in 85 citations; four citations used a topically applied CHM, with two of these citations mentioning oral plus topical CHM. Acupuncture and/or moxibustion were used in 33 citations, and other CM therapies were used in one citation which referred to a form of *qi gong* 气功. In the following analyses, the citations are divided into four groups:

- Oral CHM (87 citations);
- Topical CHM (four citations, including two oral plus topical);
- Acupuncture/moxibustion (33 citations); and
- Other CM therapy (1 citation).

Citations Related to the Definitions of the Main Terms

The definitions of the terms *ji ju* 积聚, *zheng jia* 癥瘕 and *zheng jia* 症瘕 have been discussed in detail in the volume on colorectal cancer.[15] Briefly, *ji ju* 积聚 (accumulations and aggregations) appeared in the *Huang Di Nei Jing Ling Shu* 黄帝内经灵枢 (c. first century BC) and had widespread use since that time as a term for a variety of masses, both solid and soft. The terms *zheng jia* 癥瘕 and *zheng jia* 症瘕 are cognates which could be used interchangeably and will be referred to as *zheng jia* 症/癥瘕 (concretions and agglomerations) from now on. This term appeared in the *Jin Gui Yao Lue* 金匮要略 (c. 206) and in numerous subsequent books in which it could refer to palpable masses that are fixed or moveable and located in the abdomen. It was commonly used in a gynaecological context. There was considerable overlap in the scope of meaning of the terms *ji ju* 积聚 and *zheng jia* 症/癥瘕. Both terms could encompass masses that would now be considered cancers, but not all the masses referred to by these terms were cancers, so other symptoms needed to be taken into account when making a judgement.

The term *yan* 岩 refers to 'rock' and in a medical context to lumps that are hard like a rock with a surface that is not smooth. In particular, *ru yan* 乳岩 refers to hard lumps in the breast.[16] An early description of a condition consistent with breast cancer was found in the book *Dan Xi Xin Fa* 丹溪心法 (c. 1481) which said: 'In the case of a woman who has relationship difficulties with her husband and/or in-laws; and who has anger, depression and repressed emotion, [this emotion] accumulates day by day, and damages the function of the Spleen, so the Liver can attack the Spleen [on the control (*ke* 克) cycle]. This gradually causes the development of a 'hidden kernel' (*yin he* 隐核) [in the breast] which is the size of a Chinese chess piece (*qi zi* 棋子); [the lump is] not painful and not itchy. Many decades later, it develops into an ulcer (*chuang xian* 疮陷). This is called *nai yan* 奶岩 (literally 'breast rock'); the shape of the ulcer is like a cave in a rock. This cannot be cured. If you take action early, you can eliminate the root of the disease; by clearing the mind and calming the emotions; and then treating with medicine. This way the condition can be stabilised.'

The *Dan Xi Xin Fa* 丹溪心法 did not provide any treatment for this condition and said it was not painful, at least in the early stage, but later books provided descriptions of more advanced conditions, listed more symptoms including pain and included treatments (see examples below). However, they concurred that this condition could only by treated successfully at the early stage.

The term *fan hua* 翻花 appears in the name of multiple diseases unrelated to cancer as well as in the context of breast cancer. The *Zhong Yi Da Ci Dian* 中医大辞典 gives *shi liu fan hua fa* 石榴翻花发 (literally 'open pomegranate flower') as a synonym for *ru yan* 乳岩 (p. 1072) and the entry for *shi liu fan hua fa* 石榴翻花发 (p. 443) identifies this as breast cancer (*ru ai* 乳癌).[16]

In the *Wai Ke Xin Fa Yao Jue* 外科心法要诀 (c. 1742) section on *ru yan* 乳岩 there was a detailed account of *fan hua* 翻花 as follows: 'After *fan hua* 翻花 breaks through there is angry (i.e. severe) bleeding; this disease is incurable. This is due to damage of both Liver and Spleen; *qi* stagnation (*qi yu* 气郁) and coagulation (*ning jie* 凝结) are the cause. Inside the breast there is a kernel (*jie he* 结核); at the beginning it is the size of a jujube or chestnut, but gradually it gets bigger, like a chess piece (*qi zi* 棋子). There is no redness and no fever, but sometimes there is hidden pain (*yin tong* 隐痛). Without delay use external moxa; and internally use herbal formulas to nourish Blood (*yang xue* 养血), in order to avoid internal attack (*nei gong* 内攻) [of the Spleen by the Liver]. After a long time [without treatment], the person can feel hot flashes and aversion to cold (*chao re wu han* 潮热恶寒); and start to feel severe pain that radiates and drags to the chest and axilla; and there is swelling [of the breast] that is hard like an upturned bowl (*fu man* 覆碗). The shape [of the mass] is like a pile of chestnuts, extruding like a rough rock; on the tip of the mass you can see a purple colour shining through the skin; and in the flesh you can see blood streaks (*xue si* 血丝). Firstly, it becomes putrid and then breaks through the skin; it exudes purulent liquid (*wu shui* 污水) and sometimes clear fluid (*jin* 津); sometimes bad smelling blood (*mao chou xue* 冒臭血) oozes out; there is deep decay like a cave (*yan he* 岩壑); and the *fan hua* 翻花 protrudes like the petals of a lotus. The pain is so severe it can reach the heart (*lian xin* 连心).'

Fan hua 翻花 was briefly mentioned in the *Gu Fang Hui Jing* 古方汇精 (c. 1804) section on *ru yan* 乳岩. It said: 'If [the lump] is very itchy with no pain, and a knife is used to open it, then it will become *fan hua* 翻花, this is the worst situation.' There are also examples of warnings against the use of lancing or a knife in the treatment of abscesses or lumps in the breast in other books.

In general, *fan hua* 翻花 was considered a more severe stage of *ru yan* 乳岩 or *nai yan* 奶岩 in which a cavernous lesion was present and appears consistent with late-stage breast cancer. A number of the books warned that it could not be cured and urged early treatment of breast lumps.

The term *ai* 癌 has been used to refer to the Western medicine concept of 'cancer' since at least the 19th century, but *ai* 癌 and related terms, such as *ai ji* 癌疾 and *ai chuang* 癌疮 can also be found in classical literature.[16,17] The following are some early examples.

In the *Wei Ji Bao Shu* 卫济宝书 (c. 1170) there was an explanation of the five types of *yong zu* 痈疽 (various types of open and closed sores) of which one type was called *ai* 癌. The description was as follows: '*ai ji* 癌疾 at the beginning has no special symptom, the flesh just feels hot and painful. After seven or fourteen days, the colour suddenly turns to purple-red and there is mild swelling, and the pain gradually disappears. Gradually the colour becomes a dark purple red, but it does not break through the skin.' Later in the same book the term *ai chuang* 癌疮 was used. This appears to refer to the same disease, except that the skin appears to have broken.

In the *Shi Yi De Xiao Fang* 世医得效方 volume 19 (c. 1345) there is a section which defines the five types of sores including *ju* 疽, *ai* 癌, *biao* 瘭 and *gu* 痼. *Ai* 癌 was considered one of the types that was difficult to treat. There is also a set of five diagrams (*wu fa xing tu* 五发形图) of sores of the female breast. This section said that: 'These can be swollen, red and protruding, or have a long shape, or be a large *yong* 大痈 (abscess). The five diseases depicted were *tan* 瘫, *ju* 疽, *ai* 癌, *biao* 瘭 and *gu* 痼. Following the diagram for *ai fa* 癌发, it said: 'At the beginning, there are no signs of cold or heat, the swollen area is painful, the colour is purple and dark, it does not break through the skin, but inside it is already rotten (里面坏烂).'

In the first of these two examples, the condition appears more like an abscess than a cancer, so the treatments were excluded from the analyses. In the second example, *ai* 癌 is more chronic, difficult to treat and more consistent with breast cancer, but no specific treatment was given.

The term *gu ju* 骨疽 was included as a term that was likely to have referred to metastatic diseases to the bone or bone cancer.[6,9] In the *Zhu Bing Yuan Hou Lun* 诸病源候论 (c. 610) a condition called *gu ju wei* 骨疽瘘 (literally 'bone abscess hole') was described as follows: 'This condition is due to cold and heat *qi* (*han re zhi qi* 寒热之气)

attacking the channels (*jing mai* 经脉), or it is due to parasites (*chong ju* 虫蛆) from food entering the organs (*zang fu* 腑脏). It has pus, and when it invades the bone, it is called *gu ju* 骨疽. At the beginning there is swelling (*zhong* 肿), and later it breaks through the skin; after breaking through it can heal over, but it can break through again nearby. This can repeat six or seven times; in the interior there is pus and blood (*nong xue* 脓血); the pain starts at sunset; [it is] like a needle piercing.'

The *Wai Tai Mi Yao* 外台秘要 volume 24 (c. 752) contains a similar passage in a section on the diagnosis of *fu gu ju* 附骨疽 from the *Qian Jin Fang* 千金方 as follows: 'We do not know the reason why the bone produces pus. This condition is called *fu gu ju* 附骨疽; is often located inside the large joints; married men (*zhang fu* 丈夫) and pregnant women (*chan fu* 产妇) often get it; there is swelling (*hong zhong* 洪肿) all over the body. Normally, when people feel hot they go out in the wind to get cool; but wind can enter into the bones and joints (*gu jie zhong* 骨解中); then wind and heat fight each other; this becomes *fu gu ju* 附骨疽. Symptoms are sleeplessness (*shi mian* 嗜眠) and heaviness of the body (*chen zhong* 沉重); can suddenly get tinnitus. Also, if people sleep outside in autumn and summer; and are attacked by cold; wind and heat hide and bind (*fu jie* 伏结) and produce this disease. In acute cases the heat is more than the wind, in chronic cases the wind is more than the heat. We don't know about the cause in children. Also, there is *gu ju* 骨疽 with a long-term sore (*chuang* 疮) that does not heal; it gets better and then worse; there is a hole and the bone protrudes (*gu cong kong zhong chu* 骨从孔中出).'

In these citations, the term *gu ju* 骨疽 referred to chronic deep-seated lesions that affected the bone but the causes were not clear, and it appears that lesions with multiple aetiologies would have been included under this term. Therefore, it is likely that this term would have encompassed neoplasms of the bone as well as infections such as pyogenic osteomyelitis. To enable a judgement of the likely aetiology, the classical citation would require a history of the case and/or signs and symptoms that enable differentiation of the possible diseases.

Citations Related to Aetiology and Syndromes

In addition to the above passages, further explanations of the causes, development and manifestations of *ji ju* 积聚, *zheng jia* 症/癥瘕 and *yan* 岩 were identified in the searches. The following are representative examples, some of which include treatments.

The *Zhu Bing Yuan Hou Lun* 诸病源候论 (c. 610) contains a section on *ji ju* with pain in the heart region and abdomen (*ji ju xin fu tong hou* 积聚心腹痛候) which said: '*Ji* 积 is a disorder of the *yin qi* 阴气, that arises from the five solid organs (*wu zang* 五脏); the pain does not move and has a fixed location. *Ju* 聚 is a disorder of *yang qi* 阳气, [that arises from] the six hollow organs (*liu fu* 六腑); it has no root and can move around, and the pain has no fixed location. This disorder is due to cold *qi* (*han qi* 寒气) affecting the organs (*zang fu* 脏腑); the *yin* and *yang* [of the body] resist [where the cold attacks], so there is pain in the heart region and abdomen.'

In the *Wei Sheng Bao Jian* 卫生宝鉴 (c. 1343) the use of the formula *Xi lu wan* 晞露丸 for *zheng jia* 癥瘕 was discussed as follows: '*Xi lu wan* 晞露丸 is for treating cold damaging the interior (*han shang yu nei* 寒伤于内). This causes *qi* to congeal (*qi ning* 气凝) and stops its free flowing (*bu liu* 不流). It causes binding outside the intestine. After a long time, this [binding] becomes a mass (*zheng jia* 癥瘕). Sometimes there is pain. The person cannot bend backwards at the waist [due to pain or the mass].' Then the formula ingredients (see Table 3.3) and preparation method are given. A similar citation is found in *Pu Ji Fang* 普济方 (c. 1406).

In the *Nv Ke Jing Yao* 女科精要 (c. 1694) by *Feng Zhao-zhang* 冯兆张, in the section on breast masses (*ru zheng* 乳症) is the following description of a condition consistent with breast cancer, its causes, and an approach to treatment: 'When a woman has worry, anger and depression (*you nu yi yu* 忧怒抑郁), from morning to evening there is [gradual] accumulation [of emotion]; the Spleen *qi* does not disperse (*pi qi xiao ju* 脾气消阻); the Liver *qi* attacks the Spleen (*gan qi heng ni* 肝气横逆); the *qi* and Blood are both depleted; and the sinews lose nourishment (*jin shi rong yang* 筋失荣养). The *qi* stagnation (*yu zhi* 郁滞) combines with phlegm coagulation (*tan jie* 痰结),

to produce a hidden kernel (*yin he* 隐核). At first, it is not red and there is no pain, but after a long time this mass (*ji* 积) becomes bigger. After many years, symptoms appear on the surface; since deep inside the mass there is festering (*shen lan* 深烂) [that breaks through]. This condition is called "breast rock" (*ru yan* 乳岩), because the sore (*chuang* 疮) [that appears] is like a cave. This is hard to treat. It is due to damage from the seven emotions (*qi qing* 七情); which affects the Liver channel and produces symptoms of *qi* and Blood withering (*ku gao* 枯槁). At the beginning there is burning pain (*xin tong* 焮痛), cold and heat; so treat the Branch (*biao* 表) by dispersing the pathogenic factors (*san xie* 散邪); and treat the centre by coursing the Liver (*shu gan* 疏肝); also add medicines to tonify and nourish the *qi* and Blood (*bu yang qi xue* 补养气血), such as *Yi qi yang rong tang* 益气养荣汤, *Jia we shao yao san* 加味逍遥散 or similar. These formulas have herbs with wind dispelling properties; herbs for *qi* that can move stagnation (*zhi* 滞), such as *ren shen* 人参 and *huang qi* 黄芪; *dang gui* 当归 and *shao yao* 芍药 to tonify *qi* and Blood; *wu yao* 乌药 and *mu tong* 木通 to course the mass (*shu ji* 疏积), and help remove the obstruction (*li yong* 利壅); *chai hu* 柴胡, *fang fang* 防风 and *su ye* 苏叶 to disperse the surface (*biao san* 表散); *bai zhi* 白芷 to dispel the pus and clear through the nutritive and protective *qi* (*rong wei* 荣卫); and *guan gui* 官桂 to circulate the Blood (*xing xue* 行血) and harmonise the vessels (*he mai* 和脉). If the condition is not severe, the person can recover using these kinds of formulas; but if it is severe, this treatment can only prolong life.'

The aetiology of *ru yan* 乳岩 was explained in similar terms in the *Gu Fang Hui Jing* 古方汇精 (c. 1804) as follows: '*Ru yan* 乳岩 can occur in men and women. It is due to worry depression and accumulated anger. In the beginning there is a kernel (*jie he* 结核) in the breast, with no pain and no itch. In some people after two years, in some people after four to five years [this kernel] has not disappeared. Then the kernel must break through (*kui* 溃), and when it has broken through, the disease cannot be treated.'

With regard to the aetiology of the included disorders, there was considerable diversity. The classical citations related to *ji ju* 积聚 and *zheng jia* 症/癥瘕 attributed these disorders to pathogenic cold entering deep into the body and causing blockage, leading to formation of a mass and pain. However, most citations did not give a cause for these conditions, presumably because the causes were considered well known to the reader. For *gu ju* 骨疽 in each of the two passages, the condition was due to external pathogens including cold, heat and wind which penetrated deeply, and there appears to have been a lesion that affected the bone producing pus. However, the searches of *gu ju* 骨疽 plus a term for pain did not identify any conditions consistent with bone cancer or metastasis. In the case of breast masses (*ru yan* 乳岩 and *fan hua* 翻花), numerous citations provided causes and these concurred that the origin of the disorder was emotional with depression and repressed anger affecting the relationship between Spleen and Liver to generate the original 'kernel' of the mass.

None of the citations used specific syndrome names, as do contemporary CM books, but the citations of *ji ju* 积聚 and *zheng jia* 症/癥瘕 described conditions consistent with the syndrome Wind-cold closure and obstruction (*feng han bi zu* 风寒闭阻). Also, the aetiologies included in the citations for breast masses were consistent with *qi* movement stagnation (*qi ji yu jie* 气机郁结) (see Chapter 2).

Oral Chinese Herbal Medicine

Interventions using CHM were given in 85 citations. In 84 of these the intervention was an orally administered CHM multi-herb formula and in one citation a single herb formula was used. The combination of the terms *ji ju* plus *tong* (积聚+痛) located 30 citations. The same number was located for *zheng jia* plus *tong* (症瘕+痛) with 13 for *zheng jia* plus *tong* (癥瘕+痛). Ten citations were located for *yan* plus *tong* (岩+痛), one for *fan hua* plus *tong* (翻花+痛) and one for *ai* plus *tong* (癌+痛).

Frequency of Citations of Oral CHM by Dynasty

None of the included citations were earlier than the Song 宋 dynasty (Table 3.2). The largest proportion was from the Ming 明 dynasty

Table 3.2 Dynastic Distribution of Citations of an Oral Chinese Herbal Medicine Treatment

Dynasty	No. (%) of Citations
Tang and Five dynasties (618–960) and before	0 (0)
Song and Jin dynasties (961–1271)	20 (23.2)
Yuan dynasty (1272-1368)	2 (2.4)
Ming dynasty (1369–1644)	43 (50.6)
Qing dynasty (1645–1911)	19 (22.4)
Min Guo/Republic of China (1912–1949)	1 (1.2)
Total	85 (100)

(1369–1644) followed by the Song and Jin dynasties (961–1271). Only one citation was from the Republic of China period (1912–1949).

The citations that mentioned an oral CHM treatment derived from 36 different books written between c. 992 and c. 1933. The most productive book with 24 citations was *Pu Ji Fang* 普济方 (c. 1406) followed by 11 from *Tai Ping Sheng Hui Fang* 太平圣惠方 (c. 992) and seven from *Sheng Ji Zong Lu* 圣济总录 (c. 1117).

Treatment with Oral Chinese Herbal Medicine

In the 85 citations there were mentions of 89 oral CHM interventions, since some citations mentioned more than one formula, but five of these did not mention a formula name.

Most Frequent Oral Chinese Herbal Medicine Formulas

Of the 55 named formulas, *Xi lu wan* 晞露丸 was the most frequently mentioned ($n = 6$). The formula names *Da huang wan* 大黄丸, *Fang kui wan* 防葵丸 and *Bie jia wan* 鳖甲丸 also were mentioned in three citations each but there were differences in their ingredients, so these formulas were numbered separately. Of these, only *Da huang wan* 大黄丸 no. 1 appeared in multiple citations ($n = 2$). *Xi huang wan* 犀黄丸 appeared three times but only as one component in complex formulations. Therefore, three oral formulas

Table 3.3 Most Frequent Orally Administered Formulas in Citations

Formula Name	Herb Ingredients	No. of Citations (*n*)
Xi lu wan 晞露丸	*Guang zhu* 广术, *jing shan leng* 京三棱, *gan qi* 干漆, *chuan wu* 川乌, *nao sha* 硇砂, *qing pi* 青皮, *xiong huang* 雄黄, *hui xiang* 茴香, *qing fen* 轻粉, *she xiang* 麝香, *ba dou* 巴豆 (in *Wei sheng bao jian* 卫生宝鉴 c. 1348, used for *zheng jia* 癥瘕).	6
Da huang wan 大黄丸 no. 1	*Da huang* 大黄, *tian xiong* 天雄, *xiong huang* 雄黄, *she xiang* 麝香, *zhu sha* 朱砂, *hu jiao* 胡椒, *ba dou* 巴豆, *san leng* 三棱, *bing lang* 槟榔, *dang gui* 当归, *gui xin* 桂心, *mu xiang* 木香, *gan jiang* 干姜 (in *Tai Ping Sheng Hui Fang* 太平圣惠方 c. 922, used for long-term *ji zheng jia* 积症瘕).	2
Da huang wan 大黄丸 no. 2	*Da huang* 大黄, *bie jia* 鳖甲, *chai hu* 柴胡, *wu zhu yu* 吴茱萸, *dang gui* 当归, *san leng* 三棱, *chi shao yao* 赤芍药, *niu xi* 牛膝, *bing lang* 槟榔, *gui xin* 桂心, *gan qi* 干漆 (in *Tai Ping Sheng Hui Fang* 太平圣惠方 c. 922, used for *ji ju* 积聚 in women).	1

1. Each of these formulas had detailed and complex processing requirements.
2. The use of some herbs/ingredients may be restricted in some countries. Readers are advised to comply with relevant regulations.

are listed in Table 3.3. A further 13 formulas were mentioned in two citations each.

Most Frequent Herbs in Citations of Oral Chinese Herbal Medicine

In the 85 citations there were 1,037 herbal ingredients and 166 different ingredients. Of these, the ingredients most frequently included in a formula were *rou gui* 肉桂 ($n = 45$), *san leng* 三棱 ($n = 40$), *mu xiang* 木香 ($n = 34$), *ba dou* 巴豆 ($n = 33$) and *dang gui* 当归 ($n = 32$).

One citation was of a herb used alone. This was from the book *Wei sheng yi jian fang* 卫生易简方 (c. 1410) in which *hu zhang gen*

虎杖根 was used for: 'a mass in the middle abdomen that was hard like a stone (腹中有物硬如石) with piercing pain'. The prescription used one *dou* 一斗 of dried, crushed *hu zhang* root 虎杖根, soaked in wine and taken three times a day.

Of the herbs listed in Table 3.4, the following are traditionally used for pain and are listed for this indication in the comprehensive *materia medica* book *Zhong Yao Da Ci Dian* 中药大辞典: *san leng* 三棱, *mu xiang* 木香, *ba dou* 巴豆, *e zhu* 莪术, *dang gui* 当归, *gan jiang* 干姜 and *wu tou* 乌头.[18]

Table 3.4 Most Frequent Herbs in Citations of Oral Chinese Herbal Medicine

Herb Name	Scientific Name	No. of Citations (*n*)
Rou gui 肉桂	*Cinnamomum cassia* Presl.	45
San leng 三棱	*Sparganium stoloniferum* Buch.-Ham.	40
Mu xiang 木香	*Aucklandia lappa* Decne.	34
Ba dou 巴豆	*Croton tiglium* L.	33
Dang gui 当归	*Angelica sinensis* (Oliv.) Diels	32
Gan jiang 干姜	*Zingiber officinale* Rosc.	30
E zhu 莪术	*Curcuma* spp.	27
Da huang 大黄	*Rheum palmatum* L.	26
Qing pi 青皮	*Citrus reticulata* Blanco	22
Ren shen 人参	*Panax ginseng* C. A. Mey.	21
Gan cao 甘草	*Glycyrrhiza uralensis* Fisch.	21
Bie jia 鳖甲	*Trionyx sinensis* Wiegmann	20
Wu tou 乌头	*Aconitum* spp.	19
Nao sha 硇砂	*Sal Ammoniac*	19
Chai hu 柴胡	*Bupleurum chinense* DC.	17
Jie geng 桔梗	*Platycodon grandiflorum* (Jacq.) A. DC.	17
She xiang 麝香	*Moschus*	17
Gan qi 干漆	*Toxicodendron vernicifluum* (Stokes) F. A. Barkl.	17
Hou po 厚朴	*Magnolia officinalis* Rehd. et Wils.	16
Bing lang 槟榔	*Areca catechu* L.	16

Note: The use of some herbs/ingredients may be restricted in some countries. Readers are advised to comply with relevant regulations.

Citations Related to Oral Chinese Herbal Medicine for Cancer Pain

The following are a selection of representative citations for pain associated with a range of different masses for which oral CHMs were used, including some case studies.

The formula *Bie jia wan* 鳖甲丸 was given as a treatment for various types of masses in the *Za Bing Guang Yao* 杂病广要 (c. 1853) section on *ji ju* 积聚 as follows: 'For glomus (*pi qi* 痞气) in the epigastrium (*wei guan* 胃管); with a bound mass (*jie ju* 结聚) shaped like a cup; an accumulation (*ji* 积) that has been there for a long time without dispersing; pain in the abdomen and costal region; body emaciation and exhaustion; and cannot eat and drink. Use *Bie jia wan* 鳖甲丸: *bie jia* 鳖甲, *pao fu zi* 炮附子, *jing san leng* 京三棱, *gan qi* 干漆, *mu xiang* 木香, *chuan da huang* 川大黄 and *wu zhu yu* 吴茱萸. The herbs are powdered, made into pills the size of *wu tong* seeds 梧桐子, and taken every day on an empty stomach, 20 pills with warm wine.'

Another version of *Bie jia wan* 鳖甲丸 was suggested in the *Sheng Ji Zong Lu* 圣济总录 (c. 1117) section on long-term masses (*ji zheng pi* 积症癖): 'For long term *pi* 癖 that binds and becomes hard (*jie ying* 结硬); that is below the ribs (both sides) and below the navel (i.e. whole abdomen) and is hard like a stone. When you press, it is painful; and food and drink cannot descend. Use *Bie jia wan* 鳖甲丸: *cu jiu bie jia* 醋炙鳖甲, *niu xi* 牛膝, *xiong qiong* 芎䓖, *fang kui* 防葵, *dang gui* 当归, *pao gan jiang* 炮干姜, *gui* 桂, *pao fu zi* 炮附子, *jiu gan cao* 炙甘草, *ba dou* 巴豆 and *da huang* 大黄, powdered, mixed with honey to form pills the size of *wu tong* seeds 梧桐子, and taken on an empty stomach with warm wine, five pills, twice a day.'

A case of *ru yan* 乳岩 from the *Chen Xin Tian Wai Ke Fang An* 陈莘田外科方案 (c. 1892) was described as follows: '[A woman] with the family name of Qian 钱 had a mass in the right breast. Stagnation of Liver *qi* produced blockage (*gan yu qi zu* 肝郁气阻); phlegm condensed and congealed into a mass (*xie tan ning ju* 挟痰凝聚). At first there was *ru yan* 乳岩, then gradually increasing pain of the ribs and chest. After several months, the hard lump (*kuai lei* 块磊) was protruding and hard like a stone; the colour was white and there was pain. This disease was due to the emotions. The purpose of the following herbs was to delay festering: *bei chai hu* 北柴胡, *dang gui* 当归, *shan zha* 山栀, *shi jue ming* 石决明, *yuan zhi* 远志, *zhi xiang fu* 制香附, *bai shao*, 白芍, *dan pi* 丹皮, *xiao qing pi* 小青皮 and *fu shen* 茯神.'

Another case from the *Chen Xin Tian Wai Ke Fang An* 陈莘田外科方案 (c. 1892) was as follows: '[A woman] with the family name of Wang 王 had a mass in the right breast. Liver Wood became depressed and lost its function of regulating the *qi* (*mu yu shi tiao* 木郁失条) the Liver *qi* stagnation generated fire (*yu ze sheng huo* 郁则生火); extreme fire generated phlegm (*huo shen sheng tan* 火甚生痰); the phlegm combined with the *qi* blockage (*tan sui qi zu* 痰随气阻) and became a 'rock' (*yan* 岩) in the right breast. The hard lump was protruding; the colour slowly changed to red; sometimes there was pain and sometimes no pain. The pulse was fine and choppy (*si se* 细涩); the tongue coat was coarse and white (*cao bai* 糙白). The disease was caused by the emotions. Treatment was to prevent festering and breaking through. In such cases you can use herbs and must also open up the chest (*kai huai* 开怀) and relax the emotions; and hopefully this will continuously break up the lumps (*ji qi lian po wei miao* 冀其连破为妙). Use *Xiao yao san* 逍遥散 type formulas.'

A section on cancer of the oesophagus (*shi dao ai* 食道癌), together with an example case, appeared in the Min Guo period book *Zhong Guo Nei Ke Yi Jian* 中国内科医鉴 (c. 1933). This book took a modern approach to diagnosis and treatment as follows: 'Oesophageal stricture (*shi dao xia zhai* 食道狭窄) associated with oesophageal cancer (*shi dao ai* 食道癌). Signs and symptoms: There are two kinds, benign and malignant. The benign type is due to chronic ulcer of the oesophagus, drug corrosion, mistakenly swallowing foreign matter, or from pressure outside the oesophagus, such as from goitre, aneurysms, etc. The malignant type is due to oesophageal cancer. The symptoms of this disease include difficulty swallowing, vomiting, feeling obstruction of food in a certain part of the oesophagus, etc. When the stricture is serious, only liquid food can pass through. When it is cancer, the patient often has pain, or compression and paralysis of the recurrent laryngeal nerve (*hui gui shen jing* 回归神经), which can cause dysphonia. In addition, the people develop cachexia; when the person becomes weaker day by day, there may also be cancers in other parts of the body.

Treatment: For oesophageal cancer use *Xuan fu hua dai zhe shi tang* 旋覆花代赭石汤 and a good effect can be achieved.

Case: Male, 58 years old. When I visited, he was weak, and gradually was unable to get out of bed. The main symptoms were sub-xiphoid pain, difficulty in swallowing, belching, blood in the stool for more than half a year, severe anaemia, palpitations and shortness of breath. He often vomited thick mucus and often vomited food following the mucus. After he used the *Xuan fu hua dai zhe shi tang* 旋覆花代赭石汤, the next day the pain went away. After three days, the blood in the stool stopped. After one month, the patient could have a walk in the yard. At the present, he only sometimes had difficulty swallowing and no other symptoms. But whether he was totally cured will only be known after some time has passed.'

Topical Chinese Herbal Medicine

In four citations topical interventions were included. All were for *ru yan* 乳岩. Each was from a different book, both of which were written in the Qing dynasty between 1515 and 1846. In one citation two topical formulae were mentioned, one citation mentioned a single topical ingredient and two citations were of a combination of topical plus oral CHMs.

Citations Related to Topical Chinese Herbal Medicine for Cancer Pain

Overall, the most frequently mentioned topical treatment was *da chan* 大蟾 (large toad), which was included in three citations. The main passages of text for the topical CHMs are given below.

The *Yi Xue Zheng Zhuan* 医学正传 (c. 1555) by *Yu Bo* 虞搏 contains an extended discussion on the treatment of 'breast rock' (*nai yan* 奶岩) which is attributed to a Mr. Cheng (*Cheng shi* 程氏) who appears to have been Cheng Dang 程常, a contemporary of Zhu Dan-xi 朱丹溪, who lived during the Yuan Dynasty, as follows: 'Mr. Cheng said: breast rock (*nai yan* 奶岩) starts with a kernel; then it swells and binds [to form a mass] the size of a tortoise-shell chess piece (*bie qi zi* 鳖棋子); [at this stage there is] no pain and no itch. Five or seven years later there is a sore (*chuang* 疮). At the start you can use herbs to course the *qi* and circulate the Blood (*shu qi xing xue* 疏气行血); and if the woman can relax, feel happier and regulate the emotions, she can recover. After it becomes a sore, it can become like a cave in a rock (*yan xue* 岩穴) with a sunken shape (*ao* 凹); or it is like a mouth and lip; there is red fluid (*chi ye* 赤汁), and pus (*neng shui* 脓水); it spreads to the chest and ribs, producing pain. Use *Wu hui gao* 五灰膏, and/or *Jin bao gao* 金宝膏, to remove the necrosis (*du rou* 蠹肉) and generate new flesh; and slowly the sore will heal over. This disease often occurs in middle-aged women who have melancholia (*you yu* 忧郁) and long-term accumulated anger (*ji fen* 积忿). If the mass does not break through (the skin), it can be treated, but if there is an open sore then it cannot completely recover.'

The topical use of toad skin is described in the *Yan Fang Xin Bian* 验方新编 (c. 1846) in the section on *ru yan* 乳岩: 'For breaking through with pain. Topically apply toad (*da chan* 大蟾). Take six toads, and use one every day, morning or night; open the belly; pierce [the skin] with many holes; take out the intestines, remove the gall bladder; place it over the open lesion ('suffering mouth' *huan kou* 患口) in order to draw out the toxins. Change every day; use for several days.'

A similar passage is found in *Xu Ming Yi Lei An* 续名医类案 (c. 1770) except that the external use of *da chan* 大蟾 for breast cancer with pain is combined with internal use of *Qian jin tuo li san* 《千金》托里散. But no information on the actions of the oral formula was given. Essentially the same passage appears in *Gu Fang Hui Jing* 古方汇精 (c 1804).

Discussion of Chinese Herbal Medicine

By far, the majority of the citations were for orally administered multi-ingredient CHMs. Most of these were for masses described as *ji ju* 积聚 or *zheng jia* 症/癥瘕 which were mainly in the abdomen, but there was a subgroup of breast masses. The citations relating to masses in the abdominal region varied in their level of detail, and it is likely that these included solid masses of diverse aetiologies since technologies for differentiating cancers from other types of masses were not yet available. Consequently, we cannot be certain that the herbal treatments were specific for pain due to cancer, only that actual cancers were likely to have received treatments similar to those located in the citations.

In the cases of 'breast rock' (*ru yan* 乳岩), based on the descriptions, it is highly likely that many of the cases were of breast cancer, often in an advanced stage. The descriptions of the slow development from a small lump to a large 'rock' that eventually breaks through the skin are consistent with cancer. Also, a number of books mentioned that the condition could not be cured, only managed. Nevertheless, we cannot be certain that these disorders would now be diagnosed as breast cancer.

Cancer was clearly the topic in the most recent of the citations which provided a modern description of cancer of the oesophagus. In the associated case, the oral formula appeared to have relieved the symptoms at the time of writing, but no long-term outcome was provided.

The topical CHMs were all for 'breast rock' (*ru yan* 乳岩) and three citations referred to the use of a 'large toad' (*da chan* 大蟾) which was eviscerated and applied directly to the lesion. This appears to have been treatment for a painful open lesion and one passage says the purpose was to draw out the 'toxins' but it was unclear whether it also aimed to relieve pain. In the *Ben Cao Gang Mu* 本草纲目 (c. 1578) there were many references to the use of whole toad (*chan chu* 蟾蜍) in the treatment of various toxic swellings and sores (*chuang* 疮) but the only reference to pain was as a topical powder for tooth pain. It was not used for resolving masses or for *ru yan* 乳岩. Therefore, while this appears to be a method that emerged later, the use of toad for pain was known and it is plausible that pain relief was one of the intended actions.

Acupuncture and Related Therapies

The searches identified 33 citations of treatments using acupuncture and/or moxibustion. The combination of the terms *ji ju* plus *tong* (积聚 + 痛) located 30 citations, five were located for *ji ju* plus *teng* (积聚 + 疼), which overlapped with the previous combination, and one citation was found for *yan* plus *tong* (岩 + 痛).

Frequency of Acupuncture Citations by Dynasty

The citations derived from 16 different books written between 282 AD and 1937. The most productive book was *Pu Ji Fang — Zhen Jiu* 普济方 — 针灸 (c. 1406) with six citations. Four books provided three citations each: *Sheng Ji Zong Lu* 圣济总录 (c. 1117), *Zhen Jiu Zi Sheng Jing* 针灸资生经 (c. 1220), *Zhen Jiu Da Cheng* 针灸大成 (c. 1601) and *Jin Zhen Mi Zhuan* 金针秘传 (c. 1937). The earliest book was *Zhen Jiu Jia Yi Jing* 针灸甲乙经 ($n = 2$) and the most recent was *Jin Zhen Mi Zhuan* 金针秘传 ($n = 3$).

The largest proportion of citations was from the Ming dynasty (48.5%) followed by the Song and Jin dynasties (18.2%), with the Tang dynasty and the Republic of China period providing three citations each (Table 3.5).

Table 3.5 Dynastic Distribution of Treatment Citations

Dynasty (Years)	No. (%) of Citations
Before *Tang* dynasty (before 618)	2 (6.1)
Tang and Five dynasties (618–960)	3 (9.1
Song and *Jin* dynasties (961–1271)	6 (18.2)
Yuan dynasty (1272–1368)	2 (6.1)
Ming dynasty (1369–1644)	16 (48.5)
Qing dynasty (1645–1911)	1 (3.0)
Min Guo/Republic of China (1912–1949)	3 (9.1)
Total	33 (100)

Table 3.6 Most Frequent Acupuncture Points for Cancer Pain

Acupuncture Point	No. of Citations (*n*)
KI17 *Shangqu* 商曲[1,2]	11
SP12 *Chongmen* 冲门[1,2]	9
BL18 *Ganshu* 肝俞[2]	6
CV3 *Zhongji* 中极	2
LR13 *Zhangmen* 章门[2] (also known as *Pimu* 脾募)	2

[1]Use of needle.
[2]Use of moxibustion.

Treatment with Acupuncture and Related Therapies

The 33 citations provided 35 mentions of ten different acupuncture points (Table 3.6). The most frequently mentioned point was KI17 *Shangqu* 商曲 ($n = 11$) followed by SP12 *Chongmen* 冲门 ($n = 9$) and BL18 *Ganshu* 肝俞 ($n = 6$). The use of needling was mentioned nine times for three different points, while moxibustion was mentioned 15 times for five different points. For five points there was no mention of the method of stimulation. There was no mention of *tui na* 推拿.

Citations of Acupuncture/Moxibustion for Cancer Pain

This section provides illustrative citations of treatments using acupuncture and/or moxibustion. In general, old uses of a point are retained and new uses are added over time, so the citations are given in chronological order.

The two earliest citations were from the *Zhen Jiu Jia Yi Jing* 针灸甲乙经 (c. 282 AD). Both were treatments for *ji ju* 积聚. In the section on disorders of the intestine, abdominal distension, borborygmus and shortness of breath, it said: 'For cold *qi* (*han qi* 寒气) producing abdominal distension, urinary retention, weakness of the limbs (*long yin luo* 癃淫泺), heat in the body, a mass (*ji ju* 积聚) within the abdomen with pain, a major point is CV12 *Chongmen* 冲门.'

In the section on various accumulations associated with the stomach and five solid organs, it said: 'For a mass (*ji ju* 积聚) within the abdomen, sometimes with cutting pain, a major point is KI17 *Shangqu* 商曲.'

In the Tang dynasty the same two points appeared in *Bei Ji Qian Jin Yao Fang* 备急千金要方 (c. 652), and *Qian Jin Yao Fang* 千金翼方 (c. 682) added moxa on LR13 *Zhangmen* 章门 for mass (*ji ju* 积聚) with severe fullness (*jian man* 坚满) and pain.

In the Song dynasty CV12 *Chongmen* 冲门 and KI17 *Shangqu* 商曲 were repeated. In addition, in the *Sheng Ji Zong Lu* 圣济总录 (c. 1117), in the section on the treatment of *zheng jia* 症瘕 with moxibustion, it is said that 'for fullness of the chest, abdominal distension, mass (*ji ju* 积聚) with glomus (*pi* 痞) and pain, moxa BL18 *Ganshu* 肝俞, 100 cones.' A similar passage was found in another Song Dynasty book *Zhen Jiu Zi Sheng Jing* 针灸资生经 (c. 1220).

In the Ming dynasty earlier point usages were repeated and four additional point usages were located. In the *Gu Jin Yi Tong Da Quan* 古今医统大全 (c. 1556) one of the applications given for the point SP13 *Fushe* 府舍 was '*ji ju* 积聚 with closure pain (*bi tong* 痹痛)'. The acupuncture volume of *Pu Ji Fang* 普济方 (c. 1406), in the section on pain in the lower abdomen (*xiao fu tong* 小腹痛), gave CV3 *Zhongji* 中极 for 'severe *ji ju* 积聚 that is like a stone'. It also gave the combination of BL17 *Geshu* 膈俞 and KI10 *Yinhe* 阴谷 for 'mass (*ji ju* 积聚) in the abdomen, sometimes with cutting pain'. The *Lei Jing Tu Yi* 类经图翼 (c. 1624) specified CV3 *Zhongji* 中极 as a treatment for '*ji ju* 积聚 located below the umbilicus with pain'.

In the Qing dynasty, the earlier citation of KI17 *Shangqu* 商曲 was repeated in *Zhen Jiu Feng Yuan* 针灸逢源 (c. 1822) but the reference to CV12 *Chongmen* 冲门 did not mention pain.

In the Republic of China period, all citations came from *Jin Zhen Mi Zhuan* 金针秘传 (c. 1937). These included repeats of the earlier applications of CV12 *Chongmen* 冲门 and KI17 *Shangqu* 商曲, but there was also a case of *zi gong yan* 子宫岩 (uterine mass) as follows: 'An old friend's wife had a mass in the lower abdomen that was hard, painful and could not be touched. A Western medicine doctor said it was *zi gong yan* 子宫岩. She had an examination and it confirmed this disease, and that the disease did not involve organs outside the uterus. The name *zi gong yan* 子宫岩 is a new name. Actually, it is due to *qi* and Blood coagulating (*qi xue suo ning* 气血所凝), which can produce *yan* 岩 in various locations, not only in the uterus. Therefore, you can use the *qi* to transform the mass. I used acupuncture at CV6 *Qihai* 气海, BL23 *Shenshu* 肾俞 and other points. After treatment the pain stopped, and after several days the mass disappeared.'

Discussion of Acupuncture and Related Therapies

Most of the citations for acupuncture and moxibustion were for abdominal masses described as *ji ju* 积聚 or related terms plus a mention of pain. The descriptions of these disorders were very brief, so it was not possible to judge if the mass was a cancer or due to a different disorder. Nevertheless, the description of 'severe *ji ju* 积聚 that is like a stone' found in *Pu Ji Fang* 普济方 (c. 1406) was consistent with a cancer.

Only citations in which the mention of pain appeared to be linked to the mass were included, but these links were associative rather than causal. There were no discussions of aetiology or pathogenesis or syndromes in the acupuncture citations for *ji ju* 积聚 plus pain, but this is not surprising since such discussions would typically be in other sections of the book or would have not been included since they would have been familiar to readers.

The two earliest citations from the *Zhen Jiu Jia Yi Jing* 针灸甲乙经 (c. 282) tended to be repeated in later books leading to their high frequency but sometimes the phrase on pain was omitted. Whether this was due to error or was intentional is difficult to judge. However, it is important to note that acupuncture has long been used for many kinds of pain, so its additional mention may have seemed redundant.

Only one citation was of a case. This was of a uterine mass (*zi gong yan* 子宫岩) and was recorded in the most recent of the acupuncture books. Although it had been diagnosed by a Western medicine doctor and appeared to be a cancer, its rapid improvement suggested it was more likely a benign mass. This highlights the recurrent issue of disease identity. In the past, terms such as *ji ju* 积聚 and *yan* 岩 had much broader scopes of meaning than does the modern concept of 'cancer'. Actual cancers would have been classified within the scope of *ji ju* 积聚 and *yan* 岩 but other types of masses were also included.

Other Chinese Medicine Therapies

The searches located one citation from the Qing dynasty that appeared relevant to cancer pain. This was a case recorded in *Chen Xin Tian Wai Ke Fang An* 陈莘田外科方案 (c. 1892) in which a form *of qi gong* 气功 was suggested, as follows: '*Ru yan* 乳岩 'breast rock', family name Wei 卫, located on the right side. This disease was caused by emotional depression; *qi* depression generates fire (*yu ze sheng huo* 郁则生火); extreme fire generates phlegm (*huo sheng sheng tan* 火盛生痰); phlegm accumulation blocks the *qi* mechanism (*tan ning qi zu* 痰凝气阻); and [this process] can produce lumps in the breasts. This condition was present for seven years; the mass grew and declined with the change in the *qi* (*sui qi xiao zhang* 随气消长); it was as hard as a stone (*jian ying ru shi* 坚硬如石); the colour [of the area] was pale and there was pain [on pressure]. She felt slight discomfort or soreness (*shao you suan chu* 稍有酸楚); was mentally fatigued (*shen xu* 神虚); the pulse was also deficient. In this kind of disease due to emotional disturbance, there is long time worry (*dan qing zhi zhi bing* 但情志之病) [which makes the condition worse] and the mass can eventually burst through. If it bursts through, this is *yan* 岩. In such a case, herbs cannot produce a [beneficial] effect. So, the best policy is the person must set aside their worries and do some quiet nourishing (静养) type of *qi gong* 气功.'

Classical Literature in Perspective

In classical CM there was no term that corresponded to the modern concept 'cancer pain'. This presented a difficulty when identifying citations. Pain was a clear concept with two main synonymous terms, *tong* 痛 and *teng* 疼. However, there was no classical term for 'cancer', so we used the main terms for palpable masses which were *ji ju*

积聚 and *zheng jia* 症/癥瘕 plus the term *yan* 岩 which refers to various types of rock-like lumps. These were all common terms, so when used separately they identified thousands of potential citations. Therefore, we searched for conjunctions of a term for a mass or a hard lump plus a term for pain. This identified a limited subset of the citations for masses in which the authors of the books made a direct mention of pain. An issue with this approach is not all masses produce pain, at least in the early stages. There were numerous mentions of feelings of discomfort, fullness or distension but considerably fewer of pain, so it is likely that the sample of citations identified by the searches tended to refer to more severe conditions. Conversely, some cancers such as those in the bone may produce pain without a palpable mass being evident. These could not be identified by the above approach, so to address this issue we added the term *gu ju* 骨疽, since the literature suggested it referred to bone metastasis.[6,9] However, this search term returned no citations that were clearly due to this condition.

Another issue was whether the classical terms referred to conditions that would now be diagnosed as cancer. For the terms *ji ju* 积聚 and *zheng jia* 症/癥瘕 it is likely that a considerable proportion of these masses were not cancers, but it is likely that cancers within the epigastric and abdominal regions would have been described using these terms. Hence the data set is likely to include false positives. For *yan* 岩 and especially for 'breast rock' (*ru yan* 乳岩), some citations described early-stage conditions that may have been benign lumps, but there were also descriptions consistent with late-stage painful breast cancer. Due to the nature of our search, we did not locate many treatments of early-stage breast lumps.

It is important to note that the search results do not reflect the classical treatments of cancers in general, nor do they include all the treatments for pain. What they include is the overlap between these two concepts, and it is not always evident whether the pain was a direct result of the mass or was just an accompanying symptom.

Some of the oral formulas had similar names but different ingredients. The most frequent of the oral interventions was *Xi lu wan* 晞露丸 but it only had six citations and is no longer in use. Also, it was difficult to determine whether a particular formula was intended to treat the mass, relieve the pain, or both. The oral formulas found in the classical literature were generally different to those used in contemporary books (see Chapter 2, Tables 2.1 and 2.2). One formula used in contemporary CHM was *Er chen tang* 二陈汤 which was a component of a larger formula in Table 2.2 and was combined with *Yang Le Tang* 养乐汤 in two classical citations. *Xiao yao san* 逍遥散 also appeared in two classical citations, but this was in the context of the type of formula useful to assist in relaxing the emotions rather than for the direct treatment of pain.

Considering the list of frequent formula ingredients (Table 3.4), it is evident that many had well-established applications in pain. The herbs *san leng* 三棱 and *e zhu* 莪术 were commonly used for dispersing masses and stopping pain, while *rou gui* 肉桂, *ba dou* 巴豆, *gan jiang* 干姜 and *wu tou* 乌头 were all hot herbs used for expelling pathological cold, which was considered a major cause of *ji ju* 积聚 or *zheng jia* 症/癥瘕, and for relieving pain.[18] Other herbs were often used for moving *qi* and dispersing stagnation such as *chai hu* 柴胡, *mu xiang* 木香, *qing pi* 青皮, *hou po* 厚朴 and *bing lang* 槟榔. However, the authors seldom discussed the roles of the herbs in the oral formulas, so we cannot be certain of their intended actions in the classical literature.

The two topical formulas mentioned in *Yi Xue Zheng Zhuan* 医学正传 are no longer used and the topical use of 'large toad' (*da chan* 大蟾) in late-stage breast cancer is not a common practice, but toad products remain in use in contemporary CM. These are mainly derived from the species *Bufo gargarizans* Cantor and *Bufo melanostictus* Schneider. In *Zhong Yao Da Ci Dian* 中药大辞典, the entry for the whole toad (*chan chu* 蟾蜍) mentioned that its actions included clearing toxins (*hua du* 化毒) and relieving pain (*ding tong* 定痛) (p. 2817); the entry for toad toxin (*chan su* 蟾酥) mentioned resolving toxins (*jie du* 解毒) and stopping pain (*zhi tong* 止痛); while the entry for toad skin (*chan pi* 蟾皮) mentioned resolving toxins (*jie du* 解毒) but did not mention pain. It also mentioned the topical use of toad skin for ulcers (*yong chuang* 痈疮) and toxic swellings (*zhong du* 肿毒).[18] *Chan su* 蟾酥 has been identified as a CM remedy for cancer pain[19] and toad toxins have received recent research attention for their effects in cancers and their anti-inflammatory, antimicrobial and immune regulatory actions.[20–22] *Chan su* 蟾酥 is very toxic[18,23] and must be handled with caution, so its main modern use is as one ingredient of manufactured medicines such as the oral pill *Liu shen wan* 六神丸 and the topical *Chan su gao* 蟾酥膏, both of which are included in Chapter 2.

There was very little overlap between the acupuncture points listed in contemporary books as treatments for pain in various cancers and those located in the searches of the classical literature. In Chapter 2 (Table 2.3), CV3 *Zhongji* 中极 was listed as one of the points for abdominal pain and it was listed in *Lei Jing Tu Yi* 类经图翼 (c. 1624) for mass below the navel with pain. In the classical literature, the acupuncture points were mainly on the abdomen close to the location of the mass, with some on the back at the same level as the pain, notably BL18 *Ganshu* 肝俞 and BL23 *Shenshu* 肾俞. In contrast, the modern books mainly included points on the limbs with some local points, while mentioning the additional use of local painful (*ashi* 阿是) points. Hence the classical points would all be applicable in contemporary acupuncture practice as local points for pain; the main difference is the classical literature did not mention any of the points on the limbs now used for pain relief. It is likely that this difference was due to the use of the search term *ji ju* 积聚. This limited the candidate points to those used for abdominal and epigastric masses.

The single entry for other CM therapies made mention of the importance of relaxation and regulating the emotions in the management of *ru yan* 乳岩 to prevent the condition becoming worse. The author suggested practising quiet nourishing *qi gong* 气功 but provided no further details. Other authors made similar recommendations with regard to the importance of letting go of pent-up emotions and relaxing in order to resolve this important factor in the aetiology of this condition. The use of *qi gong* 气功 remains a common practice in China to prevent disease and assist in the recovery from cancers.[24,25]

References

1. Needham J, Lu G. (2000) *Science and Civilisation in China. Volume 6, Part vi: Medicine.* Cambridge University Press, Cambridge, UK.
2. Hu R, ed. (2014) *Zhong Hua Yi Dian* [*Encyclopaedia of Traditional Chinese Medicine*], 5th ed. Hunan Electronic and Audio-Visual Publishing House, Changsha.
3. May BH, Lu CJ, Xue CCL. (2012) Collections of traditional Chinese medical literature as resources for systematic searches. *J Complement Altern Med* **18(12):** 1101–1107.
4. May BH, Lu YB, Lu CJ, *et al.* (2013) Systematic assessment of the representativeness of published collections of the traditional literature on Chinese medicine. *J Complement Altern Med* **19(5):** 403–409.
5. 中华中医药学会. (2008) 肿瘤中医诊疗指南. 北京: 中国中医药出版社.
6. 刘嘉湘. (1996) 实用中医肿瘤手册. 上海: 上海科技教育出版社.
7. 林洪生. (2014) 恶性肿瘤中医诊疗指南. 北京: 人民卫生出版社.
8. 张蓓, 周志伟. (2004) 实用中西医结合肿瘤学. 广州: 广东人民出版社.
9. 王居祥. (2009) 肿瘤内科中西医结合治疗. 北京: 人民卫生出版社.
10. 王洪武. (2010) 癌性疼痛的综合治疗. 北京: 科学普及出版社.
11. 何裕民. (2005) 现代中医肿瘤学 (普通高等教育"十五"国家级规划教材面向21世纪课程教材). 北京: 中国协和医科大学出版社.
12. 李佩文, 蔡光蓉. (2002) 癌症疼痛中西医汇通. 沈阳: 辽宁科学技术出版社.
13. 郑伟达. (1998) 肿瘤的中医防治. 北京: 中国中医药出版社.
14. May BH, Zhang A, Lu YB, *et al.* (2014) The systematic assessment of traditional evidence from the premodern Chinese medical literature: A text-mining approach. *J Complement Altern Med* **20(12):** 937–942.
15. Xue CL, Lu CJ, eds. (2019) Evidence-based Clinical Chinese Medicine. Volume 17: Colorectal Cancer. World Scientific Publishing Co., Singapore.
16. Li JW, Yu YA, Cai JF, *et al.*, eds. (2005) *Zhong Yi Da Ci Dian* [*Great Dictionary of Chinese Medicine*], 2nd ed. People's Medical Publishing House, Beijing.
17. 何华珍. (1997) "癌"字探源 [The source of the term "ai"]. *Journal of Hangzhou Teachers College* 杭州师范学院学报 **4:** 51–54.
18. Jiangsu New Medical Academy, ed. (1986) *Zhong Yao Da Ci Dian* [*Great Compendium of Chinese Medicines*]. Shanghai Scientific and Technical Publishers, Shanghai.

19. 程尧, 奚胜艳, 王彦晖, 史萌萌, 罗冠杰, 赵心悦. (2015) 癌性疼痛的中医再认识及临证用药规律探析. 中华中医药杂志 **30(11):** 3960–3964.
20. Sousa LQD, Machado KDC, Oliveira SFDC, *et al.* (2017) Bufadienolides from amphibians: A promising source of anticancer prototypes for radical innovation, apoptosis triggering and Na^+/K^+-ATPase inhibition. *Toxicon* **127:** 63–76.
21. Rodriguez C, Rollins-Smith L, Ibanez R, *et al.* (2017) Toxins and pharmacologically active compounds from species of the family bufonidae (amphibia, anura). *J Ethnopharmacol* **198:** 235–254.
22. Qi J, Zulfiker AHM, Li C, *et al.* (2018) The development of toad toxins as potential therapeutic agents. *Toxins (Basel)* **10(8):** 336.
23. Bensky D, Clavey S, Stöger E. (2004) *Chinese Herbal Medicine: Materia Medica*, 3rd ed. Eastland Press, Seattle.
24. Sze DM, Chan V, Wu MB, *et al.* (2017) Critical review in qigong and immunity cancer research. *Int J Complement Altern Med* **7(3):** 00227.
25. Oh B, Butow P, Mullan B, *et al.* (2012) A critical review of the effects of medical qigong on quality of life, immune function, and survival in cancer patients. *Integr Cancer Ther* **11(2):** 101–110.

4

Methods for Evaluating Clinical Evidence

OVERVIEW

This section describes the methods used to identify and evaluate clinical studies of Chinese medicine interventions for cancer pain. Studies identified through a comprehensive search strategy were assessed against eligibility criteria. A review of the methodological quality of the studies was undertaken using standardised methods. Results from included studies for the specified outcomes were evaluated to provide an estimate of the effects of each type of Chinese medicine therapy.

Introduction

The use of Chinese medicine (CM) for cancer pain has been extensively researched in clinical studies. In the following chapters, the efficacy, effectiveness and safety of CM interventions have been evaluated and are presented for the following main types of CM interventions:

- Chinese herbal medicine (CHM) in Chapter 5;
- Acupuncture and related therapies in Chapter 7;
- Other CM therapies in Chapter 8;
- Combination CM therapies, e.g. CHM plus *an mo* 按摩, in Chapter 9.

Published data on the clinical trials were obtained from databases and other sources and assessed by an expert review group including researchers, clinical physicians, CM experts and methodologists. All the included studies are referenced at the end of each chapter.

Randomised controlled trials (RCTs), non-randomised controlled clinical trials (CCTs) and non-controlled studies were evaluated separately. Meta-analyses were conducted for the RCTs and CCTs using the methods described below. This approach was not suitable for the evidence from the non-controlled studies. Therefore, the characteristics of the studies, details of the interventions and any adverse events were described and summarised but no assessments of outcomes were conducted.

References to included studies are indicated by a letter followed by a number. Studies of CHM are indicated by an 'H' e.g. H1; studies of acupuncture and related therapies are indicated by an 'A' e.g. A1; studies of other CM therapies are indicated by an 'O' e.g. O1; and studies of combinations of CM therapies are indicated by a 'C' e.g. C1.

Search Strategy

Comprehensive searches were conducted of multiple English- and Chinese-language databases using the methods outlined in the Cochrane Handbook of Systematic Reviews.[1] English-language databases included PubMed, Excepta Medica Database (Embase), Cumulative Index of Nursing and Allied Health Literature (CINAHL), Cochrane Central Register of Controlled Trials (CENTRAL) including the Cochrane Library, and Allied and Complementary Medicine Database (AMED). Chinese-language databases included China Biomedical Literature (CBM), China National Knowledge Infrastructure (CNKI), Chongqing VIP (CQVIP) and Wanfang. Databases were searched from their respective inceptions to April 2018. No restrictions were applied. Search terms were mapped to controlled vocabulary (where applicable) in addition to being searched as keywords.

Search terms were grouped into blocks of terms for (1) the disease (malignant tumors), (2) pain, conventional analgesic, (3) the CM intervention and (4) the type of study (clinical trial, RCT, etc.). The four search blocks were combined using "AND" (or a database-specific variant). Consequently, the following nine searches were conducted in each of the nine databases:

1. CHM — reviews;
2. CHM — controlled trials (randomised and non-randomised);
3. CHM — non-controlled studies;
4. Acupuncture and related therapies — reviews;
5. Acupuncture and related therapies — controlled trials (randomised and non-randomised);
6. Acupuncture and related therapies — non-controlled studies;
7. Other CM therapy — reviews;
8. Other CM therapies — controlled trials (randomised and non-randomised);
9. Other CM therapies — non-controlled studies.

Studies of combination CM therapies were identified from within the above searches.

In addition to the electronic databases, reference lists of systematic reviews and included studies were searched for additional publications. Clinical trial registries were searched to identify clinical trials which were ongoing or completed, and where required, trial investigators were contacted to obtain data. The searched trial registries included Australian New Zealand Clinical Trial Registry (ANZCTR), Chinese Clinical Trial Registry (ChiCTR), EU Clinical Trials Register (EU-CTR) and ClinicalTrials.gov.

Inclusion Criteria

Study Type

Controlled prospective studies with or without randomisation (including parallel groups and crossover studies) and uncontrolled studies (cohort, case series and case studies) that employed a CM therapy as a test intervention and reported an outcome of relevance to cancer pain were included.

Participants

Participants included adults aged 18 years and over who had been diagnosed with malignant tumours based on the pathology tests, or diagnosed with liver cancer based on the guidelines of the American Association for the Study of Liver Disease (AASLD)[2] or the European Association for the Study of the Liver (EASL)[3] and have chronic pain syndromes caused by cancer or cancer-related treatment e.g. surgery, chemotherapy and radiotherapy. There was no restriction on cancer stage or performance status.

Interventions

Studies that employed a CM therapy as a test intervention included the following:

- CHM: administration routes included oral and/or topical application;
- Acupuncture: with or without skin penetration, including ear acupuncture/acupressure, warm needling;
- Moxibustion: direct or indirectly applied, using various heat sources;
- Manual therapies: including *tui na* 推拿, *an mo* 按摩 (massage);
- Exercises: including *tai chi* (*tai ji* 太极) and *qi gong* 气功;
- Dietary interventions.

Table 4.1 Chinese Medicine Interventions Included in Clinical Evidence Evaluations

Category	Included Intervention
Chinese herbal medicine (CHM)	Orally administered CHM, topical CHM including fomentation (*yun tang* 熨烫) and cataplasm (*yao gao* 药膏).
Acupuncture and related therapies	Acupuncture, electro-acupuncture, ear acupressure, moxibustion, transcutaneous electrical nerve stimulation (TENS) on acupuncture points.
Other CM therapies	Chinese massage (*tui na* 推拿, *an mo* 按摩), *tai ji* 太極 and other exercise therapies, Chinese medicine (CM) diet therapy.
Combination CM	Two or more Chinese medicine interventions from different categories administered together: for example, oral CHM plus *an mo* 按摩, and combinations of other CM therapies.

Co-interventions were allowed, provided the same intervention was used in at least two arms of the study. Table 4.1 shows the CM interventions included in the clinical evidence evaluations.

Comparators in Controlled Trials (RCT, CCT)

Putatively active or inactive control interventions including the following:

- No treatment, supportive care, placebo;
- Conventional therapy recommended in guidelines (using analgesics, radiation, neurolytic block, intrathecal pump, etc. aimed at treating cancer pain);
- Studies could combine a CM intervention with a conventional therapy for cancer pain as an integrative medicine (IM) approach. Note that the combination of CM with usual supportive care and/or the co-administration of conventional therapy for non-cancer pain conditions, were not considered to be IM approaches.

Settings

In-patients or out-patients treated in hospitals or clinics or in their own homes.

Outcomes

Studies reported at least one of the following pre-specified outcome measures:

- Primary outcome assessments: studies reported at least one of the outcome measures in Table 4.2;
- Secondary outcome assessments: incidence and type of adverse events (AEs) relating to CM during the treatment.

The outcome measure instruments listed are not the only scales used for assessing people with cancer pain. Describing every scale

Table 4.2 Main Clinical Outcome Measures

Outcome Categories	Outcome Measures	Units; Direction for Improvement
Pain intensity	Numeric rating scale (NRS)[4]	Score, lower is better
	Visual Analogue Scale (VAS)	Score, lower is better
	Brief Pain Inventory (BPI), BPI-short form (BPI-SF)[5,6]	13 items, subscales for pain intensity and pain interference in life activities, lower is better
Pain duration/ frequency	Analgesic onset time	Time, sooner is better
	Duration of analgesia	Time, longer is better
	Frequency of breakthrough pain	Various, lower is better
Analgesic dose	Dosage of analgesic medications	Various, lower is better
Quality of life/ Performance status	European Organisation for Research and Treatment of Cancer Quality of Life Questionnaire (EORTC QLQ-C30, version 3)[7]	30 items (version 3), for global health status/QOL scale higher is better
	Chinese QOL scale[8]	12 items, total score is 60 points, higher is better
	NCCN impact of pain measurement[4]	7 items, total score is 70 points, higher is worse
	Karnofsky Performance Status (KPS)[9]	100 points, higher is better
	Functional Assessment of Cancer Therapy — General (FACT-G)[10,11]	27 items (version 4), higher total score is better
	Functional Assessment of Cancer Therapy Endocrine Symptoms (FACT-ES)[13,14]	18 Items (19 in version 4), higher total score is better
	The Edmonton Symptom Assessment System (ESAS)[13]	8 items, lower is better
Immune function	T-cells: CD3+, CD4+, CD8+, NK cells, CD4+/CD8+	Various
	Immunoglobulins: IgG, IgA, IgM	g/L

Table 4.2 (*Continued*)

Outcome Categories	Outcome Measures	Units; Direction for Improvement
Opioid-induced constipation (OIC)	Cleveland Clinic constipation score (CCS)[14]	8 items, total score is 30, lower is better
Adverse reactions	NCI-CTCAE criteria[15]	Number of participants, fewer is better
	WHO criteria[16]	Number of participants, fewer is better
Adverse events (AEs) associated with CM	Adverse events (as reported in studies)	Number and type of AEs and serious adverse events (SAE) in each group, fewer is better

Abbreviations: NCCN, National Comprehensive Cancer Network; QOL, quality of life; WHO, World Health Organization.

and every variation is beyond the scope of this chapter. The included scales are ones that feature in the subsequent chapters. In addition to clinical scales, outcomes in cancer research include imaging and other serological measures, but these aspects are not assessed in the following meta-analyses.

Exclusion Criteria

Study Type

Clinical studies that used the following designs:

- CM versus other CM therapy;
- CM plus other therapy versus CM;
- CM plus pharmacotherapy versus CM.

Co-interventions were allowed, provided the same intervention was used in at least two arms of the study. Retrospective RCTs or CCTs were not included in the meta-analysis or the counts for clinical trials. Such studies may be referred to in the text where relevant.

Participants

- The participant group included people with pain unrelated to cancer or cancer-related treatments, or people with postoperative pain within a short time (≤ two months), or people with phlebitis.

Interventions

- Synthetic compounds or isolated chemical compounds, homeopathic preparations, nutritional supplements and plant-based products that are not used in Chinese traditional medicine;
- Integrative medicine studies that used different therapies in the intervention group compared to the control group;
- Acupuncture anaesthesia;
- Use of pethidine or other discontinued medication.

Comparators in Controlled Trials (RCT, CCT)

- Control groups that employed an intervention that was not used in the conventional care of cancer pain (in China or other countries);
- Controls using another CM intervention, or other herbal product.

Outcomes

- For missing data and data errors in key outcomes, if we failed to obtain sufficient data after contacting authors or retrieving related articles, the studies were excluded;
- Outcome measures based on instruments of unclear origin or validity;
- Effective rate based on clinician judgement.

Risk of Bias

Risk of bias was assessed for randomised controlled trials using the Cochrane Collaboration's tool.[1] Risk of bias was assessed for the following six domains: (1) sequence generation, (2) allocation concealment, (3) blinding of participants and personnel, (4) blinding of outcome assessors, (5) incomplete outcome data, and (6) selective reporting. Each domain was assessed to determine whether the risk of bias was low, high or unclear. Risk of bias was assessed by two researchers independently, and any disagreement was resolved by discussion and consultation with a third person.

- Sequence generation: The method used to generate the allocation sequence is given in sufficient detail to allow an assessment of whether it should produce comparable groups. Low risk of bias refers to use of a random-number table or computerised randomisation. High risk of bias includes studies that describe a non-random method of sequence generation such as odd or even date of birth or date of admission;
- Allocation concealment: The method used to conceal the allocation sequence is given in enough detail to determine whether intervention allocations could have been foreseen before or during enrolment. Low risk of bias includes central randomisation or sealed envelopes and high risk of bias includes open random sequence or date of birth etc.;
- Blinding of participants and personnel: Measures are used to ensure the study participants and personnel are blind to the intervention received. In addition, information relating to whether the blinding was effective is also assessed. Studies that ensure blinding of participants and personnel are at low risk of bias. If the study is not blind or incompletely blind, it is at high risk of bias;
- Blinding of outcome assessors: Measures are used to ensure the outcome assessors are blind to knowledge of which intervention a participant received. In addition, information relating to whether the blinding was effective is also assessed. Studies that ensure blinding of outcome assessors are at low risk of bias. If the study is not blind or incompletely blind, it is at high risk of bias;
- Incomplete outcome data: Completeness of outcome data for each main outcome is examined, including drop-outs, exclusions from the analysis, with numbers missing in each group and reasons for

drop-outs or exclusions. Studies with low risk of bias would include all outcome data or, if there is missing data, it is unlikely to relate to the true outcome or is balanced between groups. Studies at high risk of bias would have unexplained missing data;

- Selective reporting: The study protocol is available and the pre-specified outcomes are included in the report. Studies with a published protocol and which include all pre-specified outcomes in their report would be at low risk of bias. Studies at high risk of bias would not include all pre-specified outcomes or the outcome data may be reported incompletely.

Statistical Analyses

Frequency of CM syndromes, CHM formulas, herbs and acupuncture points reported in included studies were presented using descriptive statistics. CM syndromes reported in two or more studies were presented. In Chapter 5, the 20 most frequently reported CHM formulas and herbs were presented where used in at least two studies. In Chapter 7, the top ten acupuncture points used in two or more studies were presented when available. Where data were limited, reports of single CM syndromes or acupuncture points were provided as a guide for the reader.

Definitions of statistical tests and results were described in the glossary. Meta-analysis of outcome measure data was performed when a sufficient number of comparable studies was available. Meta-analyses were based on reported data at the end of the treatment period (EoT). Comparisons were between the CM intervention groups and the control groups at EoT.

Dichotomous data are reported as a risk ratio (RR) with 95% confidence intervals (CI), and continuous data are reported as mean difference (MD) or standardised mean difference (SMD) with 95% CI. For dichotomous data, when the RR is greater than one and the upper and lower values of the 95% CI are both greater than one, this indicates we can be 95% certain that there is a difference between the groups and the true effect lies within these CIs. The same is true for values less than one. In such cases we say there is a 'significant difference' between the groups. For continuous data, when the MD is greater than zero and both the upper and lower values of the 95% CI are greater than zero, we say there is a 'significant difference' between the groups. The same is true on the negative side of the scale.[1]

Available case analysis with a random-effects model was used in all analyses. This provides a conservative estimate of difference between groups and is applicable to data in which heterogeneity is present. Formal tests for heterogeneity were conducted using the I^2 statistic. An I^2 score greater than 50% was considered to indicate substantial heterogeneity.[1]

Sensitivity analyses were undertaken to explore potential sources of heterogeneity, based on low risk of bias for the domain of sequence generation. Where possible and appropriate, planned subgroup analyses included type of control medication, duration of treatment, pain intensity and/or CM formula.

Summary of Findings

Summary of findings (SoF) tables are presented for major comparisons and outcomes reported by the RCTs.

Assessment Using Grading of Recommendations, Assessment, Development and Evaluation

The Grading of Recommendations, Assessment, Development and Evaluation (GRADE) approach was used.[17,18] The GRADE approach summarises and rates the strength and quality of evidence in systematic reviews using a structured process for presenting evidence summaries in terms of the 'certainty' of the evidence. The results are presented in SoF tables. These provide an overview of the evidence reported by the RCTs for the main interventions, comparisons and outcome measures for cancer pain.

A panel of experts was established to evaluate the evidence. The panel included the systematic review team, CM practitioners, integrative medicine experts, research methodologists and conventional medicine physicians. The experts were asked to rate the clinical importance of key interventions from CHM, acupuncture therapies and other CM therapies, as well as comparators and outcomes. Results were collated and based on the rating scores and subsequent discussion, a consensus on the content for the SoF tables was achieved.

The certainty of evidence for each outcome was rated according to five factors outlined in the GRADE approach. The certainty of evidence might be rated down based on:

- Limitations in study design (risk of bias);
- Inconsistency of results (unexplained heterogeneity);
- Indirectness of evidence (interventions, populations and outcomes important to the patients with the condition);
- Imprecision (uncertainty about the results);
- Publication bias (selective publication of studies).

These five factors are additive, and a reduction in one or more factors will reduce the quality of the evidence for that outcome.

The GRADE approach also includes three domains that can be rated up, including large magnitude of an effect, dose-response gradient and effect of plausible residual confounding. However, these three domains relate to observational studies including cohort, case-control, before–after and time series studies. GRADE summaries in this book only include RCTs, therefore these three domains for rating up were not assessed.

Treatment recommendations could also be assessed using the GRADE approach; however, due to the diverse nature of CM practice, treatment recommendations were not included with the SoFs. Therefore, the reader should interpret the evidence with reference to the local practice environment. It should also be noted that the GRADE approach requires judgments about the strength and quality of evidence and some subjective assessment. However, the experience of the panel members suggests the judgments are reliable and transparent representations of the certainty of evidence.

The GRADE levels of evidence are grouped into four categories:

1. High certainty: We are very confident that the true effect lies close to that of the estimate of the effect;
2. Moderate certainty: We are moderately confident in the effect estimate. The true effect is likely to be close to the estimate of the effect, but there is a possibility that it is substantially different;
3. Low certainty: Our confidence in the effect estimate is limited. The true effect may be substantially different from the estimate of the effect;
4. Very low certainty: We have very little confidence in the effect estimate. The true effect is likely to be substantially different from the estimate of effect.

References

1. Higgins JPT, Green S, eds. (2011) Cochrane Handbook for Systematic Reviews of Interventions Version 5.1.0. The Cochrane Collaboration.
2. Marrero JA, Kulik LM, Sirlin CB, *et al.* (2018) Diagnosis, staging, and management of hepatocellular carcinoma: 2018 practice guidance by the American Association for the Study of Liver Diseases. *Hepatology (Baltimore, Md)* **68(2):** 723–750.
3. European Association for the Study of the Liver, Galle PR, Forner A, *et al.* (2018) EASL clinical practice guidelines: Management of hepatocellular carcinoma. *J Hepatol* **69(1):** 182–236.
4. National Comprehensive Cancer Network. (2018) Clinical practice guidelines in oncology: Adult cancer pain, version 1. 2018. Available from: www.nccn.og.
5. Cleeland CS. (2009) Brief pain inventory: User guide. Available from: www.mdanderson.org/education-and-research/departments-programs-and-labs/departments-and-divisions/symptom-research/symptom-assessment-tools/BPI_UserGuide.pdf.
6. Wang XS, Mendoza TR, Gao SZ, Cleeland CS. (1996) The Chinese version of the brief pain inventory (bpi-c): Its development and use in a study of cancer pain. *Pain* **67(2–3):** 407–416.
7. Aaronson NK, Ahmedzai S, Bergman B, *et al.* (1993) The European Organization for Research and Treatment of Cancer QLQ-C30:

A quality-of-life instrument for use in international clinical trials in oncology. *J Natl Cancer Inst* **85(5):** 365–376.
8. 孙燕. (2001) 内科肿瘤学. 北京: 人民卫生出版社, pp. 996–997.
9. Yates JW, Chalmer B, Mckegney FP. (1980) Evaluation of patients with advanced cancer using the Karnofsky Performance Status. *Cancer* **45(8):** 2220–4.
10. Cella DF, Tulsky DS, Gray G, Sarafian B, Linn E, Bonomi A, Silberman M, Yellen SB, Winicour P, Brannon J, *et al.* The Functional Assessment of Cancer Therapy scale: development and validation of the general measure. *J Clin Oncol.* 1993 Mar;**11(3):**570–9. doi:10.1200/JCO.1993.11.3.570.
11. Cheung YB, Thumboo J, Goh C, Khoo KS, Che W, Wee J. The equivalence and difference between the English and Chinese versions of two major, cancer-specific, health-related quality-of-life questionnaires. *Cancer.* 2004 Dec 15;**101(12):**2874–80. doi:10.1002/cncr.20681. PMID: 15529310.
12. Fallowfield LJ, Leaity SK, Howell A, *et al.* (1999) Assessment of quality of life in women undergoing hormonal therapy for breast cancer: Validation of an endocrine symptom subscale for the FACT-B. *Breast Cancer Res Treat* **55(2):** 189–199.
13. Bruera E, Kuehn N, Miller MJ, Selmser P, Macmillan K. The Edmonton Symptom Assessment System (ESAS): a simple method for the assessment of palliative care patients. *J Palliat Care.* 1991 Summer;**7(2):**6–9. PMID: 1714502
14. Agachan F, Chen T, Pfeifer J, Reissman P, Wexner SD. (1996) A constipation scoring system to simplify evaluation and management of constipated patients. *Diseases of the colon and rectum* **39(6):**681–5
15. National Institutes of Health & National Cancer Institute. Common terminology criteria for adverse events (CTCAE), version 4. In: U.S. Department of Health and Human Services, editor. Bethesda. MD: National Institutes of Health; 2008.
16. Miller AB, Hoogstraten B, Staquet M, Winkler A. (1981) Reporting results of cancer treatment. *Cancer* **47(1):** 207–14
17. Schunemann H, Brozek J, Guyatt G, Oxman A, eds. (2013) Grade handbook for grading quality of evidence and strength of recommendations (the grade working group): Retrieved from http://www.guidelinedevelopment.org/handbook/ (Jan 2017).

18. Schünemann HJ, Higgins JPT, Vist GE, *et al.* (2019) Chapter 14: Completing 'summary of findings' tables and grading the certainty of the evidence. In: Higgins JPT, Thomas J, Chandler J, *et al.* (eds), Cochrane Handbook for Systematic Reviews of Interventions Version 6.0. Available from: www.training.cochrane.org/handbook.

5

Clinical Evidence for Chinese Herbal Medicine

OVERVIEW

The searches identified 30 randomised controlled trials, zero non-randomised controlled studies and four non-controlled studies of Chinese herbal medicine used in the management of pain due to cancer or directly resulting from cancer treatment. Orally administered Chinese herbal medicine was used in 14 studies; topically applied Chinese herbal medicine was used in 18 studies; and a combination of oral and topical Chinese herbal medicine was used in two studies. Therefore, the analyses of data from the RCTs are divided into these three main groups. Within each group, the meta-analyses are grouped based on the main comparisons and further subgrouped based on the outcome measure. A summary of the results for the main clinical outcomes is presented at the end of the chapter.

Introduction

Chinese herbal medicine (CHM) interventions have received research attention for their effects on pain resulting from cancer in multiple clinical studies. CHMs are typically multi-ingredient formulations which are composed of natural products of diverse origin which have been prepared and processed for medical use. These are listed in major pharmacopoeia and compendia of Chinese *materia medica.*[1,2] In cancer pain, CHMs are often administered orally and/or topically. Injection products are beyond the scope of this chapter. Studies of combinations of CHMs and other Chinese medicine (CM) therapies are included in Chapter 9.

Previous Systematic Reviews

A number of reviews of CHMs for people with cancer pain have been published. A meta-analysis of randomised controlled trials (RCTs) found that, when compared to the three-step analgesic ladder alone, CHM combined with the three-step analgesic ladder improved pain relief and quality of life (QOL) and reduced adverse reactions to conventional analgesics.[3] Another meta-analysis found that compared to indomethacin, CHM improved pain relief, analgesic onset time and duration of analgesia; and compared to tramadol, there were no significant differences between the CHM group and the tramadol group for pain relief, analgesic onset time and duration of analgesia.[4] A meta-analysis of the results of RCTs for cancer pain found that combining CHM with conventional cancer therapies reduced pain based on the visual analogue scale (VAS) but there was considerable heterogeneity in the results.[5] Another meta-analysis found that CHM combined with conventional analgesics improved pain relief and Karnofsky Performance Status (KPS), and reduced adverse reactions when compared to conventional analgesics alone.[6]

Topically applied CHMs combined with the three-step analgesic ladder improved pain relief and KPS, and reduced adverse reactions to conventional analgesics.[7] For bone cancer pain, a meta-analysis of the results of six RCTs reported that combining externally applied CHMs with conventional management resulted in improved pain relief.[8]

Identification of Clinical Studies

The searches identified 30 RCTs (H1–H30), zero non-randomised controlled clinical trials (CCTs) and four non-controlled studies (H31–H34) that met the inclusion criteria (Fig. 5.1). Oral CHM was tested in 12 RCTs (H1–H12) and two case series (H31, H32). Topical CHM was used in 17 RCTs (H13–H29) and one case report (H33).

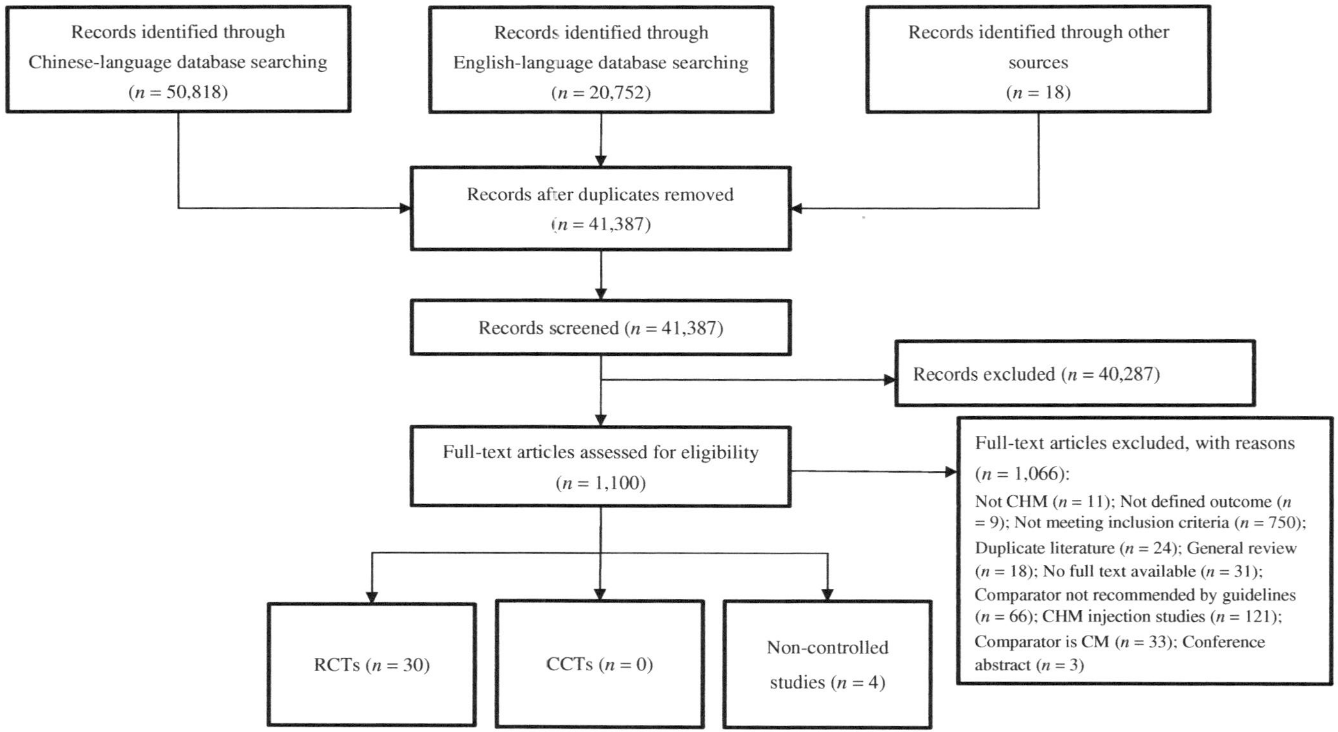

Fig. 5.1 Flowchart of study selection process: Chinese herbal medicine

Oral CHM plus topical CHM was tested in one RCT (H30) and one case report (H34).

Outline of the Data Analyses

Studies are grouped by the type of study (RCT, non-controlled study) and by the type of CHM as follows:

- Oral CHM;
- Topical CHM;
- Oral plus topical CHM.

Meta-analysis results of the RCTs are presented for each type of CHM for the following outcomes (if available):

- Pain intensity
  - Numerical rating scale (NRS),
  - Visual analogue scale (VAS);
- Analgesic onset time;
- Frequency of breakthrough pain;
- Duration of analgesia;
- Analgesic dose;
- Quality of life;
- Karnofsky Performance Status;
- Immune function;
- Cleveland Clinic constipation score; and
- Adverse reactions, adverse events.

Summary results of the non-controlled studies follow the RCTs.

Randomised Controlled Trials of Oral Chinese Herbal Medicine

The 12 RCTs of oral CHM (H1–H12) were all conducted in mainland China and enrolled 757 participants. The age of participants ranged from 18 to 88 years but the age range was not reported in four studies (H4, H6, H8, H10). Based on the reported means and standard deviations for ages, the majority of participants were aged between 46 and 77 years. Following drop-outs, 736 participants completed the studies.

Nine RCTs included comparisons with conventional analgesics:

- One RCT (H1) of oral CHM versus conventional analgesic;
- Two RCTs (H2, H3) of oral CHM plus conventional analgesic versus placebo plus conventional analgesic;
- Five RCTs (H4–H8) of oral CHM plus conventional analgesic versus conventional analgesic;
- One RCT (H9) of oral CHM plus conventional analgesic plus zoledronic acid versus conventional analgesic plus zoledronic acid.

Three RCTs included comparisons with other conventional medications:

- Two RCTs (H10, H11) of oral CHM versus calcium carbonate and vitamin D3 tablets; and
- One RCT (H12) of oral CHM versus lactulose oral solution for opioid-induced constipation (OIC).

One study (H1) had three groups, but we only included two groups since the participants in the third group were only treated with vitamin E capsules and the study did not report some results for the third group.

The groups that combined a CHM with a conventional analgesic are referred to as 'integrative medicine' groups.

Syndromes

Of the studies of oral CHM, eight RCTs used syndrome differentiation in the selection criteria, and one study (H12) used two different syndromes. In total, eight RCTs mentioned seven different syndromes. The syndrome names reported in the eight RCTs were:

- Kidney deficiency with blood stasis — *shen xu xue yu* 肾虚血瘀 (*n* = 3) (H3, H6, H9);
- *Qi* deficiency with blood stasis — *qi xu xue yu* 气虚血瘀 (*n* = 1) (H4);
- *Yin* deficiency with internal heat — *yin xu nei re* 阴虚内热 (*n* =1) (H5);
- Blood stasis due to *qi* stagnation — *qi zhi xue yu* 气滞血瘀 (*n* = 1) (H7);
- Liver depression and *qi* stagnation — *gan yu qi zhi* 肝郁气滞 (*n* = 1) (H8);
- *Qi* stagnation-type constipation — *qi bi* 气秘 (*n* = 1) (H12); and
- *Yin* deficiency with heat accumulation — *yin xu re jie* 阴虚热结 (*n* = 1) (H12).

Formula and Herb Frequencies

In the 12 RCTs there were 11 different formula names. The most frequently used formula was *Chai hu shu gan san* 柴胡疏肝散 (*n* = 2) (one used *Chai hu shu gan san* 柴胡疏肝散, and one used *Chai hu shu gan san jia wei* 柴胡疏肝散加味). Another ten formulas were tested in one study each. Of these, seven formulas were named by the authors or their hospital, one was not named, and two were commercial products (*Zhong tong an jiao nang* 肿痛安胶囊 and *Yuan hu zhi tong jiao nang* 元胡止痛胶囊).

The herbs most frequently used in the oral formulas used in the 12 RCTs were *gan cao* 甘草 (*n* = 6), *chuan xiong* 川芎 (*n* = 4), *gu sui bu* 骨碎补 (*n* = 4) and *yan hu suo* 延胡索 (*n* = 4) (Table 5.1).

Risk of Bias for Oral Chinese Herbal Medicine

The risk of bias for sequence generation was judged 'low risk' in nine RCTs since an appropriate method of randomisation was described (Table 5.2). The others were judged 'unclear risk'. Only one study

Table 5.1 Frequently Used Herbs in Randomised Controlled Trials of Oral Chinese Herbal Medicine

Herb Name	Scientific Name of Herb[1]	No. of Studies
Gan cao 甘草[2]	*Glycyrrhiza uralensis* Fisch.	6
Chuan xiong 川芎	*Ligusticum chuanxiong* Hort.	4
Gu sui bu 骨碎补	*Drynaria fortunei* (Kunze) J. Sm.	4
Yan hu suo 延胡索	*Corydalis yanhusuo* W.T. Wang	4
She she cao 蛇舌草	*Hedyotis diffusa* Willd.	3
Ban zhi lian 半枝莲	*Scutellaria barbata* D. Don	3
Bu gu zhi 补骨脂	*Psoralea corylifolia* L.	3
Di huang 地黄[3]	*Rehmannia glutinosa* Libosch.	3
Du zhong 杜仲	*Eucommia ulmoides* Oliv.	3
Shao yao 芍药[4]	*Paeonia lactiflora* Pall.; *P. veitchii* Lynch	3
Xiang fu 香附	*Cyperus rotundus* L.	3

Notes[1]: The use of some herbs may be restricted in some countries. Readers are advised to comply with relevant regulations.
[2]One RCT used *zhi gan cao* 炙甘草.
[3]Two RCTs used *shu di huang* 熟地黄 and one RCT used *sheng di huang* 生地黄.
[4]One RCT used *bai shao* 白芍 and one RCT used *chi shao* 赤芍.

Table 5.2 Risk of Bias of Randomised Controlled Trials of Oral Chinese Herbal Medicine

Risk of Bias Domain	Low Risk *n* (%)	Unclear Risk *n* (%)	High Risk *n* (%)
Sequence generation	9 (75)	3 (25)	0 (0)
Allocation concealment	1 (8.3)	11 (91.7)	0 (0)
Blinding of participants	2 (16.7)	0 (0)	10 (83.3)
Blinding of personnel	1 (8.3)	0 (0)	11 (91.7)
Blinding of outcome assessors	2 (16.7)	10 (83.3)	0 (0)
Incomplete outcome data	11 (91.7)	0 (0)	1 (8.3)
Selective outcome reporting	0 (0)	11 (91.7)	1 (8.3)

Abbreviation: *n*, number.

mentioned allocation concealment and used a proper method so it was judged 'low risk' and the remainder were judged 'unclear risk'. Two studies that used a placebo for the CHM in the control groups were judged 'low risk' for blinding of participants and outcome assessors. The remaining studies were judged 'high risk' for blinding of participants and 'unclear risk' for blinding of outcome assessors. One study described blinding of personnel, so it was judged 'low risk', and the others were 'high risk'. The three-arm study (H1) did not report some results for the third group, so it was judged 'high risk' for incomplete outcome data. In the remaining studies, there were no drop-outs or few drop-outs, so these were assessed as 'low risk'. For selective outcome reporting, no protocols could be located which led to a judgment of unclear bias, except in one study (H10) which specified it would report on calcitonin in the method but omitted these results, so it was judged 'high risk'.

Oral Chinese Herbal Medicine versus Conventional Analgesic

One RCT (H1) compared *Zhong tong an jiao nang* 肿痛安胶囊 (*san qi* 三七, *tian ma* 天麻, *jiang can* 僵蚕, *fang feng* 防风, *bai fu zi* 白附子, *qiang huo* 羌活, *tian nan xing* 天南星, etc.; two capsules, twice a day, until the end of radiotherapy) with ibuprofen capsules (0.3 g, twice a day) in head and neck cancer patients with temporomandibular joint (TMJ) disorder and pain (VAS ≥ 4) due to radiotherapy.

There were marginally significant increases in the CHM group for visual analogue scale (VAS) scores (MD 0.24 [0.001, 0.48], $n = 119$) and analgesic onset time (MD 2.50 [1.85, 3.15] hours, $n = 119$). This indicated that the oral CHM was slightly less effective than the ibuprofen. The study also reported the incidence of adverse reactions. Based on the NCI-CTCAE criteria, there were two cases of gastrointestinal reactions and one case of constipation in the CHM group, and two cases of nausea, seven cases of stomachache, five cases of constipation and three cases of itchy skin in the control group. All the adverse reactions were grade I or II. The incidence of adverse events associated with the gastrointestinal tract was lower in the CHM group versus ibuprofen (RR 0.21 [0.06, 0.69], $n = 119$).

Oral Chinese Herbal Medicine plus Conventional Analgesic versus Placebo plus Conventional Analgesic

Two RCTs (H2, H3) compared oral CHM plus conventional analgesics to placebo plus conventional analgesics.

In one study (H2), people with advanced liver cancer ($n = 50$) and moderate or severe pain (NRS ≥ 4) were treated with fentanyl transdermal system (4.2 mg every 72 hours, according to the patient's pain relief. Patients could adjust the dose to achieve NRS ≤ 3). In the CHM group, patients received *Chai hu shu gan san* 柴胡疏肝散 (*chen pi* 陈皮, *chai hu* 柴胡, *chuan xiong* 川芎, *zhi ke* 枳壳, *shao yao* 芍药, *zhi gan cao* 炙甘草, *xiang fu* 香附) one packet per day in two doses for 21 days. At the same time, people in the control group received a placebo for the CHM (ingredients were 5% dosage of *Chai hu shu gan san* 柴胡疏肝散 and powder made from dry-fried rice 炒大米 to mimic the taste of the full-strength CHM). Five people dropped out due to: death (three cases: one due to gastrointestinal bleeding and one due to septic shock in the integrative medicine group, and one due to hepatorrhexis in the control group), and cancerous fever and sweating (two cases: one in each group), so the final analysis was based on 45 participants.

In the other study (H3), participants had various advanced malignant tumours and all participants ($n = 100$) were required to have moderate or severe pain (NRS ≥ 4) and the syndrome Kidney deficiency with blood stasis (*shen xu xue yu* 肾虚血瘀). All received oxycodone HCl prolonged-release tablets for 14 days. Firstly, there was titration with short-acting opioids, then treatment was converted to oxycodone HCl extended-release tablets, taken orally, once every 12 hours. All people in the CHM group received a formula designed by the authors called *Yi shen gu kang fang* 益肾骨康方 (*shu di huang* 熟地黄, *shan yao* 山药, *mu dan pi* 牡丹皮, *ze xie* 泽泻, *fu ling* 茯苓, *gu sui bu* 骨碎补, *she she cao* 蛇舌草, *ban zhi lian* 半枝莲, *shan yu rou* 山萸肉) one packet per day in two doses from the eighth to the 14th day. The control group received a placebo for the CHM (ingredients were 10% dosage of *Yi shen gu kang fang* 益肾骨康方 to mimic the taste of the full-strength CHM, starch and dextrin) at the same time. There was no drop-out.

Both studies reported NRS scores; in one study (H2) there was no significant difference between groups (MD –0.18 [–0.68, 0.32]) while in the other study (H3) there was a significant reduction (MD –0.64 [–1.19, –0.09]) in pain in the CHM plus oxycodone HCl extended-release tablets group. The pooled result showed no difference between groups (MD –0.40 [–0.85, 0.05] I^2 = 31.7%) with moderate heterogeneity (Table 5.3).

For analgesic dose, one study (H2) reported the result for the average dose of fentanyl transdermal system on the 21st day. There was a significant reduction in the CHM group (MD –20.95 [–39.71, –2.19] ug/h, *n* = 45). The other study (H3) reported the results of the total analgesic dose in the second week of treatment. The median (interquartile range) scores were Median 175 (135, 350) mg in the CHM group, and Median 245 (173.75, 422.5) mg in the control group which the authors reported as a significant reduction (P < 0.05). This study also reported on the frequency of breakthrough pain

Table 5.3 Oral Chinese Herbal Medicine plus Conventional Analgesic versus Placebo plus Conventional Analgesic: NRS Scores

Comparator[1]	Cancer, Pain Intensity (*n* Participants), Syndrome	Effect Size MD [95% CI] I^2	Included Studies
Fentanyl transdermal system	Advanced liver cancer, NRS ≥ 4 (45) NS	–0.18 [–0.68, 0.32]	H2
Oxycodone HCl extended-release tablets	Advanced cancer, NRS ≥ 4 (100), *shen xu xue yu* 肾虚血瘀	–0.64 [–1.19, –0.09]*	H3
Total pool	2 studies (145)	–0.40 [–0.85, 0.05] 31.7%	All above

*Statistically significant.

Note: [1]The same analgesic was used in both groups.

Abbreviations: CI, confidence interval; MD, mean difference; oxycodone HCl, oxycodone hydrochloride; *n*, number; NRS, Numeric rating scale; NS, not specified.

after two weeks' treatment. There was no significant difference between groups (MD –1.52 [–3.89, 0.85] times, $n = 100$).

These two studies (H2, H3) reported on adverse reactions but did not specify which criteria were used. In one study (H3) there was a significant reduction in the incidence of constipation in the *Yi shen gu kang fang* 益肾骨康方 plus oxycodone HCl extended-release tablets group. However, there were no significant differences between groups in the incidence of any of the other adverse reactions (Table 5.4).

Oral Chinese Herbal Medicine plus Conventional Analgesic versus Conventional Analgesic

Five RCTs compared an oral CHM plus conventional analgesic(s) to conventional analgesic(s) without the use of a placebo for the CHM.

Table 5.4 Oral Chinese Herbal Medicine plus Conventional Analgesic versus Placebo plus Conventional Analgesic: Adverse Reaction (Criteria Not Specified)

Adverse Reaction[1]	Effect Size RR [95% CI] I^2	Included Studies (*n* Participants)
Nausea and vomiting	0.52 [0.11, 2.57]	H2 (45)
	0.33 [0.10, 1.16]	H3 (100)
	Pooled result: 0.39 [0.15, 1.05] 57.8%	H2, H3 (145)
Constipation	0.94 [0.47, 1.87]	H2 (45)
	0.38 [0.15, 0.998]*	H3 (100)
	Pooled result: 0.64 [0.26, 1.56] 0%	H2 (145)
Dizziness and drowsiness	1.39 [0.35, 5.53]	H2 (45)
Psychiatric symptoms	0.70 [0.13, 3.78]	
Cutaneous reactions	1.57 [0.29, 8.51]	
Dysuria	0.63 [0.17, 2.32]	
Respiratory depression	1.04 [0.24, 4.64]	
Dizziness	0.11 [0.01, 2.01]	H3 (100)
Drowsiness	0.50 [0.05, 5.34]	

*Statistically significant.

Note: [1]The same analgesic was used in both groups.

Abbreviations: CI, confidence interval; RR, relative risk; *n*, number.

Pain Intensity

All the studies reported the pain intensity using NRS scores. One study (H6) found that compared to oxycodone HCl extended-release tablets, there was a significant reduction in NRS in the integrative therapy group (MD –1.32 [–1.84, –0.80]) after 14 days, but there were no significant differences between groups for the other studies. The pooled result for all studies showed a significant reduction for CHMs combined with conventional analgesics (MD –0.59 [–1.09, –0.09] I^2 = 58%) with substantial heterogeneity (Table 5.5).

Table 5.5 Oral Chinese Herbal Medicine plus Conventional Analgesic versus Conventional Analgesic: NRS Scores

Comparator[1]	Cancer, Pain Intensity (*n* Participants), Syndrome	Effect Size MD [95% CI] I^2	Included Studies
Morphine sulfate sustained-release tablets	Malignant tumour, NRS ≥ 4 (38), *qi xu xue yu* 气虚血瘀	–0.16 [–1.07, 0.75]	H4
Conventional analgesic (Tylox®, Oxycodone HCl)	Bone metastases, NRS ≥ 4 (40), *yin xu nei re* 阴虚内热	–0.60 [–1.55, 0.35]	H5
Oxycodone HCl extended-release tablets	Bone metastases, NRS ≥ 4 (60), *shen xu xue yu* 肾虚血瘀	–1.32 [–1.84, –0.80]*	H6
Morphine sulfate sustained-release tablets	Advanced cancer, NRS ≥ 4 (60), *qi zhi xue yu* 气滞血瘀	–0.14 [–0.96, 0.68]	H7
Morphine sulphate sustained-release tablets	Liver cancer, 4 ≤ NRS ≤ 6 (46), *gan yu qi zhi* 肝郁气滞	–0.44 [–0.999, 0.12]	H8
Total pool	5 studies (244)	–0.59 [–1.09, –0.09]* 58%	All above
Sensitivity analysis 1	Bone metastases, 2 studies (100)	–1.08 [–1.74, –0.41]* 40.9%	H5, H6
Sensitivity analysis 2	Morphine sulfate sustained-release tablets, 2 studies (98)	–0.15 [–0.76, 0.46] 0%	H4, H7

*Statistically significant.

Note: [1]The same analgesic was used in both groups.

Abbreviations: CI, confidence interval; MD, mean difference; *n*, number; oxycodone HCl, oxycodone hydrochloride; NRS, Numeric rating scale.

In the sensitivity analyses, for the two studies which required patients to have bone metastases, the pooled result remained significant with reduced heterogeneity (MD –1.08 [–1.74, –0.41] $I^2 = 40.9\%$). For the two studies that used treatment with morphine sulfate sustained-release tablets, the pooled result was not significant (MD –0.15 [–0.76, 0.46] $I^2 = 0\%$) without heterogeneity.

Analgesic Onset Time

Only one study (H6) reported on analgesic onset time. Sixty-five people with bone metastases who had moderate or severe pain (NRS ≥ 4) were treated with oxycodone HCl (10 mg every 12 hours, with the dose adjusted according to the patient's pain relief) and one group of 30 people also received a formula designed by the authors called *Bu shen huo xue fang* 补肾活血方 (*yin yang huo* 淫羊藿, *tao ren* 桃仁, *hong hua* 红花, *dang gui* 当归, *xiang fu* 香附, *chuan xiong* 川芎, *niu xi* 牛膝, *bu gu zhi* 补骨脂, *gu sui bu* 骨碎补, *ban zhi lian* 半枝莲, *she she cao* 蛇舌草, *gan cao* 甘草) for 14 days. Five people dropped out due to tumour progress and received other therapy (three cases) or loss to follow-up (two cases) but the article did not report which drop-outs were in which groups. The final analysis was based on 60 participants. The results showed there was no significant difference between groups (MD 0.64 [–2.19, 3.47] minutes, $n = 60$).

Frequency of Breakthrough Pain

Only one study (H5) reported the data for frequency of breakthrough pain. The study required all participants to have bone metastases ($n = 40$) with moderate or severe pain (NRS ≥ 4) and to have the syndrome of *yin* deficiency with internal heat (*yin xu nei re* 阴虚内热). All people in the integrative therapy group received a formula designed by the authors called *Jia jian qing gu san fang* 加减清骨散方 (*yin chai hu* 银柴胡, *hu huang lian* 胡黄连, *qin jiao* 秦艽, *bie jia* 鳖甲, *di gu pi* 地骨皮, *zhi mu* 知母, *gan cao* 甘草, *tao ren* 桃仁, *ban zhi lian* 半枝莲, *mo han lian* 墨旱莲, *nv zhen zi* 女贞子, *tu bie chong* 土鳖虫, *wu gong* 蜈蚣) one packet per day for 14 days. The control group did not receive CHM therapy. All participants received the

WHO three-step analgesic ladder treatment. The results showed there was a significant reduction in the average frequency of breakthrough pain per person during the two weeks of treatment in the integrative medicine group (MD –4.30 [–8.14, –0.46] times per person, $n = 40$).

Analgesic Dose

In the three studies that reported analgesic dose, one study (H5) reported the total analgesic dose during the whole treatment and two studies (H6, H8) reported the maintenance dose so the results of these two studies could be pooled together.

In the study that reported the total analgesic dose during the whole treatment (H5) there was a significant reduction for the people with moderate pain in the integrative medicine group (MD –7.60 [–14.66, –0.54] pills of oxycodone-acetaminophen (Tylox®), ($n = 29$), but no significant difference for the participants with severe pain (MD –55.71 [–321.84, 210.42] mg of oxycodone HCl, $n = 11$) compared to the group that only received conventional analgesics.

In one study (H8), all 50 participants had liver cancer with moderate pain ($4 \leq NRS \leq 6$). All had the syndrome of Liver depression and *qi* stagnation (*gan yu qi zhi* 肝郁气滞) and received treatment with morphine sulphate sustained-release tablets (10 mg once every 12 hours, dose adjusted according to the patient's pain relief). In the integrative therapy group, patients also received *Chai hu shu gan san jia wei* 柴胡疏肝散加味 (*chen pi* 陈皮, *chai hu* 柴胡, *chuan xiong* 川芎, *zhi ke* 枳壳, *shao yao* 芍药, *gan cao* 甘草, *xiang fu* 香附, *yan hu suo* 延胡索, *bai zhi* 白芷, *zhi shi* 枳实) one packet per day in two doses for five days. The control group did not receive CHM therapy. Four people dropped out but the article did not report the reasons. The final analysis was based on 46 participants. The results showed there was no significant difference in the maintenance dose between groups (MD –2.82 [–9.25, 3.61] mg/d, $n = 46$). In contrast, the other study (H6) showed a significant reduction in analgesic dose in the *Bu shen huo xue fang* 补肾活血方 plus oxycodone HCl extended-release tablets group (MD –5.20 [–8.55, –1.85] mg/d, $n = 60$) versus oxycodone HCl extended-release tablets.

The pooled result for these two studies showed a significant reduction for the maintenance dose in the integrative medicine groups (MD –4.69 [–7.66, –1.72] mg/d, $I^2 = 0\%$, $n = 106$) with no heterogeneity.

Quality of Life

Two studies reported data on QOL. One study (H4) used a 12-item QOL scale[9] on which the total score is 60 points, with higher scores indicating better QOL. The other study (H8) used the brief pain inventory (BPI) which was developed by the Pain Research Group of the WHO Collaborating Centre for Symptom Evaluation in Cancer Care, and which has a Chinese version.[10,11] Higher scores on BPI indicate worse QOL.

The study (H4) that used the Chinese scale required all patients ($n = 38$) to have malignant tumours and to have received second-step treatment on the WHO three-step analgesic ladder without adequate pain relief. All the participants had moderate or severe pain (NRS ≥ 4), all had the syndrome of *qi* deficiency with blood stasis (*qi xu xue yu* 气虚血瘀) and all received treatment with morphine sulfate sustained-release tablets (30 mg every 12 hours). All people in the integrative therapy group received an unnamed formula (*huang qi* 黄芪, *dang shen* 党参, *bai zhu* 白术, *fu ling* 茯苓, *dan shen* 丹参, *e zhu* 莪术, *san qi* 三七, *chuan xiong* 川芎, *chi shao* 赤芍, *dang gui* 当归, *she she cao* 蛇舌草, *xian he cao* 仙鹤草, *yan hu suo* 延胡索, *jiao gu ya* 焦谷芽, *jiao mai ya* 焦麦芽, *gan cao* 甘草) one packet per day in two doses for seven days. The control group received the conventional analgesic alone. There was a significant improvement in the CHM plus morphine sulfate sustained-release tablets group (MD 4.74 [2.13, 7.35], $n = 38$).

The other study (H8) used BPI and found there was no significant difference between groups (MD 4.48 [–1.05, 10.01], $n = 46$) for *Chai hu shu gan san jia wei* 柴胡疏肝散加味 plus morphine sulphate sustained-release tablets versus morphine sulphate sustained-release tablets.

Karnofsky Performance Status

Four studies reported Karnofsky Performance Status (KPS) scores. In the study of CHM plus conventional analgesic (H5) there was no significant difference between groups, but in the other studies there was a significant improvement in the integrative medicine groups. The pooled result of four studies showed a significant improvement for CHM combined with conventional analgesic (MD 6.31 [2.28, 10.33] I^2 = 51.6%) with substantial heterogeneity (Table 5.6).

In the sensitivity analysis for the two studies which enrolled patients with bone metastases, the pooled result showed no difference between groups (MD 4.47 [–1.64, 10.58] I^2 = 58.3%);

Table 5.6 Oral Chinese Herbal Medicine plus Conventional Analgesic versus Conventional Analgesic: KPS Scores

Comparator[1]	Cancer, Pain Intensity (*n* Participants), Syndrome	Effect Size MD [95% CI] I^2	Included Studies
Morphine sulfate sustained-release tablets	Malignant tumours, NRS ≥ 4 (38), *qi xu xue yu* 气虚血瘀	7.37 [0.74, 14.00]*	H4
Conventional analgesic	Bone metastases, NRS ≥ 4 (40), *yin xu nei re* 阴虚内热	2.00 [–1.85, 5.85]	H5
Oxycodone HCl extended-release tablets	Bone metastases, NRS ≥ 4 (60), *shen xu xue yu* 肾虚血瘀	8.40 [1.27, 15.52]*	H6
Morphine sulfate sustained-release tablets	Advanced malignant tumours, NRS ≥ 4 (60), *qi zhi xue yu* 气滞血瘀	9.55 [4.06, 15.04]*	H7
Total pool	4 studies (198)	6.31 [2.28, 10.33]* 51.6%	All above
Sensitivity analysis 1	Bone metastases, 2 studies (100)	4.47 [–1.64, 10.58] 58.3%	H5, H6
Sensitivity analysis 2	Morphine sulfate sustained-release tablets, 2 studies (98)	8.66 [4.43, 12.89]* 0%	H4, H7

*Statistically significant.

Note: [1]The same analgesic was used in both groups.

Abbreviations: CI, confidence interval; MD, mean difference; *n*, number; oxycodone HCl, oxycodone hydrochloride; NRS, Numeric rating scale.

but for the studies that used treatment with morphine sulfate sustained-release tablets, the pooled result remained significant (MD 8.66 [4.43, 12.89] $I^2 = 0\%$) without heterogeneity.

Immune Function

Only one study (H7) reported data on immune function. All the participants had advanced malignant tumours ($n = 60$) with moderate or severe pain (NRS ≥ 4) and had the syndrome of *qi* deficiency with blood stasis (*qi zhi xue yu* 气滞血瘀). All received morphine sulfate sustained-release tablets. Treatment started with 10–30 mg, once every 12 hours, with the dose adjusted according to the patient's pain relief. The participants in the integrative therapy group received *Yuan hu zhi tong jiao nang* 元胡止痛胶囊 (five capsules, three times a day) for seven days, and the control group did not receive CHM therapy. There were significant differences between groups for counts of CD3+, CD8+, NK cells and the ratio CD4+/CD8+, but not for CD4+ cells (Table 5.7).

Adverse Reactions

Four studies reported adverse reactions, but one study (H4) had a data error in the results table and one study (H5) used criteria made

Table 5.7 Oral Chinese Herbal Medicine plus Conventional Analgesic versus Conventional Analgesic: Immune Function

T-cells	Effect Size MD [95% CI] I^2	Included Studies (*n* Participants)
CD3+ (%)	7.04 [3.89, 10.18]*	
CD4+ (%)	2.00 [–0.36, 4.36]	
CD8+ (%)	0.32 [0.14, 0.50]*	H7 (60)
CD4+/CD8+	2.42 [0.11, 4.73]*	
NK (%)	7.04 [3.89, 10.18]*	

*Statistically significant.

Abbreviations: CI, confidence interval; MD, mean difference; *n*, number.

by the author. So only two studies (H6, H7) were included in the meta-analysis.

One study (H7) used the WHO criteria and showed there was a significant reduction in the CHM plus morphine sulfate sustained-release tablets group for nausea, vomiting and constipation, but not for dizziness and drowsiness (Table 5.8).

Another study (H6) did not specify which criteria were used. There were no significant differences between groups for dizziness, constipation, nausea and vomiting or itchy skin (Table 5.9).

Oral Chinese Herbal Medicine plus Conventional Analgesic plus Zoledronic Acid versus Conventional Analgesic plus Zoledronic Acid

In one RCT (H9), all participants had bone metastases (n = 50) with moderate or severe pain (NRS ≥ 4) and had the syndrome of Kidney

Table 5.8 Oral Chinese Herbal Medicine plus Conventional Analgesic versus Conventional Analgesic: Adverse Reaction (WHO Criteria)

Adverse Reaction[1]	Effect Size RR [95% CI]	Included Studies (*n* Participants)
Nausea and vomiting	0.52 [0.33, 0.81]*	
Constipation	0.52 [0.32, 0.84]*	H7 (60)
Dizziness and drowsiness	0.75 [0.53, 1.06]	

*Statistically significant.
Note: [1]The same analgesic was used in both groups.
Abbreviations: CI, confidence interval; *n*, number; RR, relative risk.

Table 5.9 Oral Chinese Herbal Medicine plus Conventional Analgesic versus Conventional Analgesic: Adverse Reaction (Criteria Not Specified)

Adverse Reaction[1]	Effect Size RR [95% CI]	Included Studies (*n* Participants)
Dizziness	0.80 [0.24, 2.69]	
Constipation	0.86 [0.33, 2.25]	H6 (60)
Nausea and vomiting	0.67 [0.12, 3.71]	
Itchy skin	3.00 [0.13, 70.83]	

Note: [1]The same analgesic was used in both groups.
Abbreviations: CI, confidence interval; *n*, number; RR, relative risk.

deficiency with blood stasis (*shen xu xue yu* 肾虚血瘀). All were treated with conventional analgesics (based on the WHO three-step analgesic ladder) plus zoledronic acid (a bisphosphonate used to reduce breakdown of bone). Twenty-five people in one group also received a formula designed by the authors called *Du huo bu gu fang* 独活补骨方 (*du huo* 独活, *bu gu zhi* 补骨脂, *gu sui bu* 骨碎补, *tu si zi* 菟丝子, *du zhong* 杜仲, *tou gu cao* 透骨草, *yan hu suo* 延胡索, *ji xue teng* 鸡血藤, *ren dong teng* 忍冬藤, *tu bie chong* 土鳖虫, *xu chang qin* 徐长卿, *rou gui* 肉桂, *gan cao* 甘草, one packet per day in two doses for nine weeks).

The results showed that there was a significant reduction in NRS scores (MD –0.32 [–0.59, –0.05], $n = 50$) and a significant improvement in KPS in the integrative therapy group (MD 6.80 [4.09, 9.51], $n = 50$).

Comparisons with Other Conventional Medications

Two RCTs compared CHMs with the combination of calcium carbonate and vitamin D3 tablets as an intervention for aromatase inhibitor-associated musculoskeletal symptoms (AIMSS) and one RCT compared a CHM with lactulose oral solution as a treatment for opioid-induced constipation.

Oral Chinese Herbal Medicine versus Calcium Carbonate and Vitamin D3 Tablets

Two RCTs (H10, H11) compared oral CHM to calcium carbonate and vitamin D3 tablets. All participants were post-menopausal women with breast cancer treated with aromatase inhibitors (AIs) who had AIMSS and related pain symptoms.

One RCT (H10) compared a formula designed by the authors called *Qiang gu zhi tong fang* 强骨止痛方 (*chuan duan* 川断, *du zhong* 杜仲, *ji xue teng* 鸡血藤, *shen jin cao* 伸筋草, one packet per day in two doses for three months), with calcium carbonate plus vitamin D3 tablets (one pill per day) in breast cancer patients with AIMSS and related pain symptoms.

In the other RCT (H11) all the breast cancer patients had AIMSS and related pain symptoms. In the CHM group they received a formula named by the authors' hospital called *Bu shen qiang jin jiao nang* 补肾强筋胶囊 (*shu di huang* 熟地黄, *du zhong* 杜仲, *gu sui bu* 骨碎补, *bu gu zhi* 补骨脂, *xue jie* 血竭, *quan xie* 全蝎, two capsules, three times a day, for four weeks). In the control group, all participants were treated with calcium carbonate and vitamin D3 tablets for four weeks.

Both studies reported VAS scores (cm). In one study (H10) there was significant reduction in the CHM group (MD –0.80 [–1.26, –0.34], n = 47), and in the other study (H11) there was also a significant reduction in the CHM group (MD –1.06 [–1.48, –0.64], n = 65). The pooled result showed a significant reduction in VAS in the CHM groups (MD –0.94 [–1.25, –0.63] I^2 = 0%, n = 112) compared to calcium carbonate plus vitamin D3 tablets.

Oral Chinese Herbal Medicine versus Lactulose Oral Solution

One study (H12) compared a formula designed by the authors called *Yang yin li qi tang* 养阴理气汤 (*sheng da huang* 生大黄, *mang xiao* 芒硝, *xuan shen* 玄参, *sheng di huang* 生地黄, *mai dong* 麦冬, *wu yao* 乌药, *chen xiang* 沉香, *bing lang* 槟榔, *dang shen* 党参, *huo ma ren* 火麻仁, one packet per day in two doses for two weeks), with lactulose oral solution for constipation in cancer pain patients with opioid-induced constipation (OIC). All participants (n = 66) had the syndrome of *qi* stagnation-type constipation (*qi mi* 气秘) or *yin* deficiency with internal heat (*yin xu re jie* 阴虚热结), and OIC was diagnosed based on the Rome III Diagnostic Criteria.[12]

There was a significant reduction in the CHM group for the Cleveland Clinic Constipation Score (CCS)[13] (MD –2.66 [–4.32, –1.00], n = 66), but no significant difference between groups for NRS scores (MD –0.03 [–0.43, 0.37], n = 66).

GRADE for Oral Chinese Herbal Medicine

GRADE assessments were conducted for the pooled results for pain intensity. The comparisons were (1) oral CHM plus conventional analgesic versus placebo plus conventional analgesic (see Table 5.3), and (2) oral CHM plus conventional analgesic versus conventional analgesic (see Table 5.5).

For the first comparison, two placebo-controlled RCTs of integrative medicine (H2, H3) were available. One study found a significant reduction in NRS in the integrative group but the other study did not. The pooled result did not show a significant difference between groups with moderate heterogeneity ($I^2 = 31.7\%$). The GRADE assessment was rated down by one category to 'moderate' due to the small sample size (Table 5.10).

The second comparison was also of integrative medicine but no placebo for the CHM was used so the studies were not blinded. Five RCTs (H4–H8) were available and the pooled result showed a significant decrease in NRS scores at the end of treatment, but the heterogeneity was substantial ($I^2 = 58\%$). The GRADE of evidence was rated down by three categories to 'very low' due to lack of blinding, heterogeneity and small sample size (Table 5.11).

Table 5.10 GRADE for Pain Intensity: Oral Chinese Herbal Medicine plus Conventional Analgesic versus Placebo plus Conventional Analgesic

	Absolute Effect		Relative Effect (95% CI) *n* Studies	Certainty of Evidence
Outcome[1]	**With CHM**	**Without CHM**	**(Participants)**	**GRADE**
NRS scores	**1.46** points	**1.86** points	**MD −0.40** (−0.85 to 0.05 points) 2 (145)	⊕⊕⊕◯ MODERATE[2]
	Average difference: 0.4 points lower (95% CI: 0.85 points lower to 0.05 points higher)			

*Statistically significant result. See Table 5.3 for included studies.

Note: [1]The same analgesic was used in both groups.

[2]Two RCTs with small sample sizes.

Abbreviations: CI, confidence interval; MD, mean difference; *n*, number; NRS, numerical rating scale.

Table 5.11 GRADE for Pain Intensity: Oral Chinese Herbal Medicine plus Conventional Analgesic versus Conventional Analgesic

Outcome[1]	Absolute Effect: With CHM	Absolute Effect: Without CHM	Relative Effect (95% CI) *n* Studies (Participants)	Certainty of Evidence GRADE
NRS scores	**1.32** points	**1.91** points	**MD –0.59*** (–1.09 to –0.09 points) 5 (244)	⊕◯◯◯ VERY LOW[2,3,4]
	Average difference: 0.59 points lower (95% CI: 0.09 to 1.09 points lower)			

*Statistically significant result. See Table 5.5 for included studies.
Note: [1]The same analgesic was used in both groups.
[2]No blinding.
[3]Statistical heterogeneity was substantial.
[4]Five RCTs with small sample sizes.
Abbreviations: CI, confidence interval; MD, mean difference; *n*, number; NRS, numerical rating scale.

Randomised Controlled Trial Evidence for Individual Oral Formulas for Cancer Pain

Two studies used *Chai hu shu gan san* 柴胡疏肝散. One study (H2) used *Chai hu shu gan san* 柴胡疏肝散 plus fentanyl transdermal system versus placebo plus Fentanyl Transdermal System. The other study (H8) used *Chai hu shu gan san jia wei* 柴胡疏肝散加味 plus morphine sulphate sustained-release tablets versus morphine sulphate sustained-release tablets without a placebo for the CHM. Both reported outcomes for NRS scores (Table 5.12). In the pooled result there was no significant difference between groups (MD –0.30 [–0.67, 0.08] $I^2 = 0\%$) without heterogeneity.

Frequently Reported Herbs in Meta-analyses of Oral Chinese Herbal Medicine That Showed a Favourable Effect

In the 12 RCTs that assessed oral CHMs, the most commonly used outcome measures in the meta-analyses were pain intensity (5 RCTs)

Table 5.12 ***Chai Hu Shu Gan San*** **柴胡疏肝散 for Pain Intensity: NRS Scores**

Comparator[1]	Cancer, Pain Intensity (*n* Participants), Syndrome	Effect Size MD [95% CI] I^2	Included Studies
Placebo plus fentanyl transdermal system	Advanced liver cancer, NRS > 3 (45), NS	−0.18 [−0.68, 0.32]	H2
Morphine sulphate sustained-release tablets	Liver cancer, 4 ≤ NRS ≤ 6 (46), *gan yu qi zhi* 肝郁气滞	−0.44 [−0.999, 0.12]	H8
Total pool	2 studies (91)	−0.30 [−0.67, 0.08] 0%	All above

Note: [1]The same analgesic was used in both groups.
Abbreviations: CI, confidence interval; MD, mean difference; *n*, number; NRS, numerical rating scale; NS: not specified.

and KPS (4 RCTs). In this section, we selected one outcome of relevance to clinicians, researchers and patients. Pain intensity was selected since it is the most direct indicator of pain. KPS was not selected since it is a less specific outcome.

The herbs most frequently included as formula ingredients were *chuan xiong* 川芎, *gan cao* 甘草 and *yan hu suo* 延胡索, each of which was included in three RCTs (Table 5.13).

Randomised Controlled Trials of Topical Chinese Herbal Medicine

The 17 RCTs of topical CHM were all conducted in mainland China and enrolled 1,370 participants. The age of participants ranged from 18 to 85 years. Following drop-outs, 1,353 participants completed the studies. The studies included:

- One RCT (H13) of topical CHM versus placebo;
- One RCT (H14) of topical CHM versus conventional analgesic;
- Three RCTs (H15–H17) of topical CHM plus conventional analgesic versus placebo plus conventional analgesic;
- Eleven RCTs (H18–H28) of topical CHM plus conventional analgesic versus conventional analgesic;

Table 5.13 Frequently Reported Orally Used Herbs in Meta-analyses Showing a Favourable Effect for Pain Intensity

No. of Meta-analyses (Studies)	Herbs	Scientific Name[2]	Frequency of Use
1* (5)	*Chuan xiong* 川芎	*Ligusticum chuanxiong* Hort.	3
	Gan cao 甘草	*Glycyrrhiza uralensis* Fisch.	3
	Yan hu suo 延胡索	*Corydalis yanhusuo* W.T. Wang	3
	Bai zhi 白芷	*Angelica dahurica* (Fisch. ex Hoffm.) Benth. et Hook. f.	2
	Ban zhi lian 半枝莲	*Scutellaria barbata* D. Don	2
	Dang gui 当归	*Angelica sinensis* (Oliv.) Diels	2
	Shao yao 芍药[1]	*Paeonia lactiflora* Pall.; *P. veitchii* Lynch	2
	She she cao 蛇舌草	*Hedyotis diffusa* Willd.	2
	Tao ren 桃仁	*Prunus persica* (L.) Batsch	2
	Xiang fu 香附	*Cyperus rotundus* L.	2

*Pain intensity: refer to Table 5.5.

Notes: [1]One RCT used *chi shao* 赤芍 and one RCT used *bai shao* 白芍.

[2]The use of some herbs may be restricted in some countries. Readers are advised to comply with relevant regulations.

- One RCT (H29) of topical CHM plus conventional analgesic plus pamidronate disodium versus analgesic plus pamidronate disodium.

Of the studies of topical CHM, two RCTs used syndrome differentiation in the selection criteria. The syndrome names reported in the two RCTs were:

- Blood stasis due to *qi* stagnation — *qi zhi xue yu* 气滞血瘀 (H19); and
- *Yin* cold congealed with *qi* stagnation — *yin han ning zhi* 阴寒凝滞 (H23).

Table 5.14 Frequently Used Herbs in Randomised Controlled Trials of Topical CHMs

Herb Name	Scientific Name of Herb[5]	No. of Studies
Bing pian 冰片	*Borneolum*	9
Xi xin 细辛	*Asarum* species	9
Chuan wu 川乌[1]	*Aconitum carmichaelii* Debx.	6
Da huang 大黄[2]	*Rheum palmatum* L.; *R. tanguticum* Maxim. ex Balf.; *R. officinale* Baill.	6
Yan hu suo 延胡索	*Corydalis yanhusuo* W.T. Wang	6
Mo yao 没药	*Commiphora myrrha* Engl.; *C. molmol* Engl.	5
Quan xie 全蝎	*Buthus martensii* Karsch.	5
Ru xiang 乳香	*Boswellia carterii* Birdw.; *B. bhaw-dajiana* Birdw.	5
Cao wu 草乌[3]	*Aconitum kusnezoffii* Reichb.	4
Ding xiang 丁香	*Eugenia caryophyllata* Thunb.	4
Xue jie 血竭	*Daemonorops draco* Bl.; *Dracaena cochinchinensis* (Lour.) S.C. Chen	4
Chan su 蟾酥[4]	*Bufo bufo gargarizans* Cantor; *B. melanostictus* Schneider	3
Sheng ban xia 生半夏	*Pinellia ternata* (Thunb.) Breit.	3
Ze lan 泽兰	*Lycopus lucidus* Turcz. var. *hirtus* Regel	3

Notes: [1]Two RCTs used *sheng chuan wu* 生川乌.
[2]Two RCTs used *sheng da huang* 生大黄.
[3]Two RCTs used *sheng cao wu* 生草乌.
[4]One RCT used *gan chan pi* 干蟾皮.
[5]The use of some herbs may be restricted in some countries. Readers are advised to comply with relevant regulations.

Each study used a different formula. The herbs most frequently used in the topical formulas used in the 17 RCTs were *bing pian* 冰片 ($n = 9$), *xi xin* 细辛 ($n = 9$), *chuan wu* 川乌 ($n = 6$), *da huang* 大黄 ($n = 6$) and *yan hu suo* 延胡索 ($n = 6$) (Table 5.14).

Table 5.15 Risk of Bias of Randomised Controlled Trials of Topical Chinese Herbal Medicine

Risk of Bias Domain	Low Risk *n* (%)	Unclear Risk *n* (%)	High Risk *n* (%)
Sequence generation	9 (52.9)	8 (47.1)	0 (0)
Allocation concealment	1 (5.9)	16 (94.1)	0 (0)
Blinding of participants	4 (23.5)	0 (0)	13 (76.5)
Blinding of personnel	0 (0)	0 (0)	17 (100)
Blinding of outcome assessors	0 (0)	17 (100)	0 (0)
Incomplete outcome data	17 (100)	0 (0)	0 (0)
Selective outcome reporting	1 (5.9)	16 (94.1)	0 (0)

Abbreviation: *n*, number.

Risk of Bias for Topical Chinese Herbal Medicine

The risk of bias for sequence generation was judged 'low risk' in nine RCTs since a correct method of randomisation was described (Table 5.15). The others were 'unclear risk'. Only one study (H27) mentioned allocation concealment and used a proper method so it was judged 'low risk' and the remainder were judged 'unclear risk'. Four studies that used a placebo for the CHM in the control groups were judged 'low risk' for blinding of participants. The remaining studies were judged 'high risk' for blinding of participants. All studies were judged 'high risk' for blinding of personnel and 'unclear risk' for blinding of outcome assessors. All the studies had no drop-outs or few drop-outs so all were assessed as 'low risk' for incomplete outcome data. For selective outcome reporting, only one protocol could be located (H13) and all outcomes were reported, so it was judged 'low risk' whereas the other studies were judged 'unclear risk'.

Topical Chinese Herbal Medicine versus Placebo

One RCT (H13) enrolled liver cancer patients (n = 140) with mild pain ($1 \leq NRS \leq 3$). Seventy-three people in the CHM group received a fomentation called *Shuang bai san* 双柏散 made by the hospital from powdered *da huang* 大黄, *ce bai ye* 侧柏叶, *huang bai* 黄柏, *bo he* 薄荷 and *ze lan* 泽兰, mixed with water and honey to make a paste which was applied to the local pain area, once a day and retained for six hours, for seven days. The 67 people in the control group were treated with a placebo fomentation (main ingredients were dextrin, microcrystalline cellulose and the pigments fruit green, lemon yellow and caramel). There was a significant reduction in NRS scores in the CHM group at the end of treatment (MD –0.72 [–1.04, –0.40], $n = 140$).

Topical Chinese Herbal Medicine versus Conventional Analgesic

One RCT (H14) enrolled people ($n = 260$) with stages I to III cancer and mild to moderate pain (NRS < 7). In the CHM group, participants received *Hua jian ba du mo* 化坚拔毒膜 (*jiang huang* 姜黄, *wu gong* 蜈蚣, *da huang* 大黄, *xi xin* 细辛, *bing pian* 冰片, *chuan wu* 川乌, etc., made into a paste) three times a day for seven days which was applied to the local pain area. In the control group, people were treated with tramadol (100–200 mg per time, three times a day) for seven days.

There were no significant differences between groups for NRS scores (MD –0.15 [–0.38, 0.08], $n = 260$) or duration of analgesia (MD 0.32 [–0.26, 0.90] hours, $n = 260$), but there was a significant reduction in analgesic onset time (MD –26.02 [–27.57, –24.47] minutes, $n = 260$) in favour of the CHM group.

Topical Chinese Herbal Medicine plus Conventional Analgesic versus Placebo plus Conventional Analgesic

Three RCTs (H15–H17) compared a topical CHM plus conventional analgesic to a placebo plus conventional analgesic.

One study (H15) required all participants to have advanced malignant tumours ($n = 80$) with moderate or severe pain (NRS ≥ 4). All received morphine sulfate sustained-release tablets (after titration of a short-acting opioid, they converted to morphine sulfate sustained-release tablets, taken orally, once every 12 hours) for ten days. From the fourth to the tenth day, people in the CHM group were treated with *Bing chong zhi tong gao* 冰虫止痛膏 (*ding xiang* 丁香, *xi xin* 细辛, *ru xiang* 乳香, *mo yao* 没药, *xue jie* 血竭, *quan xie* 全蝎, *sheng ban xia* 生半夏, *gan chan pi* 干蟾皮, *da huang* 大黄, *mang xiao* 芒硝 and *bing pian* 冰片). All the above herb granules were mixed with honey and oil to make a paste that was applied on the local pain area, once a day and retained for four to six hours. The participants in the control group were treated with a placebo paste (main ingredients were yellow cornmeal, edible chocolate brown pigment, edible fruit green pigment, honey and sesame oil). Three people dropped out due to allergy (one case in the integrative medicine group due to the adhesive plaster) or when they received another therapy (two cases in the control group), so the final analysis was based on 77 participants.

Another study (H16) compared *Wu xiang tong xiao gao* 乌香痛消膏 (*chuan wu* 川乌, *bing pian* 冰片, *bai jie zi* 白芥子, etc.) which was made into a paste and put on the local pain area, once a day for seven days, with a placebo paste (ingredients not specified) in patients with malignant tumours (n = 80) who had moderate or severe pain (NRS ≥ 4). All the people received conventional analgesic treatment based on the WHO three-step analgesic ladder.

In the other study (H17), all participants (n = 60) had advanced lung cancer and severe pain (NRS ≥ 7) and were treated with oxycodone HCl, 10 mg every 12 hours, dose adjusted according to the patient's pain relief. In the CHM group, patients received *Xiao pi zhen tong gao* 消痞镇痛膏 (*chan su* 蟾酥, *cao wu* 草乌, *rou gui* 肉桂, *xi xin* 细辛, *xue jie* 血竭, *san leng* 三棱, *e zhu* 莪术, *sheng da huang* 生大黄, etc.). All the above herbs were crushed and made into a powder, mixed with honey, *huang jiu* 黄酒 and ginger juice to make a paste which was applied to the local pain area, once a day for seven days. People in the control group received a placebo paste (main ingredients were *da qing ye* 大青叶 as colouring, and peppermint volatile oil).

Pain Intensity

All studies reported NRS scores. In one study (H17) there was a significant reduction in the integrative therapy group (MD –0.87 [–1.42, –0.32]) while in the other studies there were no significant differences between groups. The pooled result showed a significant reduction in NRS scores for topical CHMs combined with conventional analgesics (MD –0.48 [–0.92, –0.05] $I^2 = 41.4\%$) with moderate heterogeneity (Table 5.16).

Analgesic Onset Time and Duration of Analgesia

One study (H16) reported data for analgesic onset time. There was no significant difference between groups (MD –0.41 [–1.12, 0.29] hours, $n = 80$). This study also reported data for duration of analgesia which showed a significant improvement in the *Wu xiang tong xiao gao* 乌香痛消膏 plus conventional analgesics group (MD 3.66 [1.13, 6.18] hours, $n = 80$) versus the conventional analgesic plus placebo group.

Table 5.16 Topical Chinese Herbal Medicine plus Conventional Analgesic versus Placebo plus Conventional Analgesic: NRS Scores

Comparator[1]	Cancer, Pain Intensity (*n* Participants)	Effect Size MD [95% CI] I^2	Included Studies
Morphine sulfate sustained-release tablets	Advanced cancer, NRS ≥ 4 (77)	–0.43 [–1.00, 0.14]	H15
Conventional analgesic	Malignant tumour, NRS ≥ 4 (80)	–0.10 [–0.71, 0.51]	H16
Oxycodone HCl extended-release tablets	Advanced lung cancer, NRS ≥ 7 (60)	–0.87 [–1.42, –0.32]*	H17
Total pool	3 studies (217)	–0.48 [–0.92, –0.05]* 41.4%	All above

*Statistically significant.

Note: [1]The same analgesic was used in both groups.

Abbreviations: CI, confidence interval; MD, mean difference; *n*, number; NRS, numerical rating scale; oxycodone HCl, oxycodone hydrochloride.

Frequency of Breakthrough Pain

For frequency of breakthrough pain, one study (H15) found there was a significant reduction in the average frequency of breakthrough pain per person during one week in the *Bing chong zhi tong gao* 冰虫止痛膏 plus morphine sulfate sustained-release tablets group (MD –1.41 [–2.20, –0.62] times per week, $n = 77$).

Analgesic Dose

For analgesic dose, one study (H15) reported the results of the maintenance dose and found it was not significantly different between groups (MD –6.24 [–20.53, 8.05] mg/d, $n = 77$). The study of *Wu xiang tong xiao gao* 乌香痛消膏 (H16) reported the total analgesic dose during the whole treatment. There was a significant reduction in the integrative therapy group (MD –138.00 [–234.22, –41.78] mg, $n = 80$) versus conventional analgesic plus placebo. The other study (H17) reported the average analgesic dose per day, which showed a significant reduction in the *Xiao pi zhen tong gao* 消痞镇痛膏 combined with oxycodone HCl extended-release tablets group (MD –60.00 [–73.77, –46.23] mg/d, $n = 60$) versus the group that received oxycodone HCl extended-release tablets plus a placebo.

Quality of Life

The above study (H15) also reported on QOL using the NCCN impact of pain measurement[14] which is a 7-item questionnaire, and the total score is 70 points with higher scores indicating worst QOL. There was a significant reduction for the topical CHM combined with morphine sulfate sustained-release tablets (MD –5.24 [–10.33, –0.15], $n = 77$).

Karnofsky Performance Status

Two studies reported data on KPS. In the study of *Bing chong zhi tong gao* 冰虫止痛膏 (H15) there was no significant difference between groups (MD 0.09 [–5.94, 6.12], $n = 77$). Similarly, in the study of *Xiao pi zhen tong gao* 消痞镇痛膏 (H17) there was no difference between groups (MD 0.73 [–2.00, 3.46], $n = 60$). Also, the pooled results of these two studies showed no significant difference between groups (MD 0.62 [–1.86, 3.11] $I^2 = 0\%$, $n = 137$).

Immune Function

The study of *Xiao pi zhen tong gao* 消痞镇痛膏 (H17) reported the results of immune function. There were significant increases for IgA (MD 1.74 [1.57, 1.90], $n = 60$), IgG (MD 4.79 [4.26, 5.31], $n = 60$) and IgM (MD 0.67 [0.53, 0.81], $n = 60$) in the CHM plus oxycodone HCl extended-release tablets group after seven days of treatment.

Adverse Reactions

Two studies (H15, H17) reported on adverse reactions. One (H15) used the NCI-CTCAE criteria, while the other (H17) did not specify which criteria were used.

The study (H15) that used NCI-CTCAE criteria showed there were no grade IV adverse reactions in either group. There was only grade I nausea, vomiting, drowsiness and allergy in both groups, and grades I to III constipation in both groups. There was a significant increase in the incidence of allergy in the *Bing chong zhi tong gao* 冰虫止痛膏 plus morphine sulfate sustained-release tablets group, but there were no significant differences between groups for any of the other adverse reactions (Table 5.17).

Table 5.17 Topical Chinese Herbal Medicine plus Conventional Analgesic versus Placebo plus Conventional Analgesic: Adverse Reaction (NCI-CTCAE Criteria)

Adverse Reaction[1]	Effect Size RR [95% CI]	Included Study (*n* Participants)
Nausea	0.83 [0.31, 2.26]	H15 (77)
Vomiting	0.65 [0.20, 2.12]	
Constipation (I + II)	1.00 [0.86, 1.17]	
Constipation (III)	0.32 [0.03, 2.99]	
Drowsiness	1.22 [0.35, 4.19]	
Allergy	7.79 [1.02, 59.37]*	

*Statistically significant.

Note: [1]The same analgesic was used in both groups.

Abbreviations: CI, confidence interval; *n*, number; RR, risk ratio.

In the study (H17) that did not specify the criteria, there was no significant difference between groups for nausea and vomiting (RR 1.00 [0.36, 2.75], $n = 60$), but there was a significant reduction in the incidence of constipation (RR 0.44 [0.28, 0.70], $n = 60$) in the *Xiao pi zhen tong gao* 消痞镇痛膏 plus oxycodone HCl extended-release tablets group.

Topical Chinese Herbal Medicine plus Conventional Analgesic versus Conventional Analgesic

Eleven RCTs compared a topical CHM plus conventional analgesic to conventional analgesic without a CHM. Two studies (H26, H28) used topical CHM on acupoints, and the others used topical CHM on the local pain area.

Pain Intensity

All the studies reported on pain intensity; one study (H21) used VAS scores and the others used NRS scores.

There were significant reductions in pain for CHMs combined with conventional analgesics in some studies, but there were no significant differences between groups in other studies. The pooled result for all studies showed a significant reduction for the integrative medicine groups (MD –0.79 [–1.07, –0.51] $I^2 = 81.7\%$) with considerable heterogeneity (Table 5.18).

In the sensitivity analysis for the seven studies which enrolled patients with moderate to severe pain (NRS ≥ 4 or VAS ≥ 4), the pooled result showed a significant difference between groups with reduced heterogeneity (MD –0.84 [–1.16, –0.51] $I^2 = 64.6\%$).

Analgesic Onset Time

Two studies (H19, H27) reported on analgesic onset time. Both studies enrolled people with malignant tumours and moderate to severe pain (NRS ≥ 4).

Table 5.18 Topical Chinese Herbal Medicine plus Conventional Analgesic versus Conventional Analgesic: Pain Intensity

Comparator[1]	Cancer, Pain Intensity (*n* Participants)	Effect Size MD [95% CI] I^2	Included Studies
Morphine sulfate sustained-release tablets	Malignant tumours, NRS ≥ 4 (65)	–0.70 [–1.57, 0.17]	H18
Oxycodone HCl extended-release tablets	Malignant tumours, NRS ≥ 4 (51)	–0.25 [–1.28, 0.78]	H19
Conventional analgesic	Malignant tumours, NRS ≥ 2 (80)	–0.62 [–1.07, –0.17]*	H20
Conventional analgesic	Malignant tumours, VAS[2] ≥ 4 (50)	–0.33 [–0.94, 0.28]	H21
Celecoxib capsules	Liver cancer, NRS ≤ 3 (36)	–1.52 [–1.77, –1.27]*	H22
Oxycodone HCl extended-release tablets	Bone metastases, NRS ≥ 4 (61)	–1.01 [–2.08, 0.06]	H23
Conventional analgesic	Ovarian cancer with pain (60)	–0.68 [–0.90, –0.46]*	H24
Conventional analgesic	Malignant tumours with pain (78)	0.05 [–0.66, 0.76]	H25
Fentanyl transdermal system	Malignant neuropathic pain, NRS ≥ 4 (34)	–0.05 [–0.91, 0.81]	H26
Morphine sulfate sustained-release tablets	Malignant tumours, NRS ≥ 4 (61)	–1.15 [–1.30, –1.00]*	H27
Intrathecal injections of morphine	Malignant tumours, NRS ≥ 4 (100)	–1.27 [–1.55, –0.99]*	H28
Total pool	11 studies (675)	–0.79 [–1.07, –0.51]* 81.7%	All above
Sensitivity analysis	NRS or VAS[2] ≥ 4, 7 studies (422)	–0.84 [–1.16, –0.51]* 64.6%	H18, H19, H21, H23, H26–H28

* Statistically significant.
Notes: [1]The same analgesic was used in both groups.
[2]One point on NRS is equivalent to 1 cm on VAS.
Abbreviations: CI, confidence interval; MD, mean difference; *n*, number; NRS, numerical rating scale; oxycodone HCl, oxycodone hydrochloride; VAS; visual analogue scale.

One study (H19) required all the participants (*n* = 51) to have the syndrome of Blood stasis due to *qi* stagnation (*qi zhi xue yu* 气滞血

瘀), and all received oxycodone HCl extended-release tablets (starting with 10 mg, once every 12 hours, with dose adjustment according to the patient's pain relief) for seven days. All people in the CHM group (*n* = 26) received a cataplasm called *Xiao zheng zhi tong gao* 消症止痛膏 (*a wei* 阿魏, *wu bei zi* 五倍子, *sheng da huang* 生大黄, *bing pian* 冰片), applied to the local pain area, once a day for seven days.

In the other study (H27), all the participants (*n* = 63) were treated with morphine sulfate sustained-release tablets (starting with 10 mg, once every 12 hours, with dose adjustment according to the patient's pain relief), and 31 people received extra treatment with a cataplasm called *Qi zheng xiao tong tie* 奇正消痛贴 (*du yi wei* 独一味, *shui bai zhi* 水柏枝, *ji dou* 棘豆, *shui niu jiao* 水牛角, *jiang huang* 姜黄, *huang jiao* 花椒) which was applied to the local pain area, once a day for seven days. Two people dropped out in the control group due to refusal of the treatment, so the final analysis was based on 61 participants.

There were significant reductions in analgesic onset time in each study, and the pooled result of these two studies showed a significantly greater reduction in the integrative medicine groups (MD −19.15 [−21.81, −16.49] minutes, I^2 = 0%) without heterogeneity (Table 5.19).

Table 5.19 Topical Chinese Herbal Medicine plus Conventional Analgesic versus Conventional Analgesic: Analgesic Onset Time (Minutes)

Comparator[1]	Cancer, Pain Intensity (*n* Participants)	Effect Size MD [95% CI] I^2	Included Studies
Oxycodone HCl extended-release tablets	Malignant tumour, NRS ≥ 4 (51)	−19.00 [−24.01, −13.99]*	H19
Morphine sulfate sustained-release tablets	Malignant tumour, NRS ≥ 4 (61)	−19.21 [−22.34, −16.07]*	H27
Total pool	2 studies (111)	−19.15 [−21.81, −16.49]* 0%	All above

*Statistically significant.

Note: [1]The same analgesic was used in both groups.

Abbreviations: CI, confidence interval; MD, mean difference; *n*, number; NRS, numerical rating scale; oxycodone HCl, oxycodone hydrochloride.

Frequency of Breakthrough Pain

Two studies (H23, H28) reported data on frequency of breakthrough pain. In one study (H23), 66 people with bone metastases and moderate or severe pain (NRS ≥ 4) were treated with oxycodone HCl extended-release tablets. All had the syndrome of *yin* cold congealed with *qi* stagnation (*yin han ning zhi* 阴寒凝滞). Five people dropped out due to loss to follow-up (one case in the integrative medicine group, and three cases in the control group), or to not taking the medicine regularly (one case in the integrative medicine group), so the final analysis was based on 61 participants. One group of 31 people also received a cataplasm designed by the authors called *Gu tong tie* 骨痛贴 (herb granules of *rou gui* 肉桂, *zhi fu pian* 制附片, *xi xin* 细辛, *gan jiang* 干姜, *xian mao* 仙茅, *quan xie* 全蝎, *wei ling xian* 威灵仙, *shan ci gu* 山慈菇 and *ding xiang* 丁香, mixed with *huang jiu* 黄酒, which was applied to the local pain area, and changed every 12 hours for 10 days). There was no significant difference between groups for the average frequency of breakthrough pain per person per day (MD –0.26 [–0.73, 0.21] times per person per day, *n* = 61).

The other study (H28) included people (*n* = 100) with malignant tumours and moderate to severe pain (NRS ≥ 4) who were treated with intrathecal injections of morphine for four weeks. All people in the integrative therapy group received an unnamed cataplasm designed by the authors (*yan hu suo* 延胡索, *ru xiang* 乳香, *mo yao* 没药, *hong hua* 红花, *xi xin* 细辛, *chuan wu* 川乌, *bing pian* 冰片). These herbs were crushed into powder and mixed with white vinegar to make a paste which was applied bilaterally to the acupoints ST36 *Zusanli* 足三里, TE6 *Zhigou* 支沟, PC6 *Neiguan* 内关 and BL13 *Feishu* 肺俞 once a day for four weeks. There was a significantly greater reduction in the average frequency of breakthrough pain per person per week in the CHM plus intrathecal morphine injection group (MD –1.21 [–1.49, –0.93] times per person per week, *n* = 100).

Duration of Analgesia

Two studies (H19, H27) reported the results for duration of analgesia. There was a significantly greater increase in the duration of analgesia

Table 5.20 Topical Chinese Herbal Medicine plus Conventional Analgesic versus Conventional Analgesic: Duration of Analgesia (Hours)

Comparator[1]	Cancer, Pain Intensity (*n* Participants)	Effect Size MD [95% CI] I^2	Included Studies
Oxycodone HCl extended-release tablets	Malignant tumour, NRS ≥ 4 (51)	1.70 [0.36, 3.04]*	H19
Morphine sulfate sustained-release tablets	Malignant tumour, NRS ≥ 4 (61)	1.32 [1.14, 1.50]*	H27
Total pool	2 studies (111)	1.32 [1.15, 1.50]* 0%	All above

*Statistically significant.

Note: [1]The same analgesic was used in both groups.

Abbreviations: CI, confidence interval; MD, mean difference; *n*, number; NRS, numerical rating scale; oxycodone HCl, oxycodone hydrochloride.

in the integrative group in each study, and the pooled result of these two studies showed a significantly greater increase in duration in the CHM combined with conventional analgesic group (MD 1.32 [1.15, 1.50] hours, I^2 = 0%) without heterogeneity (Table 5.20).

Analgesic Dose

In the five studies that reported analgesic dose, three studies (H18, H19, H26) reported the maintenance dose, one study (H23) reported the total analgesic dose during the whole treatment, and one study (H28) reported the average analgesic dose per day.

The results of the three studies that reported the maintenance dose were pooled together. There was a significant reduction in each of the studies, and the pooled result of these three studies showed a significantly greater reduction in maintenance dose in the integrative therapy groups (MD −32.47 [−57.11, −7.82] mg/d, I^2 = 79%) with considerable heterogeneity (Table 5.21). This was mainly due to the study that enrolled patients with malignant neuropathic pain (H26). When this study was removed, the pooled result showed a significant

Table 5.21 Topical Chinese Herbal Medicine plus Conventional Analgesic versus Conventional Analgesic: Analgesic Maintenance Dose (mg/d)

Comparator[1]	Cancer, Pain Intensity (*n* Participants)	Effect Size MD [95% CI] I^2	Included Studies
Morphine sulfate sustained-release tablets	Malignant tumour, NRS ≥ 4 (65)	−17.52 [−25.60, −9.44]*	H18
Oxycodone HCl extended-release tablets	Malignant tumour, NRS ≥ 4 (51)	−22.68 [−43.36, −1.99]*	H19
Fentanyl transdermal system	Malignant neuropathic pain, NRS ≥ 4 (34)	−72.94 [−107.30, −38.58]*	H26
Total pool	3 studies (150)	−32.47 [−57.11, −7.82]* 79%	All above
Sensitivity analysis	Malignant tumour, NRS ≥ 4, 2 studies (116)	−18.20 [−25.73, −10.68]* 0%	H18, H19

*Statistically significant.

Note: [1]The same analgesic was used in both groups.

Abbreviations: CI, confidence interval; MD, mean difference; *n*, number; NRS, numerical rating scale; oxycodone HCl, oxycodone hydrochloride.

reduction in the CHM plus conventional analgesic groups (MD −18.20 [−25.73, −10.68] mg/d, $I^2 = 0\%$) without heterogeneity.

One study (H23) reported the total analgesic dose during the whole treatment and found there was no significant difference between groups (MD 91.57 [−226.40, 409.54] mg, $n = 61$). Another study (H28) showed there was a significantly greater reduction in the average analgesic dose per day (MD −3.37[−3.77, −2.97] mg/d, $n = 100$) in the CHM plus intrathecal morphine injection group.

Quality of Life

Eight RCTs reported on QOL. Data from the following three different QOL scales were included in the meta-analysis.

- The European Organisation for Research and Treatment of Cancer Quality Of Life Questionnaire (EORTC QLQ-C30, version 3) is a 30-item questionnaire available in multiple languages that includes five functional scales, a scale for global health status/QOL and scales for multiple symptoms.[15] Scoring is normed at 100 with higher scores indicating better QOL for the first six scales with the reverse for the symptoms. In the following analysis, only the global health status/QOL scale was used.

- A Chinese QOL scale[9] on which higher scores indicate better QOL; and
- The NCCN impact of pain measurement[14] on which lower scores indicate less pain.

The meta-analysis results are presented separately for each questionnaire. Three RCTs (H19, H26, H28) reported on QLQ-C30. In one study (H26), all participants (n = 34) had malignant neuropathic pain with moderate to severe pain (NRS ≥ 4) and were receiving fentanyl transdermal system (starting with 4.2 mg, once every 72 hours, with dose adjustment according to the patient's pain relief). One group (n = 17) also received a cataplasm designed by the authors called *Zhi tong san* 止痛散 (herb granules of *ma qian zi* 马钱子, *wu gong* 蜈蚣, *quan chong* 全虫, *bi hu* 壁虎, *shui zhi* 水蛭, *chuan wu* 川乌, *cao wu* 草乌, *nan xing* 南星, *xi xin* 细辛 and *bing pian* 冰片), mixed with vinegar or zanthoxylum oil to make a paste which was applied on the acupoint CV8 *Shenque* 神阙 and on local tender points (*ashi* points 阿是穴), once a day and retained for 4–6 hours, for seven days. The other studies (H19, H28) have been described above.

There was a significantly greater improvement for CHMs combined with conventional analgesics in each study, and the pooled result of these three studies showed a significant improvement in global health status (MD 6.85 [1.80, 11.89], I^2 = 65.5%) with substantial heterogeneity (Table 5.22). When the study which used intrathecal injections of morphine (H28) was removed in the sensitivity analysis, the pooled result was similar with reduced heterogeneity (MD 9.97 [2.18, 17.76], I^2 = 51.4%).

Four RCTs reported results for QOL using the Chinese scale.[9] One study (H27) showed a significantly greater improvement in QOL in the *Qi zheng xiao tong tie* 奇正消痛贴 plus morphine sulfate sustained-release tablets group, but the other studies showed no

Table 5.22 Topical Chinese Herbal Medicine plus Conventional Analgesic versus Conventional Analgesic: Quality of Life (QLQ-C30)

Comparator[1]	Cancer, Pain Intensity (*n* Participants)	Effect Size MD [95% CI] I^2	Included Studies
Oxycodone HCl extended-release tablets	Malignant tumour, NRS ≥ 4 (51)	15.05 [5.38, 24.72]*	H19
Fentanyl transdermal system	Malignant neuropathic pain, NRS ≥ 4 (34)	6.86 [1.24, 12.48]*	H26
Intrathecal injections of morphine	Malignant tumour, NRS ≥ 4 (100)	3.91 [2.40, 5.42]*	H28
Total pool	3 studies (185)	6.85 [1.80, 11.89]* 65.5%	All above
Sensitivity analysis	NRS ≥ 4, 2 studies (85)	9.97 [2.18, 17.76]* 51.4%	H19, H26

*Statistically significant.

Note: [1]The same analgesic was used in both groups.

Abbreviations: CI, confidence interval; MD, mean difference; *n*, number; NRS, numerical rating scale; oxycodone HCl: oxycodone hydrochloride.

significant differences between groups. The pooled results showed no significant difference between groups (MD 1.18 [–0.57, 2.93], I^2 = 79.8%), but there was considerable heterogeneity in these results. In the sensitivity analysis that included the three studies with NRS ≥ 4 or VAS ≥ 4, there was less heterogeneity and a significant improvement (MD 1.86 [0.32, 3.40], I^2 = 61.3%) (Table 5.23).

One study (H23) that used the NCCN impact of pain measurement showed no significant difference between groups (MD –5.84 [–13.92, 2.24], *n* = 61).

Karnofsky Performance Status

Seven RCTs reported data for KPS scores. Four studies showed greater improvements in the integrative medicine groups. The pooled result showed a significant improvement in the topical CHM plus conventional analgesic groups (MD 5.40 [1.43, 9.36], I^2 = 84.2%), but the heterogeneity was considerable (Table 5.24). In a sensitivity analysis for the studies

Table 5.23 Topical Chinese Herbal Medicine plus Conventional Analgesic versus Conventional Analgesic: Quality of Life (Chinese Scale)

Comparator[1]	Cancer, Pain Intensity (n Participants)	Effect Size MD [95% CI] I^2	Included Studies
Morphine sulfate sustained-release tablets	Malignant tumours, NRS ≥ 4 (65)	–0.52 [–3.61, 2.57]	H18
Conventional analgesic	Malignant tumours, VAS[2] ≥ 4 (50)	1.68 [–0.17, 3.53]	H21
Conventional analgesic	Malignant tumours with pain (78)	–0.22 [–1.92, 1.48]	H25
Morphine sulfate sustained-release tablets	Malignant tumours, NRS ≥ 4 (61)	2.74 [2.24, 3.25]*	H27
Total pool	4 studies (254)	1.18 [–0.57, 2.93] 79.8%	All above
Sensitivity analysis	Malignant tumours, NRS ≥4 or VAS[2] ≥ 4, 3 studies (176)	1.86 [0.32, 3.40]* 61.3%	H18, H21, H27

*Statistically significant.

Notes: [1]The same analgesic was used in both groups.

[2]One point on NRS is equivalent to 1 cm on VAS.

Abbreviations: CI, confidence interval; MD, mean difference; *n*, number; NRS, numerical rating scale; VAS, Visual Analogue Scale.

which enrolled patients with moderate to severe pain (NRS ≥ 4 or VAS ≥ 4), the pooled result showed a significant difference between groups with reduced heterogeneity (MD 4.25 [0.19, 8.30] I^2 = 67%).

Adverse Reactions

Four studies (H18, H21, H25, H28) reported on adverse reactions, but did not specify which criteria were used. In the CHM plus conventional analgesic medication groups there were significant reductions in the incidence of people experiencing nausea and vomiting (RR 0.48 [0.28, 0.81] I^2 = 0%), and constipation (RR 0.57 [0.36, 0.91] I^2 = 0%). There were no differences between groups for urinary retention, dizziness, thirst, itchy skin and headache (Table 5.25).

Table 5.24 Topical Chinese Herbal Medicine plus Conventional Analgesic versus Conventional Analgesic: KPS

Comparator[1]	Cancer, Pain Intensity (*n* Participants)	Effect Size MD [95% CI] I^2	Included Studies
Morphine sulfate sustained-release tablets	Malignant tumour, NRS ≥ 4 (65)	3.14 [−3.97, 10.25]	H18
Oxycodone HCl extended-release tablets	Malignant tumour, NRS ≥ 4 (51)	7.97 [0.52, 15.42]*	H19
Conventional analgesic	Malignant tumour with pain (80)	4.16 [0.23, 8.09]*	H20
Conventional analgesic	Malignant tumour, VAS[2] ≥ 4 (50)	8.40 [1.55, 15.24]*	H21
Oxycodone HCl extended-release tablets	Bone metastases, NRS ≥ 4 (61)	5.35 [−0.42, 11.12]	H23
Conventional analgesic	Ovarian cancer with pain (60)	10.22 [6.82, 13.62]*	H24
Morphine sulfate sustained-release tablets	Malignant tumour, NRS ≥ 4 (61)	0.05 [−1.37, 1.46]	H27
Total pool	7 studies (428)	5.40 [1.43, 9.36]* 84.2%	All above
Sensitivity analysis	NRS or VAS ≥ 4, 5 studies (288)	4.25 [0.19, 8.30]* 67%	Excluding H20, H24

*Statistically significant.

Notes: [1]The same analgesic was used in both groups.

[2]One point on NRS is equivalent to 1 cm on VAS.

Abbreviations: CI, confidence interval; MD, mean difference; *n*, number; NRS, numerical rating scale; oxycodone HCl, oxycodone hydrochloride; VAS, Visual Analogue Scale.

Topical Chinese Herbal Medicine plus Conventional Analgesic plus Pamidronate Disodium versus Analgesic plus Pamidronate Disodium

In one RCT (H29), all participants had bone metastases ($n = 60$) and had their pain treated with oxycodone HCl extended-release tablets (dose adjusted according to the patient's pain relief) plus pamidronate disodium. Thirty people in the integrative therapy group also received a cataplasm designed by the authors called *Die da gao* 跌打膏 (*da luo san* 大罗伞, *tou gu xiao* 透骨消, *diu le bang* 丢了棒, *da huan*

Table 5.25 Topical Chinese Herbal Medicine plus Conventional Analgesic versus Conventional Analgesic: Adverse Reaction

Adverse Reaction[1]	No. of Studies (No. of Participants)	Effect Size RR [95% CI]	Included Studies
Nausea and vomiting	4 (293)	0.48 [0.28, 0.81]* 0%	H18, H21, H25, H28
Constipation	4 (293)	0.57 [0.36, 0.91]* 0%	H18, H21, H25, H28
Urinary retention	2 (165)	0.53 [0.19, 1.50] 0%	H18, H28
Dizziness	1 (50)	0.67 [0.12, 3.65]	H21
Thirst	1 (50)	2.00 [0.19, 20.67]	H21
Itchy skin	1 (100)	0.50 [0.05, 5.34]	H28
Headache	1 (100)	0.50 [0.05, 5.34]	H28

*Statistically significant.
Note: [1]The same analgesic was used in both groups.
Abbreviations: CI, confidence interval; RR, relative risk.

hun 大还魂, *xiao huan hun* 小还魂, *guo jiang long* 过江龙, *liu e ling* 六耳菱, *ze lan* 泽兰, *hei lao hu* 黑老虎, *liao dao zhu* 寮刀竹, etc.) which was applied to the local pain area once a day for 28 days.

There was no significant difference between groups for NRS scores (MD –0.30 [–0.64, 0.04], $n = 60$). The study also reported an incidence of 10 points or more increase in KPS. There was a significantly higher incidence of KPS improvement in the combination therapy groups (RR 1.27 [1.005, 1.61], $n = 60$).

GRADE for Topical Chinese Herbal Medicine

GRADE assessments were conducted for the pooled results of pain intensity for the following comparisons: (1) Topical CHM plus conventional analgesic versus placebo plus conventional analgesic (NRS scores) (see Table 5.16), and (2) Topical CHM plus conventional analgesic versus conventional analgesic (NRS ≥ 4 or VAS ≥ 4) (see Table 5.18).

For the first comparison there were three placebo-controlled RCTs available. The meta-analysis found a significantly greater reduction in the integrative medicine groups with only moderate

Table 5.26 GRADE for Pain Intensity: Topical Chinese Herbal Medicine plus Conventional Analgesic versus Placebo plus Conventional Analgesic

Outcome[1]	Absolute Effect: With CHM	Absolute Effect: Without CHM	Relative Effect (95% CI) *n* Studies (Participants)	Certainty of Evidence GRADE
NRS scores (NRS ≥ 4 or NRS ≥ 7)	**1.26** points	**1.74** points	**MD –0.48*** (–0.92 to –0.05 points) 3 (217)	⊕⊕⊕◯ MODERATE[2]
	Average difference: 0.48 points lower (95% CI: 0.05 to 0.92 points lower)			

*Statistically significant result. See Table 5.16 for included studies.

Note: [1]The same analgesic was used in both groups.

[2]Three RCTs with small sample sizes.

Abbreviations: CI, confidence interval; MD, mean difference; *n*, number; NRS, numerical rating scale.

heterogeneity (I^2 = 41.4%). The GRADE of evidence was rated down by one category to 'moderate' due to the small total sample size (*n* = 217) (Table 5.26).

For the second comparison, the seven included RCTs all had participants with pain intensity of NRS ≥ 4 or VAS ≥ 4. These were not placebo-controlled. In the meta-analysis there was a significantly greater reduction in pain intensity in the integrative medicine groups with substantial heterogeneity (I^2 = 64.6%). Therefore, the GRADE of evidence was rated down by two categories to 'low' due to the lack of blinding and the statistical heterogeneity (Table 5.27).

Frequently Reported Herbs in Meta-analyses of Topical Chinese Herbal Medicine that Showed a Favourable Effect

In the 17 RCTs that assessed topical CHMs, the most commonly used outcome measures in the meta-analyses were pain intensity (14 RCTs) and KPS (7 RCTs). In this section, we selected pain intensity as the outcome of most relevance to clinicians, researchers and patients.

In order to assess which herbs were likely to have contributed to meta-analyses that showed significant benefits for the use of topical

Table 5.27 GRADE for Pain Intensity: Topical Chinese Herbal Medicine plus Conventional Analgesic versus Conventional Analgesic

Outcome[1]	Absolute Effect With CHM	Absolute Effect Without CHM	Relative Effect (95% CI) *n* Studies (Participants)	Certainty of Evidence GRADE
Pain intensity (NRS ≥ 4 or VAS ≥ 4)	**1.73** points Average difference: 0.84 points lower (95% CI: 0.51 to 1.16 points lower)	**2.57** points	**MD –0.84*** (–1.16 to –0.51 points) 7 (422)	⊕⊕○○ LOW[2,3]

*Statistically significant result. See Table 5.18 for included studies.
Notes: [1]The same analgesic was used in both groups.
[2]No blinding.
[3]Statistical heterogeneity was substantial.
Abbreviations: CI, confidence interval; MD, mean difference; *n*, number; NRS, numerical rating scale; VAS, visual analogue scale.

CHMs, we selected the meta-analysis pools that showed significant differences in favour of the topical CHM test groups and calculated the frequencies of the individual herbal ingredients included in the CHM interventions. Each study was counted once only.

The most frequently used herbs in the topical CHMs were *bing pian* 冰片, *xi xin* 细辛 and *yan hu suo* 延胡索, followed closely by *chuan wu* 川乌, *mo yao* 没药 and *ru xiang* 乳香 (Table 5.28).

Randomised Controlled Trials of Oral plus Topical Chinese Herbal Medicine

One RCT (H30) combined an oral and a topical CHM. The oral CHM was designed by the authors and called *Ai tong zheng gu fang* 癌痛正骨方 (*sheng huang qi* 生黄芪, *dang gui* 当归, *shu di huang* 熟地黄, *bai zhu* 白术, *bu gu zhi* 补骨脂, *gu sui bu* 骨碎补, *chi shao* 赤芍, *chuan xiong* 川芎, *yan hu suo* 延胡索, *xiang fu* 香附, *san qi* 三七, *ban zhi lian* 半枝莲, *quan chong* 全虫, *sang piao xiao* 桑螵蛸 and *gan cao* 甘草). One packet per day was decocted and divided into two doses.

Table 5.28 Frequently Reported Topical Herbs in Meta-analyses Showing a Favourable Effect for Pain Intensity

No. of Meta-analyses (Studies)	Herbs	Scientific Name[4]	Frequency of Use
2* (14)	*Bing pian* 冰片	*Borneolum*	8
	Xi xin 细辛	*Asarum* species	8
	Yan hu suo 延胡索	*Corydalis yanhusuo* W. T. Wang	6
	Chuan wu 川乌[1]	*Aconitum carmichaelii* Debx.	5
	Mo yao 没药	*Commiphora myrrha* Engl.; *C. molmol* Engl.	5
	Ru xiang 乳香	*Boswellia carterii* Birdw.; *B. bhaw-dajiana* Birdw.	5
	Cao wu 草乌[2]	*Aconitum kusnezoffii* Reichb.	4
	Da huang 大黄[3]	*Rheum palmatum* L.; *R. tanguticum* Maxim. ex Balf.; *R. officinale* Baill.	4
	Ding xiang 丁香	*Eugenia caryophyllata* Thunb.	4
	Quan xie 全蝎	*Buthus martensii* Karsch.	4
	Xue jie 血竭	*Daemonorops draco* Bl.; *Dracaena cochinchinensis* (Lour.) S. C. Chen	4

*Pain intensity: Refer to Tables 5.16 and Table 5.18.

Notes: [1]Two RCTs used *sheng chuan wu* 生川乌.

[2]Two RCTs used *sheng cao wu* 生草乌.

[3]Two RCTs used *sheng da huang* 生大黄.

[4]The use of some herbs may be restricted in some countries. Readers are advised to comply with relevant regulations.

The topical CHM was a cataplasm designed by the hospital called *Yi ai zhi tong gao* 抑癌制痛膏 (*e zhu* 莪术, *san leng* 三棱, *yan hu suo* 延胡索, *ru xiang* 乳香, *mo yao* 没药, *shan ci gu* 山慈菇, *wei ling xian* 威灵仙, *bing pian* 冰片, *chan su* 蟾酥, etc.) which was made into a paste which was applied to the local pain area, once a day and retained for 24 hours.

Both treatments continued for five days followed by a two-day break, and then were repeated. The study was conducted in mainland China. The participants (n = 111) were aged 41 to 69 years and all had bone metastases with moderate or severe pain (4 ≤ NRS ≤ 9). All had the syndrome of *qi* deficiency with blood stasis (*qi xu xue yu* 气虚血瘀) and all received oxycodone HCl extended-release tablets (4 ≤ NRS ≤ 6 started with 5 mg, 7 ≤ NRS ≤ 9 started with 10 mg; once every 12 hours, with the dose adjusted according to the patient's pain relief) for the duration of the study (two weeks).

For sequence generation the risk of bias was judged 'low risk' due to the description of the details of the method used. There was no mention of a method of allocation concealment, so the risk of bias was judged as 'unclear risk'. There was no mention of blinding of participants, personnel or outcome assessors so these domains were all judged as 'high risk' for blinding of participants and personnel and 'unclear risk' for blinding of outcome assessors. Since there were no drop-outs, the study was judged 'low risk' for incomplete outcome data. No protocol could be located but all the outcomes appear to have been reported, so the study was judged 'unclear risk' for selective outcome reporting.

There were no significant differences between groups for NRS scores (MD –0.29 [–0.88, 0.30], n = 111) or QOL (MD –3.36 [–8.72, 2.00], n = 111) based on the NCCN impact of pain measurement, but there was a significantly greater reduction for analgesic maintenance dose in the integrative therapy group (MD –16.26 [–29.70, –2.82] mg/d, n = 111). The study also reported on adverse reactions but did not specify which criteria were used. The results showed there was no significant difference between groups in the incidence of any of the adverse reaction categories (Table 5.29).

Controlled Clinical Trials of Chinese Herbal Medicine

No non-randomised controlled clinical trials of oral CHM, topical CHM or CHM enema were identified.

Table 5.29 Combination Oral plus Topical Chinese Herbal Medicine plus Oxycodone HCl versus Oxycodone HCl: Adverse Reaction

Adverse Reaction[1]	Effect Size RR [95% CI]	Included Studies (*n* Participants)
Nausea and vomiting	0.28 [0.06, 1.29]	H30 (111)
Constipation	0.45 [0.17, 1.20]	
Thirsty	0.25 [0.03, 2.13]	
Dizziness or headache	0.14 [0.01, 2.65]	
Drowsiness and fatigue	0.09 [0.005, 1.58]	
Respiratory depression	Both groups = 0 events	
Others	0.74 [0.17, 3.14]	

Note: [1]The same analgesic was used in both groups.
Abbreviations: CI, confidence interval; *n*, number; RR, relative risk.

Non-controlled Clinical Trials of Chinese Herbal Medicine

Two case-series studies (H31, H32) of oral CHM, one case report (H33) of topical CHM and one case report (H34) of oral plus topical CHM for cancer pain were identified.

One case-series (H32) reported all participants had the syndrome Kidney and *yin* dual deficiency (*shen yin kui xu* 肾阴亏虚) or static blood obstruction (*yu xue zhu zhi* 瘀血阻滞), and one case report (H34) mentioned the syndrome was Blood stasis due to *qi* stagnation (*qi zhi xue yu* 气滞血瘀). All studies were conducted in mainland China. Each study used a different CHM formula.

One study (H31) included 56 people with malignant tumours and moderate or severe pain (VAS ≥ 4) who received morphine sulfate sustained-release tablets (30–60 mg every 12 hours) plus the commercial CHM product *Da huang jiao nang* 大黄胶囊 (2–3 pills/day) orally for seven days. After treatment, the VAS scores in the moderate pain group decreased from 5.3±0.8 to 0.9±1.1, and in the severe pain group the VAS scores decreased from 8.8±1.2 to 1.1±1.3. This study also reported on adverse reactions but did not specify which criteria were used. By the end of treatment the main adverse events were constipation (15 people), abdominal distention (13 people), nausea (11 people) and vomiting (7 people).

In another case-series study (H32), 65 people with malignant tumours and moderate or severe pain (NRS ≥ 4) received oxycodone HCl extended-release tablets (firstly titrated on a short-acting opioid, then converted to oxycodone HCl extended-release tablets taken orally, once every 12 hours) for two weeks and were also given an oral formula designed by the authors called *Yi shen gu kang fang* 益肾骨康方 (*shu di* 熟地, *gu sui bu* 骨碎补, *she she cao* 蛇舌草, *bai zhi lian* 半枝莲, *bai jiang can* 白僵蚕, *shan yao* 山药, *shan yu rou* 山萸肉, *dan pi* 丹皮, *ze xie* 泽泻 and *fu ling* 茯苓), one packet per day decocted and divided into two doses, from the eighth to the 14th day. Compared to the outcome after one week of analgesic treatment, there were additional reductions after two weeks of treatment for NRS scores, analgesic dose and average frequency of breakthrough pain per person per day, and there were improvements in QOL (NCCN impact of pain measurement) and KPS scores.

In one case report (H33), a 59-year-old woman with lung cancer and bone metastases had received Indometacin tablets but this was not effective for pain relief. She received a cataplasm called *Chan su xiao zhong gao* 蟾酥消肿膏 (*chan su* 蟾酥, *xi xin* 细辛, *sheng chuan wu* 生川乌, *qi ye yi zhi hua* 七叶一枝花, *hong hua* 红花, *bing pian* 冰片, etc. — 20 herbs in total) which was applied to the local pain area once per day. After 15 minutes the pain was relieved, and the relief could continue for 24 hours. After two weeks, the pain had almost disappeared.

Another case report (H34) was a 67-year-old man with stage IV lung cancer and bone metastasis-related pain who had the syndrome of Blood stasis due to *qi* stagnation (*qi zhi xue yu* 气滞血瘀). He was treated with oxycodone HCl extended-release tablets (120 mg every 12 hours) but the pain relief was unsatisfactory. He was prescribed the oral formula *Ai tong zheng gu fang* 癌痛正骨方 (*sheng huang qi* 生黄芪, *dang gui* 当归, *shu di huang* 熟地黄, *bai zhu* 白术, *bu gu zhi* 补骨脂, *gu sui bu* 骨碎补, *chi shao* 赤芍, *chuan xiong* 川芎, *yan hu suo* 延胡索, *xiang fu* 香附, *san qi* 三七, *ban zhi lian* 半枝莲, *quan xie* 全蝎, *hai piao xiao* 海螵蛸, *gan cao* 甘草), one packet per day in two doses; plus topical *Yi ai zhi tong gao* 抑癌制痛膏 (*e zhu* 莪术, *san leng* 三棱, *yan hu suo* 延胡索, *ru xiang* 乳香, *mo yao* 没药, *shan ci gu* 山慈菇, *wei ling xian* 威灵仙, *bing pian* 冰片, *chan su* 蟾酥, etc.) made into a paste which was applied to the local pain area, once a day and retained for 24 hours. The treatment was for more than two months. After treatment the pain had been relieved, the symptoms improved, and the oxycodone HCl dose was reduced to 40 mg every 12 hours.

Safety of Chinese Herbal Medicine

In 12 RCTs there was no mention of the safety of the CHMs (oral and/or topical). Ten RCTs stated there were no adverse events (AEs) associated with the CHMs. In eight studies the AEs and/or reasons for drop-outs were stated for the CHM groups. Six (H13, H15, H18, H20, H22, H25) were of topical CHM and two (H2, H12) were of oral CHM. The AEs and reasons for drop-outs in the CHM and control groups are listed in Table 5.30. Except for two studies (H2, H15), the

Table 5.30 Adverse Events and Reasons for Drop-outs in Randomised Controlled Trials of Chinese Herbal Medicine

CHM Group[1]	Without CHM Group	Included Studies
Death (2 dpo); cancerous fever and sweating (1 dpo)[2]	Death (1 dpo); cancerous fever and sweating (1 dpo)	H2
Diarrhoea (1 AE)[2]	NS	H12
Rash (2 AE)[3]	NS	H14
Skin allergy due to the adhesive plaster (1 AE)[3]	NS	H15
Rash and pruritus (2 AEs)[3]	NS	H18
Skin flushing (3 AEs)[3]	NS	H20
Skin flushing (1 AE)[3]	NS	H22
Skin allergy (5 dpo)[3]	NS	H25

Notes: [1]The same conventional analgesic was used in both groups.
[2]Oral CHM.
[3]Topical CHM.
Abbreviations: CHM, Chinese herbal medicine; dpo, drop-out, AE, adverse event but did not drop out; NS, not specified.

AEs in the other six studies were likely due to the CHMs. Overall, there were three serious adverse events (SAEs), all of which were in the same study (H2) which mentioned that these deaths were not related to the CHM or the conventional analgesic.

In the four non-controlled studies, one study (H32) stated there were no AEs associated with the CHMs, and in the others there were no mentions of the safety of the CHMs.

Evidence for Chinese Herbal Medicine Treatments Commonly Used in Clinical Practice

One formula commonly used in clinical practice and included in Chapter 2 is *Chai hu shu gan san* 柴胡疏肝散 (including modified versions). It was also the formula most frequently investigated in the RCTs (see previous sections). It was tested in two RCTs. One RCT (H2) used *Chai hu shu gan san* 柴胡疏肝散 plus fentanyl transdermal system versus placebo plus fentanyl transdermal system for advanced liver cancer patients with NRS ≥ 4. The other RCT (H8) used *Chai hu shu gan san jia wei* 柴胡疏肝散加味 plus morphine sulphate sustained-release tablets versus morphine sulphate sustained-release tablets without a placebo for the CHM in liver cancer patients with 4 ≤ NRS ≤ 6. The results of these two studies are summarised in Table 5.31. The only significant difference between groups was for reduction in analgesic dose.

Yuan hu zhi tong jiao nang 元胡止痛胶囊 is a manufactured medicine mentioned in Chapter 2 as *Yuan hu zhi tong ke li* 元胡止痛颗粒. *Yuan hu zhi tong jiao nang* 元胡止痛胶囊 was investigated in one RCT (H7) for people who had advanced malignant tumours with moderate or severe pain (NRS ≥ 4) and had the syndrome of *qi* deficiency with Blood stasis (*qi zhi xue yu* 气滞血瘀). The results of this study are summarised in Table 5.32. When combined with morphine sulfate sustained-release tablets there was no significant improvement in NRS scores in the integrative group but KPS scores improved. There were improvements in some T-cell subsets and significant reductions in nausea and vomiting, and constipation.

Clinical studies of the other CHMs mentioned in Chapter 2 in participants with cancer pain were not located in the searches.

Table 5.31 ***Chai Hu Shu Gan San*** **柴胡疏肝散 (Including Modified Versions): Results**

Outcome	Comparison	Effect Size [95% CI]	Included Study (*n* Participants), Type
NRS scores	Oral CHM plus FTS versus placebo plus FTS	MD –0.18 [–0.68, 0.32]	H2 (45), RCT
	Oral CHM plus MSRT versus MSRT	MD –0.44 [–0.999, 0.12]	H8 (46), RCT
	Pooled result	MD –0.30 [–0.67, 0.08] 0%	H2, H8 (91)
Analgesic dose (ug/h)	Oral CHM plus FTS versus placebo plus FTS	MD –20.95 [–39.71, –2.19]*	H2 (45), RCT
Analgesic maintenance dose (mg/d)	Oral CHM plus MSRT versus MSRT	MD –2.82 [–9.25, 3.61]	H8 (46), RCT
Quality of life (BPI)		MD 4.48 [–1.05, 10.01]	
	Adverse reaction (criteria NS)		
Nausea and vomiting	Oral CHM plus FTS versus placebo plus FTS	RR 0.52 [0.11, 2.57]	H2 (45), RCT
Constipation		RR 0.94 [0.47, 1.87]	
Dizziness and drowsiness		RR 1.39 [0.35, 5.53]	
Psychiatric symptoms		RR 0.70 [0.13, 3.78]	
Cutaneous reactions		RR 1.57 [0.29, 8.51]	
Dysuria		RR 0.63 [0.17, 2.32]	
Respiratory depression		RR 1.04 [0.24, 4.64]	

*Statistically significant.

Abbreviations: BPI, brief pain inventory; CHM, Chinese herbal medicine; CI, confidence interval; FTS, fentanyl transdermal system; MD, mean difference; MSRT, morphine sulphate sustained-release tablets; *n*, number; NS, not specified; RR, relative risk; ug, microgram; mg, milligram; d, day; h, hour.

Table 5.32 *Yuan Hu Zhi Tong Jiao Nang* 元胡止痛胶囊: Results

Outcome		Comparison	Effect Size [95% CI]	Included Study (*n* Participants), Type
NRS scores		Oral CHM plus morphine sulfate sustained-release tablets versus morphine sulfate sustained-release tablets	MD −0.14 [−0.96, 0.68]	H7 (60), RCT
KPS scores			MD 9.55 [4.06, 15.04]*	
T-cell subsets	CD3+ (%)		MD 7.04 [3.89, 10.18]*	
	CD4+ (%)		MD 2.00 [−0.36, 4.36]	
	CD8+ (%)		MD 0.32 [0.14, 0.50]*	
	CD4+/CD8+		MD 2.42 [0.11, 4.73]*	
	NK (%)		MD 7.04 [3.89, 10.18]*	
Adverse reaction (WHO criteria)	Nausea and vomiting		RR 0.52 [0.33, 0.81]*	
	Constipation		RR 0.52 [0.32, 0.84]*	
	Dizziness and drowsiness		RR 0.75 [0.53, 1.06]	

*Statistically significant.
Abbreviations: CHM, Chinese herbal medicine; CI, confidence interval; KPS, Karnofsky Performance Status; MD, mean difference; *n*, number; NRS, numerical rating scale; RR, relative risk; WHO, World Health Organisation.

Summary of the Clinical Evidence for Chinese Herbal Medicine

This summary covers the key points of Chapter 5 and it is followed by a dot-point summary of all the main pain and QOL-related results found in the chapter.

For orally administered CHMs, most of the evidence was based on 12 RCTs with some supporting data from two case-series studies. In the single RCTs that provided a direct comparison with the nonsteroidal anti-inflammatory drug (NSAID) ibuprofen, the CHM was less effective at relieving pain but there were also fewer adverse reactions.

Two blinded studies combined a CHM with an opioid. In one study, the combination showed no significant improvement in pain reduction while the other study showed a significant reduction, but the pooled result showed no significant reduction in pain when the CHMs were combined with opioids (Table 5.3). The GRADE assessment was 'moderate' (Table 5.10).

A further five RCTs used the same comparison but without blinding. In the pooled result there was a significantly greater reduction in pain in the group that used CHMs combined with conventional analgesic medications (mainly opioids) but the result was heterogeneous (Table 5.5). This was likely due to variations in the cancer types, drugs used and the different CHMs. When only studies that included bone metastasis were included, there was still an improvement in the combined therapy group and the statistical heterogeneity was reduced (Table 5.5). The GRADE assessment was 'very low' (Table 5.11).

Besides effects on pain, the pooled data from four oral RCTs found a significant improvement in KPS scores (Table 5.6). The two case-series studies (H31, H32) also reported improvements in pain when CHMs were combined with opioids.

In two RCTs the comparison was with calcium carbonate and vitamin D3 tablets for aromatase inhibitor-associated musculoskeletal symptoms (AIMSS). The pooled result found a significantly greater reduction in VAS for the oral CHM groups.

Only one oral CHM was used in two separate RCTs. This was *Chai hu shu gan san* 柴胡疏肝散 in combination with opioids. The pooled result showed no significant benefit for adding the CHM to the opioid therapy for pain (Table 5.12), but one study reported a reduction in analgesic dose.

Topically applied CHMs were used in 17 RCTs and one case study. One RCT (H13) compared a topical CHM with placebo in mild pain and found a significant reduction in pain in the CHM group. An open-label RCT (H14) compared a topical CHM with the opioid tramadol in mild to moderate pain and found no differences in measures of pain but the topical CHM showed faster onset in analgesia.

Topical CHMs were combined with conventional analgesic medications in three blinded RCTs. The pooled results found reduced pain in the combination therapy groups (Table 5.16). The GRADE assessment was 'moderate' (Table 5.26).

In a further 11 RCTs the same comparison was used but without blinding. The pooled result found a greater reduction in pain in the groups that used topical CHMs plus conventional analgesic medications, but the heterogeneity was considerable (Table 5.18). When only the seven studies of moderate to severe pain were included, the heterogeneity was reduced and a significant reduction in pain remained. The GRADE assessment was 'low' (Table 5.27). There was also improvement in the pooled result for analgesic onset time (Table 5.19) which was likely due to the relatively longer time required for opioids to induce analgesia. Moreover, the pooled results for the combination of topical CHMs with opioids showed increased duration of analgesia (Table 5.20) and reduction in the analgesic maintenance dose (Table 5.21). The single case report found pain relief following the use of a cataplasm that contained *chan su* 蟾酥 (H33).

For measures of QOL, the RCTs found combining a topical CHM with conventional analgesic medications produced significantly greater improvements in the pooled results for QLQ-C30 (Table 5.22) but not for the Chinese QOL scale (Table 5.23), but both showed heterogeneity. There was significant improvement in KPS but heterogeneity was considerable (Table 5.24).

In the single RCT (H30) of oral plus topical CHMs in combination with an opioid, there was no improvement in pain intensity but there was a greater reduction in analgesic maintenance dose. The case report (H34) found improvement in pain and reduction in medication dose.

Discussion of Main Results

When interpreting the data, it is important to note that the search only included studies in which all the enrolled participants had pain due to the cancer or the cancer treatment at the beginning of the study. We did not include studies in which pain was due to the surgery, since post-surgical pain can occur in many diseases, and pain can be due to other causes, mixed causes or unclear causes. Nevertheless, the exact cause of pain can be difficult to determine, so it is possible that some of the people included in the studies may have had pain that appeared due to the cancer but may have had a mixed etiology. When pain was one component of a broader QOL measure, this outcome was excluded since QOL scales were not considered specific measures of pain intensity. However, QOL outcomes were assessed for the included studies.

Overall, it seems reasonable to conclude that most, if not all, participants were experiencing cancer pain at baseline, so the changes in the pain scores and other outcomes reflected the relative effects, specific and non-specific, of the interventions. In the studies of oral CHM combined with conventional analgesics, the reduction in pain intensity was not significant in the placebo-controlled studies but it was significant in the unblinded studies. This may have been induced by non-specific effects due to lack of blinding. However, the direction of the effect was the same in both meta-analysis pools while the size of the placebo-controlled pool was smaller.

Regarding the safety of the interventions, only 12 of the 30 RCTs mentioned safety. Analysis of drop-outs suggested that some of the topical CHMs produced skin reactions that led to drop-outs, but there was a lack of comparative data for the control groups so statistical assessment was not feasible (Table 5.30). A few studies mentioned adverse reactions associated with pain medications and there were some improvements in pooled rates of constipation, and nausea and vomiting (Table 5.25). Overall, the safety data were too scarce for complete assessments to be made.

Summary of Results of Randomised Clinical Trials for Main Clinical Outcomes

The available evidence on CHMs used in the management of cancer pain was analysed above in three main categories:

- Oral CHM (12 RCTs, 0 CCT, two non-controlled studies);
- Topical CHM (17 RCTs, 0 CCT, one non-controlled study); and

- Oral plus topical CHM (one RCT, 0 CCT, one non-controlled study).

The following summary includes the main results of the RCTs on CHM for cancer pain. These are based on the findings of significance tests between groups at the end of the treatment period for each of the comparisons and for the main clinical outcome measures reported within each comparison. Adverse reactions and safety are not included here. For further details see the relevant sections of this chapter.

Oral Chinese Herbal Medicine

Oral Chinese herbal medicines were investigated in 12 RCTs (757 participants). The results are summarised under the following comparisons.

Oral CHM versus conventional analgesic (one RCT)

- Less effect than ibuprofen on VAS for pain (one RCT, $n = 119$);
- Less effect than ibuprofen for analgesic onset time (one RCT, $n = 119$).

Oral CHM plus conventional analgesic versus placebo plus conventional analgesic (two RCTs)

- No difference in NRS scores for pain (two RCTs, $n = 145$);
- No difference in frequency of breakthrough pain (one RCT, $n = 100$);
- Reduction in average dose of opioid medication (one RCT, $n = 45$);
- Reduction in total analgesic dose (one RCT, $n = 100$).

Oral CHM plus conventional analgesic versus conventional analgesic (five RCTs)

- Reduction in NRS scores for pain (five RCTs, $n = 244$) but the heterogeneity was substantial;
- No difference in analgesic onset time (one RCT, $n = 65$);
- Reduction in the average frequency of breakthrough pain per person (one RCT, $n = 40$);

- Reduction in the maintenance dose of analgesic medication (two RCTs, *n* = 106);
- Reduction in total analgesic dose in people with moderate pain but not severe pain (one RCT, *n* = 40);
- Improvement on Chinese QOL scale (one RCT, *n* = 38);
- No difference on brief pain inventory (BPI) (one RCT, *n* = 46);
- Improvement on KPS (four RCTs, *n* = 198) but the heterogeneity was substantial.

Oral CHM plus conventional analgesic plus zoledronic acid versus conventional analgesic plus zoledronic acid (one RCT)

- Reduction in NRS scores for pain (one RCT, *n* = 50);
- Improvement on KPS (one RCT, *n* = 50).

Oral CHM versus calcium carbonate and vitamin D3 tablets (two RCTs)

- Reduction in VAS for pain due to aromatase inhibitors (two RCTs, *n* = 112), no heterogeneity.

Oral CHM versus lactulose oral solution (one RCT)

- No difference in NRS scores for pain (one RCT, *n* = 66);
- Reduction in the Cleveland Clinic Constipation Score (CCS) (one RCT, *n* = 66).

Topical Chinese Herbal Medicine

Topical Chinese herbal medicines were investigated in 17 RCTs (1,370 participants). The results for each comparison are summarised below.

Topical CHM versus placebo (one RCT)

- Reduction in NRS for pain (one RCT, *n* = 140).

Topical CHM versus conventional analgesic (one RCT)

- No difference in NRS for pain (one RCT, $n = 260$);
- No difference in duration of analgesia (one RCT, $n = 260$);
- Reduction in analgesic onset time (one RCT, $n = 260$).

Topical CHM plus conventional analgesic versus placebo plus conventional analgesic (three RCTs)

- Reduction in NRS for pain (three RCTs, $n = 217$), with moderate heterogeneity;
- No reduction in analgesic onset time (one RCT, $n = 80$);
- Reduction in the average frequency of breakthrough pain per person (one RCT, $n = 77$);
- No difference in the analgesic maintenance dose (one RCT, $n = 77$);
- Reduction in total analgesic dose (one RCT, $n = 80$);
- Reduction in the average analgesic dose per day (one RCT, $n = 60$);
- Improvement in QOL using the NCCN impact of pain measurement (one RCT, $n = 77$);
- No difference on KPS (two RCTs, $n = 137$), without heterogeneity.

Topical CHM plus conventional analgesic versus conventional analgesic (11 RCTs)

- Reduction in NRS or VAS for pain (11 RCTs, $n = 675$), with considerable heterogeneity;
- Reduction in analgesic onset time (two RCTs, $n = 111$), without heterogeneity;
- No difference for average frequency of breakthrough pain per person per day (one RCT, $n = 61$);
- Reduction in average frequency of breakthrough pain per person per week (one RCT, $n = 100$);
- Increase in the duration of analgesia (two RCTs, $n = 111$), without heterogeneity;
- Reduction in the analgesic maintenance dose (three RCTs, $n = 150$), without heterogeneity;

- No difference in total analgesic dose (one RCT, $n = 61$);
- Reduction in the average analgesic dose per day (one RCT, $n = 100$);
- Improvement in QOL on QLQ-C30 (three RCT, $n = 185$), with substantial heterogeneity;
- No difference on Chinese QOL scale (four RCTs, $n = 254$), with considerable heterogeneity;
- No difference on NCCN impact of pain measurement (one RCT, $n = 61$);
- Improvement on KPS (seven RCT, $n = 428$), with considerable heterogeneity.

Topical CHM plus conventional analgesic plus pamidronate disodium versus analgesic plus pamidronate disodium (one RCT)

- No difference in NRS for pain (one RCT, $n = 60$);
- Improvement in KPS (one RCT, $n = 60$).

Oral plus Topical Chinese Herbal Medicine

Combination of oral plus topical CHM plus oxycodone HCl extended-release tablets versus oxycodone HCl extended-release tablets (one RCT):

- No difference in NRS for pain (one RCT, $n = 111$);
- Reduction in analgesic maintenance dose (one RCT, $n = 111$);
- No difference on NCCN impact of pain measurement (one RCT, $n = 111$).

References

1. Chinese Pharmacopoeia Commission. (2015) *Zhong Hua Ren Min Gong He Guo Yao Dian* [*Pharmacopoeia of the People's Republic of China*]. China Medical Science Press, Beijing.
2. Jiangsu New Medical Academy, ed. (1986) *Zhong Yao Da Ci Dian* [*Great Compendium of Chinese Medicines*]. Shanghai Scientific and Technical Publishers, Shanghai.

3. 段凯男, 马文华, 孟茂斌, 冯敏, 张瑞明. (2009) 中药配合三阶梯止痛治疗癌痛随机对照试验的 meta 分析. 华西医学 **24(1):** 9–13.
4. 王庆全. (2010) 中药复方治疗癌性疼痛的系统评价及用药规律分析. 新疆医科大学: 新疆医科大学.
5. Lee JW, Lee WB, Kim W, *et al.* (2015) Traditional herbal medicine for cancer pain: A systematic review and meta-analysis. *Complement Ther Med* **23(2):** 265–274.
6. 杜志华, 王菊勇, 董昌盛, 王青, 王方圆. (2015) 中西医结合治疗癌痛临床疗效及安全性 meta 分析. 辽宁中医杂志 **42(12):** 2290–2296.
7. 吴驻林, 谭婉君, 连宝涛, 彭立生. (2016) 中药外敷联合三阶梯止痛法治疗癌性疼痛的系统评价. 辽宁中医杂志 **43(9):** 1816–1821.
8. Yan X, Yan Z, Liu W, *et al.* (2016) External application of traditional Chinese medicine in the treatment of bone cancer pain: A meta-analysis. *Support Care Cancer* **24(1):** 11–17.
9. 孙燕. 内科肿瘤学. (2001) 北京: 人民卫生出版社 pp. 996–997.
10. Cleeland CS. (2009) Brief pain inventory: User guide. Available from: www.mdanderson.org/education-and-research/departments-programs-and-labs/departments-and-divisions/symptom-research/symptom-assessment-tools/BPI_UserGuide.pdf.
11. Wang XS, Mendoza TR, Gao SZ, Cleeland CS. (1996) The Chinese version of the brief pain inventory (BPI-C): Its development and use in a study of cancer pain. *Pain* **67(2–3):** 407–416.
12. Shih DQ, Kwan LY. (2007) All roads lead to Rome: Update on Rome iii criteria and new treatment options. *Gastroenterol Rep* **1(2):** 56–65.
13. Agachan F, Chen T, Pfeifer J, *et al.* (1996) A constipation scoring system to simplify evaluation and management of constipated patients. *Dis Colon Rectum* **39(6):** 681–685.
14. National Comprehensive Cancer Network. (2018) Clinical practice guidelines in oncology: Adult cancer pain, version 1. Available from: www.nccn.org.
15. Aaronson NK, Ahmedzai S, Bergman B, *et al.* (1993) The European Organization for Research and Treatment of Cancer QLQ-C30: A quality-of-life instrument for use in international clinical trials in oncology. *J Natl Cancer Inst* **85(5):** 365–376.

References to Included Studies

Study Number	Reference
H1	陈琦, 吴芸. (2015) 肿痛安治疗癌症放射治疗后颞下颌关节疼痛的疗效评价. 国际口腔医学杂志 **42(1):** 24–27.
H2	吴敏华, 周月芬, 陈旭烽, 朱月娇, 谢艳茹, 涂建飞. (2013) 柴胡疏肝散辅助芬太尼透皮贴治疗肝癌疼痛. 中西医结合肝病杂志 **23(2):** 83–85.
H3	宋洪丽, 殷玉琨, 周磊, 冯利. (2018) 益肾骨康方联合盐酸羟考酮缓释片治疗中重度癌性躯体痛肾虚血瘀证患者随机对照双盲临床研究. 中医杂志 **59(15):** 1300–1303.
H4	黄敏. (2007) 益气化瘀法配合美施康定治疗中重度癌性疼痛的临床研究. 学位论文. 南京中医药大学 13–21.
H5	李伟锋. (2016) 加减清骨散治疗阴虚内热型骨转移癌痛的临床研究. 学位论文. 广州中医药大学 20–28.
H6	宋程. (2016) 补肾活血方治疗骨转移癌痛临床疗效及镇痛机制研究. 学位论文. 湖南中医药大学 2–10.
H7	王卫华, 周小伟. (2012) 活血行气化瘀法治疗癌性疼痛疗效分析. 山东中医杂志 **31(10):** 725–727.
H8	阿依宝塔·努腊勒木. (2018) 柴胡疏肝散加味治疗肝癌肝郁气滞型癌痛的临床研究. 学位论文. 新疆医科大学 5–13.
H9	白平, 陈皎皎, 胡陵静, 张国铎. (2017) 独活补骨方联合唑来膦酸治疗恶性肿瘤骨转移的临床观察. 南京中医药大学学报 **33(5):** 133–135.
H10	赵炜, 关念波, 周蕴明, 张美英. (2018) 强骨止痛方治疗芳香化酶抑制剂所致乳腺癌骨丢失性疼痛. 中国中西医结合外科杂志 **24(1):** 15–20.
H11	钟莹, 郭智涛, 黄映飞, 梁喆盈, 吴玢. (2017) 补肾强筋胶囊治疗乳腺癌芳香化酶抑制剂相关骨关节症状的临床观察. 中医药导报 **23(8):** 38, 39, 43.
H12	张翔, 李和根, 顾芳红. (2016) 养阴理气汤治疗阿片性便秘的临床研究. 山东中医杂志 **35(2):** 104–107.
H13	冯丽红. (2012) 双柏散外敷为主治疗肝癌轻度癌痛的疗效观察. 学位论文. 广州中医药大学 10–24.
H14	张莹. (2004) 化坚拔毒膜对癌性疼痛的干预作用及其机理研究. 学位论文. 天津中医学院 253–267.
H15	唐倩. (2013) 冰虫止痛膏外用辅助治疗局部癌性疼痛的临床研究. 学位论文. 北京中医药大学 53–70.

(*Continued*)

(*Continued*)

Study Number	Reference
H16	王院春, 王希胜, 李仁廷, 惠建荣. (2014) 乌香痛消膏外治癌性疼痛 40 例. 山东中医杂志 **33(3):** 188–189.
H17	宋琳, 蒋益兰, 王容容. (2017) 消痞镇痛膏外敷联合奥施康定片治疗肺癌重度疼痛30例临床观察. 中医杂志 **58(21):** 1846–1849.
H18	丁致熏. (2015) 消积止痛贴联合美施康定治疗中重度癌痛的临床研究. 学位论文. 湖北中医药大学 10–22.
H19	黄逸姣. (2013) 消症止痛膏联合羟考酮控释片对中重度癌性疼痛的临床研究. 学位论文. 南京中医药大学 16–30.
H20	李成银, 罗秀丽, 王琦苑, 邹顺霞, 赵井苓. (2016) 见肿消巴布剂治疗癌性疼痛的临床研究. 湖北中医药大学学报 **18(3):** 87–89.
H21	李高杨. (2006) 中药镇痛 I 号外用辅助三阶梯止痛方案治疗中重度癌痛的疗效研究. 学位论文. 广州中医药大学 13–20.
H22	刘峥峥. (2017) 双柏散外敷治疗肝癌轻度癌痛的临床疗效评价. 中国现代药物应用 **11(3):** 177–179.
H23	田娇. (2015) 骨痛贴外用治疗阴寒凝滞型癌性躯体痛的临床观察. 学位论文. 北京中医药大学 31–49.
H24	王于真, 李妍妍, 魏征. (2016) 癌痛消外用贴治疗卵巢癌疼痛 60 例临床观察. 中国民间疗法 **24(8):** 29–30.
H25	许蕾. (2013) 中药五生酊外用治疗癌性疼痛临床疗效观察. 学位论文. 广州中医药大学 12–18.
H26	赵玮璿. (2016) 中药止痛散脐敷治疗癌性疼痛的临床研究. 学位论文. 北京中医药大学 27–38.
H27	钟星. (2009) 奇正消痛贴联合美施康定治疗癌性疼痛的临床研究. 学位论文. 北京中医药大学 20–29.
H28	车瑾, 徐洋, 曹蔚, 洪帆, 秦婷婷. (2018) 鞘内注射阿片类药物联合自拟中药穴位贴敷对中重度癌性疼痛、睡眠和生活质量的影响. 现代中西医结合杂志 **27(18):** 1949–1953.
H29	刘平庄. (2015) 跌打膏外敷联合帕米磷酸二钠治疗骨转移疼痛的临床研究. 实用中西医结合临床 **15(1):** 31–32.
H30	苏新平, 邓天好, 谭达全. (2016) 中医内外兼治气虚血瘀型骨转移癌痛 56 例临床观察. 中医药导报 **22(1):** 33–35.
H31	张志芳, 张浩. (2007) 美施康定合大黄胶囊治疗中重度癌性疼痛 56 例. 湖南中医杂志 **23(1):** 43, 46.

(*Continued*)

Study Number	Reference
H32	周磊. (2015) 益肾骨康方缓解癌性躯体痛的临床研究. 学位论文. 中国中医科学院 39–50.
H33	刘嘉湘, 郁诗玲, 徐振晔, 施志明. (1985) 蟾酥消肿膏治疗晚期恶性肿瘤疼痛 187 例疗效观察. 辽宁中医杂志 **4:** 30–31.
H34	邓天好. (2016) 中药内服外用治疗骨转移癌痛的经验. 广西中医药 **39(2):** 57–59.

6

Pharmacological Actions of the Common Herbs

OVERVIEW

This section reviews the available experimental evidence for the 11 Chinese herbs most frequently used in the formulas that showed reductions in cancer pain when tested in the randomised controlled clinical trials included in Chapter 5. Their biological activities of relevance to pain are summarised and discussed.

Introduction

Chinese herbal formulas exert their actions in cancer pain via the constituent compounds contained in the formula ingredients. To investigate the effects of specific herbs on pain and their mechanisms of action, experimental studies using *in vitro* and/or *in vivo* models have been conducted using whole extracts of herbs, fractions and/or purified components of the herbs.

The meta-analyses of the results of randomised clinical trials (RCTs) in Chapter 5 indicated that the addition of topical Chinese herbal medicine (CHM) to conventional cancer pain management produced significant reductions in pain intensity (Table 5.16, Table 5.18) but the results were less clear for the orally administered CHMs (Table 5.3, Table 5.5). Therefore, the herbs selected for this chapter were the most frequently used herbs in the topical preparations: *bing pian* 冰片, *xi xin* 细辛, *yan hu suo* 延胡索, *da huang* 大黄, *chuan wu* 川乌, *cao wu* 草乌, *mo yao* 没药, *ru xiang* 乳香, *ding xiang* 丁香, *quan xie* 全蝎 and *xue jie* 血竭 (Table 5.14). Of these, *yan hu suo* 延胡索 was also used frequently in orally administered formulas. Since both *chuan wu* 川乌 and *cao wu* 草乌 are from *Aconitum* species, these were combined.

Searches were conducted in PubMed for each of the 11 herbs to identify studies relevant to their actions on pain, hyperalgesia and related symptoms, and any studies of the herbs used in conjunction with opioids. Search terms included the scientific names for the herb and its principal compounds. Where required, search results were limited by the addition of pain-related terms such nociception, analgesia and hyperalgesia. Included studies could relate to any type of pain, not just cancer pain, and were mainly *in vivo* studies, but clinical studies of herbs, extracts or compounds were also included. Since the herbs were administered topically, studies relating to their effects on barrier function were included.

Bing Pian 冰片

Bing pian 冰片 is also called *long nao* 龙脑. The pharmaceutical name is Borneolum (PPRC) and it is commonly known as borneol. The traditional source of natural *bing pian* 冰片 (*tian ran bing pian* 天然冰片) is the tropical tree *Dryobalanops aromatica* Gaertn. [synonym: *Dryobalanops sumatrensis* (J. F. Gmel.) Kosterm.] but other sources include *Blumea balsamifera* (L.) DC. and *Cinnamomum camphora* (L.) Presl.[1,2] Borneol can be synthesised from turpentine or camphor; synthetic *bing pian* 冰片 is known as *he cheng long nao* 合成龙脑 and the pharmaceutical name is Borneolum Syntheticum.[1]

Synthetic borneol derived from the reduction of (±)-camphor is mainly composed of (–)-borneol, (+)-borneol, (+)-isoborneol and (–)-isoborneol. Semi-synthetic borneol from natural (+)-camphor is mainly (–)-isoborneol and (+)-borneol. Natural borneol from *Dryobalanops aromatica* mainly contains (+)-borneol plus other compounds whereas natural borneol from *Blumea balsamifera* contains mainly (–)-borneol plus other compounds. Natural borneols do not contain substantial amounts of isoborneol.[2–4]

Effects on Pain

In a series of mouse models of inflammation and pain, intraperitoneal (i.p.) injection of borneol reduced acetic acid-induced writhing; reduced pain due to injection of formalin in the hind paw (which produces both acute and chronic inflammatory responses); and increased latency in a hot plate test. There were no effects in the rotarod and grip strength tests indicating borneol did not produce a sedative effect.[5]

The excitatory transient receptor potential ankyrin 1 (TRPA1) ion channel is involved in acute nociception and inflammatory pain. In a cell-based screen of camphor analogues, borneol was a stronger antagonist of human TRPA1 than camphor.[6] In a mouse model of neuropathic pain induced by intrathecal injection of oxaliplatin which produced mechanical hyperalgesia and cold hyperalgesia, (+)-borneol dose-dependently increased the paw withdrawal threshold. Its actions involved blocking the TRPA1 channels.[7] In mice with chronic neuropathic pain due to segmental spinal nerve ligation, the paw withdrawal threshold to mechanical stimulus was increased by systemic and local administration of (+)-borneol. In inflammatory pain induced by complete Freund's adjuvant (CFA), (+)-borneol increased paw withdrawal threshold. It had no effect on motor function in a rotarod test.[8]

In *Xenopus* oocytes stimulated by mustard oil, d-(+)-borneol blocked TRPA1 activity and the effect was greater than for camphor. In cultured mouse trigeminal neurons, it blocked activation by nicotine but there were resistant subpopulations of neurons.[9] In frog sciatic nerves, the effects of various aromatics on compound action potentials (CAPs) were assessed. CAP amplitude was concentration-dependently reduced by (+)-borneol and (–)-borneol at similar concentrations.[10]

In mice subjected to capsaicin injection into the hind paw, the pre-application of topical 25% borneol reduced lifting and licking responses. In formalin-induced pain, dose-dependent analgesia was evident and in a CFA-induced hyperalgesia model, 15% borneol reduced both mechanical and thermal hyperalgesia. It was proposed that the analgesic effect was mediated via transient receptor potential melastatin-8 (TRPM8) receptors in sensory neurons. This receptor is also activated by menthol.[11,12] A placebo-controlled clinical study of postoperative patients reported that a single topical application of 25% borneol for approximately 30–60 minutes reduced postoperative pain based on VAS.[12]

Skin and Blood Brain Barrier Permeation Effects

Transdermal delivery of drugs is inhibited by the barrier function of the stratum corneum, so substances that improve skin permeation are added to enhance drug delivery. A study of the effects of borneol and menthol on the permeation of ligustrazine (LTZ), an active compound from *Ligusticum chuanxiong* Hort., employed Franz diffusion cell experiments using the abdominal skin of rats to study the *in vitro* permeation-enhancing effects of borneol and menthol at different concentrations. In previous experiments, borneol had shown greater permeation-enhancing effects on the hydrophilic drug 5-fluorouracil[13] whereas menthol was stronger for the hydrophobic drug osthole,[14] although borneol showed enhanced permeation of osthole at higher temperatures.[15] For ligustrazine, both borneol and menthol enhanced penetration but the effects were related to concentration and they showed some differences in mechanism of action. While both permeated the lipid layer, menthol was more effective at lower concentrations, but at higher concentrations borneol also induced the lipid layer to form transient water channels which enhanced penetration of ligustrazine.[16] In a comparison with the standard skin penetration enhancer laurocapram (Azone®), borneol showed low skin irritation potential and promoted penetration of 5-fluorouracil, antipyrine, aspirin, salicylic acid and ibuprofen.[17]

The blood-brain barrier (BBB) is another membrane that is a major obstacle in drug delivery. Traditionally, *bing pian* is an 'orifice opening' herb that affects the brain.[2] Orally administered borneol is absorbed rapidly into the brain and its co-administration with a number of drugs has enhanced drug transportation and bioavailability.

Its mechanisms of action appear to be via efflux protein function, transmembrane tight-junction proteins and vasodilatory neurotransmitters.[18] One study in rats found borneol could decrease the expression of the tight junction protein Zonula occludens-1 (ZO-1) and increase expression of adenosine receptors.[19] In a study in rats, intragastric administration of borneol in corn oil enhanced the penetration of the dye Evans blue through the BBB; however, the mechanism appeared to be via increasing the expression of intercellular cell adhesion molecule-1 (ICAM-1), rather than effects on tight-junction proteins such as occludin.[20] A review of *in vivo* studies found 58 studies of various drugs, including anti-neoplastic drugs, which generally found improved drug delivery when the drugs were combined with borneol.[21]

Xi Xin 细辛

The herb *xi xin* 细辛 consists of the roots and rhizomes of certain *Asarum* species. The pharmaceutical name is Asari Radix et Rhizoma. It is officially sourced from *Asarum heterotropoides* Fr. Schmidt var. *mandshuricum* (Maxim) Kitag. (*bei xi xin* 北细辛), *Asarum sieboldii* Miq. var. *seoulense* Nakai (*han cheng xi xin* 汉城细辛) and *Asarum sieboldii* Miq. (*hua xi xin* 华细辛), but many other *Asarum* species are used regionally.[1,2,22] The leaves should not be used and non-official *Asarum* species can contain toxic constituents including aristolochic acids.[2,23,24]

Many compounds have been identified in the roots of *Asarum* species and these vary according to the species. In the volatile oils of *Asarum heterotropoides* var. *mandshuricum* and *Asarum sieboldii* var. *seoulense* the following main components have been reported at 3% in at least one of these two species: alpha and beta-pinene, 3-carene, eucalyptol, eucarvone, alpha-terpineol, 3,5-dimethoxytoluene, safrole, methyl eugenol (3-4-5-trimethoxytoluene), 2,3,5-trimethoxytoluene, croweacin, pentadecane, 1-pentadecene, asaricin; and the following have been reported at 1% to less than 3%: camphene, sabinene, alpha-phellandrene, p-cymene, limonene, borneol, estragole, alpha-guaiene.[25] Other compounds have also been reported.[2]

Effects on Pain

A 70% methanol extract of *Asarum sieboldii* roots was administered to rats intraperitoneally in a series of assessments of its antinociceptive and anti-inflammatory actions. In the tail flick test and acetic acid-induced writhing, the extract showed dose-dependent antinociceptive effects which were inhibited by pre-administration of naloxone. In carrageenan-induced paw oedema the extract showed anti-inflammatory actions.[26] When a powdered aqueous *Asarum* extract was orally administered to mice, there was no effect in the tail flick, tail pressure, or hot plate tests of nociception. In hind paw formalin injection, there was no effect in the first phase but the extract significantly reduced behaviours in the second phase. It also reduced the nociceptive behaviours induced by intrathecal injection of N-methyl-d-aspartic acid (NMDA). The result suggested that the peripheral antinociceptive actions may be mediated by NMDA receptors.[27]

Methyl Eugenol

Methyl eugenol is a major component of *xi xin* 细辛. In mouse models of formalin-induced and NMDA-induced pain, oral administration of methyl eugenol inhibited licking and biting behaviours in the second but not the first phase. It also reduced NMDA-induced pain-related behaviours. These effects were inhibited by the GABA-A antagonist bicuculline. Methyl eugenol showed no effect on cyclooxygenase (COX-1, COX-2) activity, suggesting the analgesic effects were via GABA-A receptors and not via reduction of inflammation.[28] A whole-cell patch clamp technique using transfected Chinese hamster ovary (CHO) cells that transiently express the human peripheral sodium (Nav1.7) channel isoform found that methyl eugenol inhibited peripheral sodium (Na+) channels, which may account for the antinociceptive and anaesthetic effects.[29]

Yan Hu Suo 延胡索

The herb *yan hu suo* 延胡索 (also called *yuan hu* 元胡) is sourced from the rhizomes of *Corydalis yanhusuo* W.T. Wang. Its pharmaceutical name is Corydalis Rhizoma.[1,2] Major constituents of the roots are the alkaloids tetrahydrocolumbamine, glaucine, d,l-tetrahydropalmatine, corydaline, palmatine, berberine, epiberberine, tetrahydroberberine, dehydrocorydaline, L-corydalmine, canadine, fumaricine, columbamine, dehydrocorybulbine, protopine, alpha-allocryptopine, allocryptopin, coptisine, tetrahydrocoptisine, jatrorrhizine, and others.[2,30–33]

Effects on Pain

In a cold pressor test in healthy humans, a single dose of an extract of *Corydalis yanhusuo* (*yan hu suo* 延胡索) plus *Angelica dahurica* (*bai zhi* 白芷) reduced pain in a placebo-controlled RCT.[34] An extract of total alkaloids was found to significantly inhibit pain-related behaviours in rats induced by the formalin test at both the early and late phase. Of the compounds, protopine, glaucine, tetrahydropalmatine and corydaline had all crossed the BBB and were identified in the striatum.[30] Of the alkaloids from *yan hu suo* 延胡索, tetrahydroprotoberberine and levo-tetrahydropalmatine (l-THP) have received considerable research attention as analgesics and as treatments for opioid addiction.[35,36]

A water extract of *Corydalis yanhusuo* 延胡索 which contained the alkaloids levo-tetrahydropalmatine and dehydrocorybulbine (DHCB) was tested in a series of models of nociception in mice at dosages that showed no sedative effects on the rotarod. In the formalin paw assay, mice showed responses in both the early phase and late phase which were reduced by the extract. Similar effects were found in the tail flick assay, in a model of mechanical allodynia tested with von Frey filaments and in a model of thermal hyperalgesia in a hot box test. Further experiments suggested that the analgesic effects in acute and neuropathic pain were at least partially mediated by dopamine D2 receptors.[37]

Levo-tetrahydropalmatine

In a mouse model of mechanical hyperalgesia induced by oxaliplatin, i.p. injection of l-THP reduced responses to von Frey filaments dose dependently. This anti-hyperalgesic effect was significantly attenuated by administration of the selective dopamine D1 receptor antagonist SCH23390.[38] The effects of l-THP were tested in a spinal nerve ligation-induced model of neuropathic pain in mice. At ten days post-surgery, mechanical hypersensitivity was dose-dependently reduced by l-THP (i.p.). In inflammatory pain induced by CFA, l-THP reduced mechanical hypersensitivity. It had no effect on the rotarod test. The selective dopamine D1 receptor antagonist SCH23390, blocked the anti-hyperalgesic effects suggesting involvement of dopamine D1 receptors.[39]

A series of blinded experiments assessed the effects of l-THP on mouse models of pain. Intraperitoneal administration prior to hind paw formalin injection did not affect the first phase but showed a dose-dependent reduction in the second phase of nociceptive responses. There was a reduction in mechanical allodynia induced by direct activation of sigma-1 (Sig-1) receptor which was blocked by the Sig-1R antagonist BD1047. In neuropathic pain induced by ligation of the common sciatic nerve, mechanical allodynia, assessed via von Frey filaments, was reduced and there was improvement in the CatWalk Automated Gait Analysis. These antinociceptive effects of l-THP were not affected by naloxone and there was no motor impairment on the rotarod. Further tests suggested that these antinociceptive effects were primarily mediated by Sig-1R activation in the spinal cord.[40] When whole-cell patch-clamp and voltage-clamp recordings were conducted using dorsal root ganglion neurons from rats to determine the effects of l-THP on acid-sensing ion channels (ASICs), it was found to inhibit functional activity suggesting a possible mechanism for its peripheral analgesic actions.[41]

A model of bone cancer pain was induced in rats by injecting Walker 256 rat mammary gland carcinoma cells into the right tibia intramedullary space. Intragastric administration of l-THP showed dose-dependent reductions in thermal hyperalgesia (hot plate test) and mechanical allodynia (electronic von Frey). In the rat L4–L5 spinal cord, repeated administration of l-THP attenuated model-induced increases in TNF-alpha and IL-18 but did not reduce IL-1beta.

There were significant reductions in activated microglial cells in the spinal cord but no changes in astrocyte activation.[42]

Dehydrocorybulbine

Dehydrocorybulbine showed dose-dependent antinociceptive activity in the tail flick assay in mice without showing sedative effects on the rotarod and can penetrate the BBB. Like l-THP, DHCB showed antagonism at dopamine receptors and its analgesic effects were not antagonized by naloxone. The selective dopamine 1 receptor agonist SKF-38393 did not block the effect of DHCB but the selective dopamine 2 receptor agonist quinpirole significantly reduced the antinociceptive effects of DHCB. Moreover, in dopamine 2 receptor knockout mice, DHCB did not show antinociceptive effects, suggesting its effect in acute pain was via dopamine 2 receptors. In the formalin test, DHCB showed effects on behaviours at both the early phase (acute pain) and late phase (inflammatory pain). In neuropathic pain induced by spinal nerve ligation, it reduced sensitivity to von Frey filaments and reduced thermal sensitivity in a hot box test. Repeated applications of DHCB did not induce tolerance.[43]

Levo-corydalmine

A rat model of bone cancer pain was induced by tibia bone cavity implantation of Walker 256 mammary gland carcinoma cells, which produced mechanical hypersensitivity. After 14 days experimenter-blind tests of mechanical nociception were conducted on rat feet using von Frey filaments. Following intrathecal injections of different concentrations of levo-corydalmine (l-CDL), there were increased paw withdrawal thresholds in a dose-related manner from day 14 to day 20 without tolerance and resistance. Further tests in spinal neurons suggested the mechanism of action involved inhibition of NMDA and group I metabotropic glutamate (mGlu1/5) receptors.[44]

In a model of tumour compression-induced pain in mice, S180 sarcoma cells were injected close to the sciatic nerve. Palpable masses were evident by day 6. Levo-corydalmine, levo-tetrahydropalmatine and the combination of oxycodone and acetaminophen (positive control) were administered intragastrically from day 6 to day 14. Paw latency in a hot box test was decreased and responses to mechanical stimulation with von Frey filaments were reduced in the active treatment groups compared to negative controls. In mouse spinal cords there was decreased expression of TNF-alpha mRNA and IL-1beta mRNA in the active groups, and tumour-induced activation of spinal microglia and astrocytes were reduced. In cell cultures of primary mouse astrocytes, l-CDL reduced the protein and mRNA expression of CC chemokine ligand 2 (CCL2) and chemotactic cytokine receptor 2 (CCR2), suggesting that the reductions in pain and hypersensitivity involved regulation of proinflammatory cytokines.[45]

In a mouse model of vincristine-induced neuropathic pain, intragastric l-CDL reduced mechanical allodynia tested with von Frey filaments and reduced heat sensitivity in the tail flick test. In mouse spinal cord, upregulation of chemokine (C-X-C motif) ligand 1 (CXCL1) and NFkB activation due to vincristine treatment were attenuated by l-CDL.[46]

Dehydrocorydaline

The alkaloid dehydrocorydaline (DHC) showed dose-dependent reductions in acetic acid-induced writhing in mice. In the formalin paw test, DHC showed the greatest reductions in phase 2 and only showed an effect in phase 1 at the highest dose. Naloxone abolished the phase 1 effect and reduced but did not prevent effects at phase 2. There were no significant effects on locomotor activity or any adverse effects on behaviour, body weight or physical appearance.[47]

In a mouse model of bone cancer pain induced by right femoral implantation with osteosarcoma NCTC 2472 cells, DHC or vehicle control was administrated intraperitoneally on day 14 after surgery. All tests of nociception were experimenter blind. Pain was assessed by the number of spontaneous flinches of the right hind paw in a two-minute interval, and assessment of mechanical allodynia used von Frey filaments. Measures of pain increased following implantation but were significantly reduced at one and four hours following DHC administration compared to control. In the spinal cord, DHC reduced elevated levels of IL-1beta and IL-10 and shifted microglial polarization toward the M2 phenotype, suggesting reductions in proinflammatory responses.[48]

Da Huang 大黄

Th official sources of *da huang* 大黄 are the roots and rhizomes of the following species of rhubarb: *Rheum palmatum* L. (*zhang ye da huang* 掌叶大黄); *Rheum tanguticum* Maxim. ex Balf. (*tang gu te da huang* 唐古特大黄) and *Rheum officinale* Baill. (*yao you da huang* 药用大黄). The pharmaceutical name is Rhei Radix et Rhizoma.[1,2]

A large number of compounds have been identified including the anthraquinones emodin, aloe-emodin, chrysophanol, physcion, sennidin, palmidin, rhein and rheidin; and their glycosides including sennosides A-F; phenylbutanone glycosides including lindleyin and isolindleyin; and tannins including gallic acid, catechin, epicatechin, epicatechin-gallate, and others.[2,49]

Effects on Pain

A number of compounds found in *da huang* 大黄 and their metabolites have been studied in animal models and some have been tested in clinical trials.

Emodin

In primary cultures of rat dorsal root ganglia (DRG) neurons, neuronal cells were isolated and the effects of emodin on the pain-associated ion channel TRPV1 were assessed. At concentrations of emodin that did not affect cell viability, the mRNA expression of TRPV1 was downregulated and emodin downregulated increases in intracellular calcium evoked by capsaicin. However, this effect was not blocked by pre-treatment of the neurons with the TRPV1 antagonist capsazepine (CPZ), suggesting the effect may be via a non-TRPV1 channel pathway.[50]

A rat model of neuropathic pain was induced by chronic constriction injury (CCI) to the sciatic nerve. Emodin or vehicle (control) was injected intraperitoneally once a day for two weeks. Mechanical hyperalgesia threshold was assessed using von Frey filaments and thermal hyperalgesia was assessed by a hot box method. Reductions in thermal hyperalgesia were evident from day 3 in the emodin-treated group compared to vehicle alone and mechanical hyperalgesia showed significant reductions from day 7. In neurons from the DRG of vertebrae L4–L5 at day 14, immunohistochemistry showed reduced expression of the P2X2 and 2X3 receptors in the emodin group compared to control. *In situ* hybridisation showed reduced P2X2 and P2X3 mRNA expression in the emodin group. These results suggested that emodin downregulated the level of P2X2/3 mRNA, thereby decreasing the expression P2X2/3 protein leading to reduction in DRG primary afferent transmission and reduction in pain.[51]

The antinociceptive effects of emodin, encapsulated in nanoparticles to improve targeting and bioavailability, were assessed in a rat model of type 2 diabetes with diabetic peripheral neuropathy that was induced by streptozocin and a high-calorie diet. Assessments were blinded. Paw withdrawal threshold in response to stimulation using von Frey filaments was increased in the emodin injection group compared to control, suggesting an increase in the mechanical hyperalgesia threshold. The increased response latency to thermal stimulus indicated elevated threshold for thermal hyperalgesia in the nano-emodin injection group. Analysis of DRG from L4–L5 rat vertebrae showed lower expression levels of the P2X3 receptor at the protein and mRNA levels and lower expression levels of the receptor TNF-R1, which is activated by TNF-alpha. This suggests that the action of emodin may be via inhibition of excitatory transmission in DRG neurons which is mediated by P2X3 receptors.[52]

Rhein and Diacerein

Diacerein is transformed to its active metabolite rhein during absorption. In an ascetic acid-induced model of visceral pain in mice, diacerein showed antinociceptive effects when administered by multiple routes (i.p., intragastric, supraspinally, spinally or peripherally).[53] In a rat model of knee joint inflammation and pain induced by CFA, diacerein inhibited mechanical and thermal hypersensitivity, vocalization, spontaneous pain score and joint swelling. In spinal cords, astroglial activation was inhibited, as were increases in MMP-9 and TRPV1 expression.[54]

A large open-label study (7,923 participants) of osteoarthritis of the knee conducted in India found that 12 weeks of treatment with diacerein improved pain scores on a visual analogue scale (VAS) with good tolerance of the medication.[55] In a single blind RCT of adults with early symptomatic osteoarthritis of the knee, diacerein significantly reduced pain scores on VAS and scores on the Western Ontario and McMaster Universities Osteoarthritis Index (WOMAC) compared to placebo.[56] The European Society for Clinical and Economic Aspects of Osteoporosis and Osteoarthritis (ESCEO) found an acceptable benefit-risk balance for diacerein in the symptomatic treatment of hip and knee osteoarthritis despite its association with soft stools and diarrhoea.[57]

Gallic Acid

The polyphenolic compound gallic acid is present in many plants including rhubarb. Gallic acid and its derivatives have been investigated for analgesic activity.[58] In a series of mouse models of pain, orally administered gallic acid reduced the following: pain responses following injection of TRPA1 agonists; paw oedema and mechanical allodynia; inflammatory pain and oedema induced by carrageenan; mechanical allodynia and cold allodynia induced by CCI of the sciatic nerve; and an assay of mouse spinal cord synaptosomes that indicated activity via TRPA1. The researchers concluded that gallic acid was a TRPA1 antagonist.[59]

Catechin and Epicatechin

In arthritis induced by CFA in rats, the intragastric administration of catechin improved scores on the polyarthritis index and pain in a foot bend test. There were also reductions in TNF-alpha, interleukin-1 and prostaglandin E2 (PGE2), suggesting an anti-inflammatory effect.[60] In the glutamate model of nociception in mice, (–) epicatechin reduced pain behaviours without impairing motor activity. The effect was abolished by pre-administration of naloxone (an opioid antagonist), glibenclamide (a potassium channel antagonist), yoimbina (an alpha 2 receptor antagonist), pindolol (a beta-adrenergic and serotonergic (5HT1) antagonist) and atropine (a muscarinic antagonist), suggesting involvement of multiple pathways in this model.[61]

In rats with diabetes induced by streptozotocin and pain induced by the formalin test, pre-treatment with epicatechin (i.p.) significantly prevented nociceptive behaviours in the second phase with a lesser effect in the first phase. This effect was reduced by serotonergic (5-HT) receptor antagonists but not by naloxone.[62] In addition, there have been numerous studies of the related compound epigallocatechin-3-gallate (which is not found in rhubarb) in models of nociception.[63]

Rutin and Quercetin

The flavonoid rutin is found in numerous plants including rhubarb. When rutin enters the blood stream it is converted to quercetin.[64] The effects of rutin and quercetin on pain have long been known[65] and the antinociceptive activity of extracts of several plants has been attributed to rutin.[66–68]

In a mouse model, painful neuropathy was induced by oxaliplatin injection into the hind paws resulting in reductions in the mechanical and cold nociceptive thresholds up to the 49th day. Both rutin and quercetin reduced tail withdrawal from cold water and increased paw withdrawal threshold in response to electronic von Frey. In dorsal horn neurons, rutin and quercetin reduced the oxaliplatin-induced increases in neuronal cell atrophy and increase in the number of glial cells. In paw skin, oedema of conjunctive tissue was reduced. Both flavonoids inhibited iNOS expression in the dorsal horn region, suggesting protective effects against oxaliplatin neurotoxicity via their antioxidant actions.[64] Mice were treated with oxaliplatin i.p. to produce mechanical allodynia and hepatic steatosis; and rutin, resveratrol, quercetin and a quercetin nanoemulsion (NQT) were administered daily by gavage. The mechanical hyperalgesia threshold measured using von Frey filaments was improved by all four interventions and there were reductions in liver weight and other features of hepatic steatosis.[69]

In a model of acute pancreatitis induced by l-arginine injections, the mice developed abdominal hyperalgesia. Administration of rutin reduced response to an electronic von Frey device and improved measures of acute pancreatitis. The authors interpreted the results as due to reductions in the oxidative stress induced by l-arginine.[70]

The effects of rutin were investigated in a model of diabetic neuropathy in rats injected with streptozotocin to induce diabetes. Rutin, the non-steroidal anti-inflammatory drug (NSAID) nimesulide, and a combination of the two were administered i.p. and pain was assessed at weeks 4 to 8 using models of mechanical allodynia, cold allodynia, mechanical hyperalgesia and thermal hyperalgesia. All treatment groups showed improvement with greater reductions in pain in the combination group.[71] In a similar model, rats developed hyperglycaemia, cognitive dysfunction and hyperalgesia. Administration of rutin by oral gavage for 30 days from onset of hyperglycaemia decreased nociception in the formalin test at both phase 1 and phase 2 compared to vehicle control, and there were improvements in learning acquisition and memory retention.[72]

The effects of rutin, tramadol or morphine, administered alone or in combination with naltrexone were tested in rats after systemic i.p. administration and intracerebral administration via cannula to the periaqueductal grey (PAG). In the formalin test, rutin and tramadol showed significant antinociceptive effect in both phases and naltrexone blocked these effects of rutin. Administration via cannula to the PAG produced antinociceptive effects in both phases for rutin and morphine. Naltrexone did not modify the phase 1 effect of rutin but abolished the phase 2 effect. The results suggest that the effect of rutin involves partial opioidergic participation but it also acts via a non-opioidergic mechanism.[68]

Chuan Wu 川乌 and Cao Wu 草乌

Chuan wu 川乌, and its prepared forms *zhi chuan wu* 制川乌 and *fu zi* 附子 which have lower toxicity, are sourced from the roots of *Aconitum carmichaelii* Debx. The pharmaceutical name of the prepared root is Aconiti Radix Cocta. The related herb *cao wu* 草乌, and its prepared form *zhi cao wu* 制草乌, is sourced from the roots of *Aconitum kusnezoffii* Reichb. The pharmaceutical name of the prepared root is Aconiti Kusnezoffii Radix Cocta.[1,2]

The major constituents of these aconitum species are the alkaloids aconitine, hypaconitine, songorine, mesaconitine, benzoylmesaconine, neoline, karakoline, fuziline, aconine, 14-benzoylaconine, talati samine, chasmanine and higenamine.[2,73,74]

Effects on Pain

Aconitum species have been used for multiple conditions including pain in Asia, India and Europe but the roots are highly toxic and require careful processing to render them suitable for medicinal use.[75,76]

The effects of oral administration of unprocessed and three processed extracts of the root of *Aconitum carmichaeli* were assessed in the tail flick test in mice and rats. The median lethal dose (LD50) was from seven to 14 times greater in the unprocessed herb compared to the processed forms which had reduced aconitine content. In rats, all extracts showed longer tail flick latencies with the strongest effect from the unprocessed extract. These effects were reduced by naloxone. In opioid mu-receptor knockout mice latencies were reduced compared to wild-type mice.[77]

A placebo-controlled study investigated the effects of an extract of processed *Aconitum carmichaeli* (TJ-3022) in rats following ligation of the common sciatic nerve. In models of mechanical allodynia and thermal hyperalgesia, the orally administered extract increased paw withdrawal thresholds dose dependently. The effects were reversed by the selective kappa-opioid receptor antagonist, nor-BNI, but not by naloxone.[78] In the same model of sciatic nerve ligation in mice, oral administration of another extract of processed *Aconitum* (TJ-3023 — *bushi/fu zi* 附子) showed reductions in tests of mechanical and thermal hyperalgesia, and this effect continued after administration ceased. In the spinal cord, the extract inhibited activation of astrocytes in the dorsal horn in the late maintenance phase of pain.[79]

Processed *Aconitum carmichaeli* mother root (*zhi chuan wu* 制川乌) extract was tested in mouse models of CFA-induced chronic inflammatory pain. The extract reduced mechanical hypersensitivity without showing drug tolerance; did not affect baseline thresholds in normal mice; and did not impair motor activity. Similar antinociceptive effects were found for hypersensitivity to heat in a hot plate test. These effects were reversed by nor-BNI, suggesting involvement of kappa-opioid receptors. The antinociceptive effects of the extract were also reduced in TRPV1 –/– knockout mice suggesting the effects were via inhibition of the TRPV1 ion channel in the spinal cord.[80]

In a mouse model of peripheral neuropathic pain induced by oxaliplatin, a boiled water extract of *zhi chuan wu* 制川乌 and a number of fractions of this extract were tested for effects on mechanical hyperalgesia and cold hyperalgesia in response to acetone. Oral administration of the extract significantly increased the paw withdrawal threshold to von Frey filaments and reduced response to acetone. In DRG neurons, the oxaliplatin produced cytotoxicity and inhibited neurite elongation. The extract prevented inhibition of neurite elongation in DRG neurons in a concentration-dependent manner and the fractions that showed this effect contained neoline. It did not produce sedation. Moreover, neoline showed significant effects in the mouse models of mechanical hyperalgesia and cold hyperalgesia.[81]

In mice with acetic acid-induced abdominal pain, pre-administration of the aconitum alkaloids napelline, songorine, hypaconitine, mesaconitine and 12-epinapelline N-oxide all reduced the onset of pain and the number of writhings, with hypaconitine showing the greatest activity. In a similar model in which abdominal cramps were induced by acetylcholine hydrochloride, the results were similar with songorine and hypaconitine showing the greatest latencies to pain onset and reductions in the numbers of cramps. In inflammatory arthritis induced by injection of Freund's complete adjuvant, pain was induced by passive bending of the joint. Napelline, 12-epinapelline N-oxide, and hypaconitine showed the greatest analgesic effects. The effects of these alkaloids were cancelled by naloxone injection suggesting the involvement of opioid receptors.[82] In carrageenan-induced acute inflammation and oedema, the preventative effect was greatest for napelline and hypaconitine but for the alleviation of inflammation one hour following injection, 12-epinapelline N-oxide and mesaconitine showed the greatest effects, while songarine showed similar effects on prevention and alleviation. Unlike NSAIDs, none of the alkaloids damaged the gastrointestinal tract.[83] A review of the effects of songarine noted its antiarrhythmic, antianxietic, antinociceptive, anti-inflammatory and wound healing properties.[84]

Effects on Morphine Tolerance

In mice, the repeated administration of morphine injections produced analgesic tolerance, as measured in a tail pressure test. Oral administration of processed aconitum (TJ-3022 — *fu zi* 附子) at doses below those required to have antinociceptive effects dose-dependently attenuated morphine tolerance. There was no acute antinociceptive interaction between processed aconitum and morphine. The effect was mainly due to mesaconitine but the total extract was more effective.[85] The effect appeared to be mediated by kappa-opioid receptors.[86] At doses that produce analgesic effects, the combination of processed aconitum and morphine reduced the antinociceptive effects of morphine in the tail pressure and tail flick tests in morphine-naïve mice in the short term. However, with longer term administration the effects of morphine were potentiated due to attenuation of morphine tolerance.[87]

Mo Yao 没药

The medicinal substance *mo yao* 没药 is an aromatic resin called myrrh which exudes from trees of some species in the genus

Commiphora in response to injury of the bark and sapwood. The pharmaceutical name is Myrrha.[1] The official sources are *Commiphora myrrha* Engl. and *Commiphora molmol* Engl.[1] These names are given as synonyms in some sources.[2] The species *Commiphora gileadensis* (L.) C. Chr, [synonym *Balsamodendron ehrenbergianum* O. Berg] is also given as a source of *mo yao* 没药.[2,22] Myrrh from *Commiphora mukul* (Hook. ex Stocks) Engl [synonym: *Commiphora wightii* (Arnott) Bhandari; *Balsamodendron mukul* (Hook. ex Stocks)] are not official sources of *mo yao* 没药.

The phytochemistry of myrrh is complex and appears to vary considerably between and within species.[88–90] Major constituents of the resin include alpha, beta and gamma commiphoric acids; commiphorinic acid; alpha and beta heerabomyrrhol; heeraboresene; and commiferin.[2,22] Components of the essential oil include furanoeudesma-1,3-diene, curzerene, lindestrene, germacrone, dihydrolinderalactone, acetoxy-furanodiene, eugenol, pinene, limonene, heerabolene, cinnamic aldehyde, cumin aldehyde and m-cresol.[2,22,91–93]

Effects on Pain

Myrrh has long been used for the relief of pain and for the management of other disorders in the Middle East, Europe and Asia.[89,91,94,95] When powdered commercial myrrh was administered to mice it increased latency to paw licking in a hot plate test. Fractionation identified the analgesic effects as due to a fraction that contained the sesquiterpenes furanoeudesma-1,3-diene (over 90%), curzerene and furanodiene. Of these compounds, furanoeudesma-1,3-diene and curzerene showed significant antinociceptive activity while furanodiene did not. Furanoeudesma-1,3-diene (i.p) reduced acetic acid-induced writhing. Its analgesic effects were reversed by naloxone in both models, suggesting effects via central opioid pathways.[91]

In humans, an extract of *Commiphora myrrha,* which was rich in the furanodienes, curzerene, furanoeudesma-1,3-diene and lindestrene, was tested for its effects on various types of (non-cancer) pain in a placebo-controlled RCT. Oral administration reduced headache, fever-related headache and muscular pain, joint pain, muscle aches, lower back pain and menstrual cramps, with dose-related effects for some symptoms.[92]

When *mo yao* 没药, identified as resin from *Commiphora myrrha,* was extracted using different solvents and tested for anti-inflammatory and analgesic activity in mice, the petroleum ether and ethanol extracts showed the most significant reductions in formalin-induced paw oedema and were associated with reduced prostaglandin E2 (PGE2) levels. Acid-induced writhing was significantly reduced by both extracts but there was no effect in the hot plate test.[96] It is notable that the analysis of the *mo yao* 没药 reported different compounds to the above studies.[91,92] The same research group tested water extracts of *mo yao* 没药, *ru xiang* 乳香 (see below), and a combination of *mo yao* 没药 plus *ru xiang* 乳香. For the water extract of *mo yao* 没药, in mice it inhibited formalin-induced paw edema and carrageenan-induced paw oedema; reduced levels of PGE2 and nitric oxide; and reduced writhing in oxytocin-induced dysmenorrhea.[97]

A 90% ethanol extract of Somali myrrh, identified as deriving from *C. molmol,* was concentrated and orally administered to mice at three dosage levels. In a hot plate test, the extract dose-dependently increased response latency. In acetic acid-induced writhing, the number of abdominal writhings was reduced by the two higher doses. Hind paw formalin-induced oedema was significantly reduced by the two higher dosages at 3 to 12 hours. In addition, the extract reduced body weight and serum lipids in obese mice.[98]

Germacrone

The sesquiterpene germacrone is present in *Commiphora myrrha* [93] and other plants. A study of the effects of extracts of *Curcuma aeruginosa* Roxb in mouse models of inflammation and nociception, found the fraction that contained germacrone reduced oedema induced by carrageenin and reduced writhes induced by acetic acid, suggesting anti-inflammatory and analgesic effects.[99] Another study that aimed to isolate the main antinociceptive compound from the methanol extract of *Curcuma aeruginosa,* identified germacrone as showing activity against acetic acid-induced writhing in mice, suggesting peripheral antinociceptive activity. In formalin-induced licking, germacrone showed inhibition of early-phase and late-phase licking, suggesting both central and peripheral antinociceptive actions.[100]

Ru Xiang 乳香

Ru xiang 乳香 is an aromatic resin which is derived from the sap of trees in the genus *Boswellia* which grow in desert regions in the Middle East and north-eastern Africa. It is commonly called frankincense or olibanum. In the pharmacy it is called Gummi Olibanum or Olibanum.[1] The official sources of *ru xiang* 乳香 are *Boswellia carterii* Birdw. and *Boswellia bhaw-dajiana* Birdw. [synonym: *B. sacra* Flueck.].[1] Other *materia medica* books also list *B. neglecta* S. Moore as a source.[2,22] Another major commercial species is *Boswellia serrata* Roxb. ex Colebr. which is called Indian frankincense.[101]

Major components of the resin are boswellic acids and their derivatives alpha-boswellic acid, 0-acetyl-alpha-boswellic acid, beta-boswellic acid, 0-acetyl- beta-boswellic acid, 11-keto-b-boswellic acid (KBA) and 3-acetyl-11-keto-β-boswellic acid (AKBA); olobanorecene; dihydroroburic acid; epilupeol acetate; tirucallol and its derivatives 3-oxo-tirucallic acid, 3-acetoxy-tirucallic acid and 3-hydroxy-tirucallic acid; and incensole acetate.[2,22,102,103] Major volatiles in *Boswellia carterii* include alpha-pinene, beta-myrcene, limonene and beta-carophyllene.[104] There are considerable differences in the constituents of different *Boswellia* species but boswellic acids are typical of the genus and *Boswellia serrata* contains multiple boswellic acids including KBA and AKBA.[101,105,106]

Effects on Pain

Frankincense has had a wide range of applications since ancient times, including the relief of inflammation and pain.[105] In Chinese medicine (CM) it is often combined with *mo yao* 没药 for the alleviation of pain.[2]

Water extracts of *ru xiang* 乳香, *mo yao* 没药 and the combination of the two extracts were tested in mouse models of inflammation and pain. All three extracts inhibited formalin-induced paw oedema and inhibited PGE2 production. Carrageenan-induced paw oedema was reduced by all three extracts at three hours post-injection but earlier effects (one and two hours) were only evident for the myrrh extract and the combined extract. In an oxytocin-induced dysmenorrhea model, writhing was most markedly reduced by CWE which the authors interpreted as indicating that the combination of *mo yao* 没药 plus *ru xiang* 乳香 had a superior analgesic effect.[97] A water extract of equal weights of frankincense and myrrh administered to mice by intragastric gavage reduced sensitivity to heat in a tail flick test and alleviated capsaicin-induced licking and biting. In a mouse model of neuropathic pain due to CCI, high and low doses of the extract resulted in improvements in mouse responses to mechanical allodynia and thermal hypersensitivity. When the effects on transient receptor potential vanilloid 1 (TRPV1) was investigated, there were decreases in the percentage of TRPV1 immunoreactive neurons in the DRG of L4–L5 and S1–S3. In isolated DRG neurons, WFM reduced response to capsaicin.[107]

In mice with 12-O-tetradecanoylphorbol-13-acetate (TPA)-induced ear inflammation, a range of triterpene acids (notably boswellic acids) and other compounds from *Boswellia carteri* resin showed marked anti-inflammatory activity.[108] An acetone extract of *Boswellia carteri* resin was tested in a CFA model of persistent, inflammatory pain in rats using a randomised blinded design. Intragastric administration of three dosage levels of the extract was used but the highest dose level was terminated due to adverse effects. The other two doses showed reductions in hind paw thermal hyperalgesia and oedema. Fos protein (c-Fos) expression induced by CFA in dorsal horn neurons was lower in the extract-treated groups.[109] When a medium level dose of the same extract was tested in a randomised trial of a rat model of polyarthritis induced by CFA, the extract significantly reduced arthritis score and paw oedema. There were also significant reductions in TNF-alpha and IL-1beta in local tissue samples.[110]

Topical Application

In order to overcome the unwanted gastrointestinal effects of the oral administration of frankincense and boswellic acids, microemulsions of a bioactive fraction rich in AKBA were developed for transdermal delivery. Permeation of rat skin by AKBA was in the range of 30% to 97% for the different preparations and skin irritancy was low. In carrageenan-induced rat paw oedema the small globule-sized microemulsion showed the greatest reduction in oedema.[103] A study of the topical application of frankincense oil or a water extract in mice showed no effect for the water extract but the oil reduced xylene-induced ear oedema and formalin-induced hind paw oedema, and increased pain threshold. Of the constituents of the oil, alpha-pinene, linalool and 1-octanol all improved the anti-inflammatory and analgesic effects.[111]

Clinical Studies

In a registry study, people with symptomatic knee osteoarthritis received a standardised Boswellia extract in addition to standard care or standard care alone for four weeks. The combined group showed greater improvements in pain, stiffness and physical functions, greater walking distance, and normal blood test results.[112] In a subsequent study, an extract containing 90% boswellic acid, 20% curcumin and 0.8% valeric acid was used in conjunction with best standard management for four weeks resulting in greater improvement in pain-free walking distance and less use of rescue medication.[113] For acute knee pain and inflammation in healthy rugby players, a *Boswellia serrata* extract improved local pain and pain-free walking.[114] In a double-blind RCT, 201 patients with osteoarthritis of the knee received (1) a preparation containing boswellic acids and curcuminoids; (2) a preparation containing curcuminoids; or (3) a placebo for three months. Physical performance and joint pain improved within both active preparations and boswellic acids, plus curcuminoids was superior to placebo.[115] In a registry study of ankle sprain due to sports injury in 72 cases, an extract containing boswellic acids derived from *B. serrata* in addition to usual management showed improvements in pain after three and seven days of treatment.[116]

A meta-analysis of four placebo-controlled RCTs of *Boswellia* preparations found significant improvement in pain and function without serious adverse events,[117] and a meta-analysis of various dietary supplements for osteoarthritis found clinically important short-term effects for pain reduction for *Boswellia* extracts.[118]

Ding Xiang 丁香

Ding xiang 丁香 is sourced from the flower buds of *Eugenia caryophyllata* Thunb. which is also called *Syzygium aromaticum* (L.) Merrill & Perry. The common name is clove and the pharmaceutical name is Caryophylli Flos.[1,2]

The main component of the oil from the flower buds is eugenol (50–80%), eugenyl acetate/acetyl eugenol (2–20%), beta-caryophyllene (3.5–35%), alpha-humulene (1–3%) and a large number of minor components.[2,119]

Effects on Pain

Clove oil has long been used topically to relieve pain and produce analgesia, especially in dental procedures where its constituent eugenol continues to be in use. It also has antibacterial, antiviral and antitumour activities.[120,121]

In a single blind study in adult volunteers, a gel preparation of clove oil administered to the buccal mucosa produced reductions in pain assessed by VAS that were equivalent to benzocaine 20% gel, suggesting its possible use as a topical dental anaesthetic.[122]

In the tail flick and formalin tests in mice, i.p. administration of clove oil reduced formalin-induced pain in both phases at the highest dose but only showed effects in the second phase at lower doses. A similar result was found in the tail flick test and the effect was reversed by naloxone. In addition, clove oil reduced scopolamine-induced impairment in learning and memory in a maze test.[123]

In mice, i.p. pre-injection of a preparation of clove oil reduced acetic acid-induced writhing, increased response latencies in a hot plate test, and reduced carrageenan-induced paw oedema, indicating antinociceptive and anti-inflammatory effects.[124] A similar effect was found for an ethanol extract with dose-dependent reductions in pain behaviours in the acetic acid and formalin tests.[125]

In a rat model of acute corneal pain induced by NaCl, subcutaneous administration of an essential oil of cloves reduced eye-wiping responses and a reduction in mechanical sensation induced by von Frey filaments. In addition, topical administration of clove produced a local anaesthetic effect and a similar effect was obtained for eugenol. The antinociceptive effects induced by cloves were inhibited by pre-administration of naloxone and atropine, suggesting mediation via opioidergic and cholinergic systems.[126]

Eugenol

In a model of osteoarthritis in rats induced by monoiodoacetate, administration of low- or high-dose eugenol by gavage improved gait in the CatWalk test in the high-dose condition. For tests of mechanical allodynia using von Frey filaments there was a small reduction in the low-dose group and a significant improvement in the high-dose group. No toxic effects were evident. The eugenol did not improve joint histology, suggesting that its effects were analgesic.[127]

In mice with acetic acid-induced writhing, pre-treatment with eugenol orally produced a dose-dependent reduction in abdominal constrictions. In glutamate-induced paw pain, eugenol produced dose-dependent reductions. Pre-treatment with naloxone prevented the effects on eugenol. In an open field test, the highest dose of eugenol affected locomotor activity but not the lower therapeutic doses.[128] In a similar model in mice, oral eugenol dose-dependently attenuated the acetic acid-induced writhing and reduced pain behaviours in the formalin test in the second phase only. Administration of opioidergic receptor antagonists reduced the analgesic effects of eugenol but a serotonergic receptor antagonist had no effect.[129]

An assessment of the anaesthetic activity of eugenol in rats when administered by injection showed dose-dependent, reversible anaesthetic activities.[130] In a model of neuropathic pain in rats induced by sciatic nerve ligation, repeated administration of eugenol by gavage gradually reduced thermal sensitivity over the five days of treatment but there were no significant differences between groups in mechanical sensitivity assessed using Frey filaments. Eugenol concentration in blood and plasma peaked rapidly after oral administration and persisted through the experiment.[131] In the same model, intrathecal injections of eugenol reduced responses to thermal hyperalgesia and mechanical allodynia. There was no toxicity to eugenol and a pharmacodynamic study showed that eugenol penetrated the CNS of rats and showed a preferential distribution in the spinal cord.[132]

Studies of the mechanisms of action of eugenol have suggested that its nociceptive functions are mediated by GABA-A receptors[133] and/or TRPA1.[134]

Effects on Skin Permeation

A study investigated the effects of clove oil on the enhancement of skin penetration by ibuprofen, which has poor skin permeation. In rabbit abdominal skin a gel containing clove oil and ibuprofen significantly enhanced permeation. In live rabbits the plasma concentrations of ibuprofen following topical delivery were higher for ibuprofen plus clove oil and ibuprofen plus Azone compared with ibuprofen, but there was no significant difference between the clove and Azone groups.[135] In a comparison of five essential oils as penetration enhancers for the transdermal delivery of ibuprofen in a rat skin model, the most effective was *chuan xiong* oil followed closely by clove oil.[136] A similar study also found *chuan xiong* oil to have the best penetration enhancement effects for ibuprofen, but clove oil was also effective.[137]

Quan Xie 全蝎

Quan xie 全蝎 is the whole body of the scorpion *Buthus martensii* Karsch. The pharmaceutical name is Scorpio.[1,2]

The main active components are peptides from the venom of *Buthus martensii* (BmK) including BmK antitumour-analgesic peptide (BmK AGAP);[138–144] BmK AGAP-SYPU2,[145] BmK AGP-SYPU1;[146] anti-neuroexcitation peptide (ANEP);[147] BmK AS;[148,149] BmK9;[150] BmK AngM1;[151,152] BmK IT2;[153,154] BmK IT-AP;[155,156] BmK dITAP3;[157] and BmK AngP1.[158]

Other components include multiple amino acids and organic acids as well as other compounds including trimethylamine, betaine, hydroxylamine, picrate, cholesterol, lecithin and taurin.[2]

Effects on Pain

Although *Buthus martensii* (BmK) is not severely toxic to humans, a large number of insect toxins (IT) have been isolated from the venom.[156,159]

One of the first of the toxins to show analgesic effects in mammals was BmK insect toxin-analgesic peptide (BmK IT-AP). In mice, pre-administration reduced acetic acid-induced writhing without neurotoxicity.[156] Its crystal structure has been determined.[155] Using the same methods, another two peptides (dITAP3 and BmK AngP1) were isolated and both showed analgesic effects without toxicity in the acetic acid model in mice.[157,158]

In the formalin pain model, rats received a different peptide BmK IT2 prior to, or after, formalin injection and their behaviour was evaluated. Pre-treatment significantly inhibited the number of flinches at both the first and second phase. Post-treatment produced a similar but lesser result.[153] It also suppressed carrageenan-evoked thermal hyperalgesia, and suppressed formalin-induced spinal c-Fos expression in L4–L5 segments.[154]

Another peptide, BmK AngM1, showed dose-dependent inhibition in the acetic acid test in mice without toxicity. Whole-cell patch clamp recordings of rat hippocampal pyramidal neurones showed inhibition on voltage-dependent Na^+ current and voltage-dependent delayed rectifier K^+ current.[151,152]

For the peptide BmK9, a series of site-specific mutants were developed to explore their effects on nociception. The peptide and all mutants at position 54 (Ser54) showed inhibition in the acetic acid model but the effect was reduced in some mutants suggesting a functional role for Ser54 in its antinociceptive effects.[150] In another study, the acetic acid model was used to guide separation and identify another peptide with analgesic effects, BmK AGP-SYPU1.[146]

Pre-injection (i.p.) of the peptide BmK AS inhibited acetic acid-induced writhing in mice and injection into the tail vein reduced responses in a hot plate test. The effects were dose dependent.[148] In the formalin test in rats, intrathecal pre-injection of BmK AS dose-dependently reduced nociceptive behaviours in both phases without impairment in motor function. In rat spinal cords at L4–L5, formalin-induced c-Fos expression was suppressed.[149]

A study of anti-neuroexcitation peptide (ANEP), which showed inhibition in the acetic acid model in mice, molecular dynamics simulations of mouse sodium channel 1.7 (mNav1.7) suggested its activity may be via binding to this voltage-gated sodium channel.[147]

Of the peptides isolated so far, perhaps the most studied is BmK antitumour-analgesic peptide (BmK AGAP). It showed significant reductions in acetic-acid induced writhings in mice and inhibited responses in a hot plate test. It also showed antitumour activity.[141] An investigation of mutant forms enabled location of the domain responsible for its analgesic activity.[142] In the formalin test in mice, pre-injection of BmK AGAP decreased pain-related behaviours at both phases dose-dependently. In the spinal cord at L4–L5, the expression of the activated MAPKs (p-JNK p-ERK, p-p38) were downregulated and BmK AGAP inhibited the formalin-induced expression of Fos protein in the dorsal horn.[143] In a mouse model of CCI-induced neuropathic pain, intrathecal injection of BmK AGAP inhibited thermal hyperalgesia due to radiant heat, and mechanical allodynia measured using von Frey filaments. In mouse spinal cord, BmK AGAP significantly attenuated the CCI-induced increases in expression of spinal Fos protein and phosphorylated MAPKs (p-JNK p-ERK, p-p38), suggesting the inhibition of neuropathic and inflammation-associated pain was via a MAPK-mediated mechanism.[144] In a related study, a new peptide with analgesic and antitumour activities, BmK AGAP-SYPU2, was identified by bioassay-driven chromatographic purification. It showed inhibition in the acetic acid and hot plate tests in mice and had long-lasting effects when compared with morphine.[145]

Xue Jie 血竭

Xue jie 血竭, which is commonly called dragon's blood, is a red resin or latex derived from the sap of certain species of tree which is secreted in response to tissue damage.[160] Various types of dragon's blood are used in Europe, the Middle East, Africa, Asia and the Americas. In Europe, the Middle East and Africa the main sources are *Dracaena cinnabari* Balf. f. and *Dracaena draco* (L.) L. In Asia, *Daemonorops draco* (Willd.) Blume and a number of *Dracaena* species are used. In the West Indies *Pterocarpus draco* L. is used and *Croton* species are used in Mexico, Central and South America.[161] In traditional medicine it is known as Sanguis Draxonis.

Daemonorops draco is listed in the Chinese pharmacopoeia as the official source of *xue jie* 血竭.[1] However, three source species are given in *Zhong Hua Ben Cao* 中华本草: *Daemonorops draco* (Willd.) Blume (*qi lin jie* 麒麟竭), *Dracaena cochinchinensis* (Lour.) S.C. Chen (*jian ye long xue shu* 剑叶龙血树) and *Dracaena angustifolia* (Medik.) Roxb. (*zhang hua long xue shu* 长花龙血树).[162] So, all three species were searched for this review.

For *xue jie* 血竭 derived from *Daemonorops draco,* the Chinese pharmacopoeia lists the compound dracorhrodin (血竭素) as a marker for quality control and requires a minimum of 1.0%.[1] One analysis reported 6.6 mg of dracorhrodin from a 100 mg sample derived from *D. draco.*[163] Other compounds are dracorubin and nordracorubin; flavonoids including (2S)-5-methoxy-6-methylflavan-7-ol, (2S)-5-methylflavan-7-ol, dracoflavan A, 2,4-dihydroxy-6-methoxychalcone and 2,4-dihydroxy-5-methyl-6-methoxychalcone; organic acids including pimaric acid, isopimaric acid, sandaracopimaric acid, abietic acid, dehydryabietic acid, benzoylacetic acid and benzoic acid; dracoalban, dracoresene, pterocarpol, dracooxepine; and others.[2,161,162]

A large number of compounds have been identified in *xue jie* 血竭 derived from *Dracaena cochinchinensis* including the chalcones and dihydrochalcones: 2,4,4′-trihydroxychalcone, 2′-methoxy-4,4′-dihydroxychalcone; loureirin A, loureirin B, loureirin C, loureirin D, 2,4,4′-trihydroxydihydrochalcone, cochinchinenin A, 4-hydroxy-2-methoxy-dihydrochalcone, 4,4′-dihydroxy 2,6-methoxydihydrochalcone; the flavonoids: 7,4′-dihydroxyflavone, 7,4′-dihydroxy-dihydroflavone, 4′-methoxy-3′,7-dihydroxyflavone, 4′,7-dihydroxyflavan, 7-hydroxy-4′-methoxyflavane, 4′,7-dihydroxy-3′-methoxyflavan, cochinchinenin B, and others; stilbenes: resveratrol, pterostilbene; steroids and triterpenoids; lignans; phenolics; alkanes; acids; esters; and aromatics.[164–166]

Traditionally, *xue jie* 血竭 has been orally and topically used to dispel Blood stasis, relieve pain, stop bleeding and heal sores.[2] Research has reported that *xue jie* 血竭 from *Daemonorops draco* could induce apoptosis in cancer cells, inhibit platelet aggregation, and inhibit viruses and bacteria.[161,165] *Xue jie* 血竭 from *Dracaena cochinchinensis* has shown the following effects: improving blood flow, reducing thrombus formation, inhibiting platelet aggregation, reducing blood glucose and blood lipids, inhibiting bacterial and fungal growth, promoting wound healing, reducing inflammation and reducing pain.[161,165,166]

Effects on Pain

Experiments have been conducted on the analgesic effects of *xue jie* 血竭 from *Dracaena cochinchinensis* and its constituent compounds, notably loureirin A, loureirin B, cochinchinenin A and cochinchinenin B. A pharmacokinetic study in rats of loureirin A and loureirin B administered by gavage found rapid absorption and a wide distribution in tissues including the brain. These compounds appear to be metabolised in the liver and eliminated by the kidneys.[167]

Early studies of *xue jie* 血竭 showed inhibitory effects in animal models of inflammation and pain including acetic-acid induced writhing and carrageenan-induced joint pain but it was unclear whether the observed effects were due to reductions in inflammation or to analgesic effects.[168] Subsequently, a series of experiments focused directly on pain models, the effects of specific compounds and their possible mechanisms of action.

A whole-cell patch clamp recording method was used to record tetrodotoxin-sensitive (TTX-S) sodium currents in isolated rat DRG neurons. The results showed dose-dependent inhibitory effects of a whole extract and loureirin B on sodium peak current amplitudes.[168] In a similar experiment, tetrodotoxin-resistant (TTX-R) sodium currents were inhibited by the extract and by cochinchinenin A, cochinchinenin B and loureirin B, but with greater effect for the combination of the three compounds.[169] Using the same method in rat trigeminal ganglion (TG) neurons, inhibitory effects were found for the whole extract and loureirin B on both tetrodotoxin-sensitive (TTX-S) and tetrodotoxin-resistant (TTX-R) sodium currents.[170] To further investigate these effects, extracellular microelectrode recordings were made in anaesthetised rats, in wide dynamic range (WDR) neurons in the spinal dorsal horn (SDH) in response to stimulation of the sciatic nerve. Dose-dependent inhibition was evident for the extract and all three compounds with maximal inhibition at about ten minutes following administration. The combination of the three compounds in the same concentrations as in the extracts, cochinchinenin A (0.38 nmol/L), cochinchinenin B (0.19 nmol/L) and loureirin B (0.08 nmol/L), produced an effect equivalent to the whole extract.[171]

Using a similar whole-cell patch clamp recording method, the effects of cochinchinenin B on capsaicin-activated currents in rat DRG neurons were investigated. The results showed inhibition that was concentration dependent, reversible and not competitive, and suggested a TRPV1-mediated effect.[172] To further investigate the possible role of TRPV1 channels, the effect of loureirin B on Ca2+ concentration was investigated in isolated rat DRG neurons. This experiment found that loureirin B dose-dependently induced a slow rise in Ca2+ in DRG neurons, but only about 40% of DRG neurons responded to loureirin B.[173]

In a further series of experiments in rats, i.p. injection of a *xue jie* 血竭 extract showed an antinociceptive effect in a hot plate test, a tail flick test and in acetic acid-induced writhing. Whole-cell patch clamp recordings were conducted in acutely dissociated DRG neurons to assess the effects of the extract and the three compounds in capsaicin-induced TRPV1 receptor currents to determine an optimal combination of the compounds. All three compounds produced concentration-dependent effects, with loureirin B being the most effective, but the three compounds also showed a synergistic effect. The authors found that the IC50 (half maximal inhibitory concentration) value of the extract which inhibited TTX-R sodium current was three times higher than that required to inhibit capsaicin-induced TRPV1 receptor currents, suggesting that the first target of *xue jie* 血竭 in DRG neurons was TRPV1 receptors rather than TTX-R sodium channels.[174]

A similar series of experiments was conducted to investigate the inhibitory effects of the three flavonoids (loureirin B, cochinchinenin A and cochinchinenin B) on acid-sensing ion channels (ASIC). Firstly, in a rat model of chronic inflammatory hyperalgesia that was induced by injecting CFA, cochinchinenin B did not show analgesic efficacy in response to thermal stimulus but the other two compounds showed similar analgesic effects, without having any effect on paw oedema. Then, when the flavonoids were tested in rat DRG neurons using whole-cell patch clamp recordings, only loureirin B inhibited the transient ASIC currents with IC50 but all three compounds inhibited the sustained ASIC currents, and the combination showed more than 50% inhibition.[164]

To investigate the effect on inflammatory pain in a rat model of carrageenan-induced paw oedema, an extract of *xue jie* 血竭 was administered intragastrically. Two hours after injection the extract had attenuated the oedema and increased the pain threshold in response to thermal stimulation. The hind paw skins of the rats showed reduction in carrageenan-induced COX-2 expression. In a CCI model of neuropathic pain, intragastric *xue jie* 血竭 dose-dependently reduced mechanical allodynia. In the DRG of L-5 of the treated rats sacrificed at day 28, immunofluorescence showed inhibition of COX-2 protein expression and preprotachykinin-A

(PPTA) mRNA expression. To further investigate the mechanism, cultured rat DRG cells were treated with capsaicin and bradykinin to induce substance P release. Inhibitory effects were found for both the *xue jie* 血竭 extract and cochinchinenin B. In cultured DRG neurons, both the extract and cochinchinenin B blocked capsaicin-evoked increases in the intracellular calcium ion concentration and this effect was blocked by a selective TRPV1 agonist.[175]

In a rat model of neuropathic pain resulting from spared nerve injury (SNI) to the sciatic nerve resulting in mechanical hypersensitivity, an extract of total flavonoids from *D. cochinchinensis*, was administered intragastrically after surgery for 14 days. The extract mainly contained loureirin A, loureirin B, pterostilbene, resveratrol and 7,4-dihydroxyhomoisoflavonoid. Paw withdrawal mechanical threshold (PMWT) in response to stimulation with von Frey filaments was increased dose-dependently. There was no effect on time on a rotarod. After 15 days, in the spinal dorsal horn, the levels of nitric oxide (NO), nitric oxide synthase (NOS), tumour necrosis factor-α (TNF-α) and interleukin-1β (IL-1β) were reduced in the *xue jie* 血竭 group while the level of interleukin-10 (IL-10) was upregulated. Also, Western blotting and immunofluorescence showed reduced expression of fibroblast growth factor receptor 3 (FGFR3), phosphorylated cyclic AMP response element-binding protein (p-CREB) and glial fibrillary acidic protein (GFAP). This suggested the extract inhibited astrocyte release of proinflammatory cytokines and inhibited the NO/p-CREB pathway.[176]

Summary of Evidence

These brief reviews of the herbs used most frequently in the topical CHMs investigated in RCTs of cancer pain were focused on their actions on any type of pain in experimental models and in humans. We did not limit the topic to cancer pain or to topical application, but we have noted any effects on barrier permeability with regard to skin and/or BBB. The included studies were all derived from PubMed searches for which full text papers in English were available. Searches did not include other databases, so these reviews did not include all available literature and should be considered as overviews.

Although the herbs were selected based on their frequency of inclusion in topical preparations, it is notable that all have received research attention for pain even when they may have had other roles in the formula. For example, *bing pian* 冰片 (borneol) is well known for enhancing skin penetration in topical formulations, and clove oil (*ding xiang* 丁香) can also enhance the skin penetration. Therefore, the addition of these herbs to a formula may have aimed to facilitate the antinociceptive effects of other herbs. In addition, both are known to reduce pain independently when applied topically. We did not locate any studies of their effects in combination with other herbs, but both *bing pian* 冰片 and *ding xiang* 丁香 have been shown to enhance the skin penetration of certain conventional medications.

Perhaps the herb that has received the most research is *yan hu suo* 延胡索 (corydalis). An extract reduced pain in humans and its extracts and/or constituent compounds have been tested in a range of experimental studies in animals including models of cancer pain. In contrast, *xi xin* 细辛 (asarum) and its extracts have received relatively little research attention for pain although one of its major constituents, methyl eugenol, which is found in a large number of plants,[177] has received more attention. In the case of *da huang* 大黄 (rheum), we did not locate studies of its extracts for pain but many of its constituent compounds, which are also present in other plants, have been investigated in experimental models.

The related herbs *chuan wu* 川乌 and *cao wu* 草乌 (aconitum) are well known for their analgesic properties but they are highly toxic unless processed adequately. This limits their use as orally administered analgesics, but we were not able to identify studies of their analgesic effects when applied topically. Notably, the processed herb attenuated morphine tolerance in an animal model.

Mo yao 没药 (myrrh) and *ru xiang* 乳香 (frankincense) are often used in combination in CM for pain.[2] They are also used widely in the Middle East, Europe and India but can derive from multiple species. Both have been tested in animal models and have shown antinociceptive properties. In addition, extracts of Indian frankincense have been developed into commercial preparations for pain due to osteoarthritis.

In recent decades, toxins from invertebrates have received considerable attention in pain research. Toxins from the marine snail *Conus magus* have been developed into the non-opioid intrathecal drug ziconotide which is used for neuropathic pain.[178,179] In addition, peptides derived from the venom of various species of scorpion have been investigated for a range of disorders.[159] In the case of *quan xie* 全蝎, the venom has yielded peptides with antinociceptive effects, which may form the basis for new drugs.

Various types of dragon's blood derived from multiple plant species have been used from Europe to the Americas. We limited our discussion to three species used as *xue jie* 血竭 in CM. Evidence for effects in multiple pain models was found for *Dracaena cochinchinensis* but studies of the other species for pain could not be located in the English language literature.

In summary, each of the herbs identified from the clinical studies has been shown to reduce pain in experimental models. However, most animal experiments administered single herbal extracts or compounds orally or i.p. rather than topically, so their relevance to the clinical effects of these herbs when used in complex topical formulations is questionable. Further research is needed on this aspect.

Abbreviations

AKBA	3-acetyl-11-keto-β-boswellic acid
ANEP	anti-neuroexcitation peptide
ASIC	acid-sensing ion channel
BBB	blood-brain barrier
BmK AGAP	BmK antitumour-analgesic peptide
BmK IT-AP	BmK insect toxin-analgesic peptide
BmK	*Buthus martensii*
CAP	compound action potential
CCI	chronic constriction injury
CCL2	CC chemokine ligand 2
CCR2	chemotactic cytokine receptor 2
CFA	complete Freund's adjuvant
c-Fos	Proto-oncogene c-Fos

CHO	Chinese hamster ovary
COX	cyclooxygenase
CPZ	capsazepine
CXCL1	chemokine (C-X-C motif) ligand 1
DHCB	dehydrocorybulbine
DRG	dorsal root ganglia
ESCEO	European Society for Clinical and Economic Aspects of Osteoporosis and Osteoarthritis
Fos	Proto-oncogene c-Fos
GABA-A	gamma-aminobutyric acid A
i.p.	intraperitoneal
ICAM-1	intercellular cell adhesion molecule-1
IL-10	interleukin-10
IL-1beta	interleukin-1 beta
KBA	11-keto-b-boswellic acid
l-CDL	levo-corydalmine
LD50	Lethal median dose
l-THP	levo-tetrahydropalmatine
LTZ	ligustrazine
MAPK	mitogen-activated protein kinase
MMP-9	Matrix metalloproteinase-9
mRNA	Messenger RNA ribonucleic acid
NFkB	nuclear factor kappa-light-chain-enhancer of activated B cells
NMDA	N-methyl-d-aspartic acid
NSAID	non-steroidal anti-inflammatory drug
P2X3 receptor	P2X purinoceptor 3
PAG	periaqueductal grey
p-ERK	phosphorylated extracellular-signal-regulated kinase
PGE2	prostaglandin E2
p-JNK	phosphorylated c-Jun N-terminal kinase
p-p38	phosphorylated P38 mitogen-activated protein kinases
PPTA	preprotachykinin-A gene (that encodes Substance P)
Sig-1	sigma-1

Sig-1R	sigma-1 receptor
TNF-alpha	tumour necrosis factor-alpha
TPA	12-O-tetradecanoylphorbol-13-acetate
TRPA1	transient receptor potential ankyrin 1
TRPV1	transient receptor potential cation channel subfamily V member 1 (aka capsaicin receptor; vanilloid receptor 1)
TTX-R	tetrodotoxin-resistant
TTX-S	tetrodotoxin-sensitive
VAS	visual analogue scale
WOMAC	McMaster Universities Osteoarthritis Index
ZO-1	Zonula occludens-1
5-HT	serotonin

References

1. Chinese Pharmacopoeia Commission. (2015) *Zhong Hua Ren Min Gong He Guo Yao Dian* [*Pharmacopoeia of the People's Republic of China*]. China Medical Science Press, Beijing.
2. Bensky D, Clavey S, Stöger E. (2004) *Chinese Herbal Medicine: Materia Medica*, 3rd ed. Eastland Press, Seattle.
3. Yang MY, Khine AA, Liu JW, *et al.* (2018) Resolution of isoborneol and its isomers by GC/MS to identify "synthetic" and "semi-synthetic" borneol products. *Chirality* **30(11):** 1233–1239.
4. Zou L, Zhang Y, Li W, *et al.* (2017) Comparison of chemical profiles, anti-inflammatory activity, and UPLC-Q-TOF/MS-based metabolomics in endotoxic fever rats between synthetic borneol and natural borneol. *Molecules* **22(9):** 1446.
5. Almeida JRGdS, Souza GR, Silva JC, *et al.* (2013) Borneol, a bicyclic monoterpene alcohol, reduces nociceptive behavior and inflammatory response in mice. *Sci World J* **2013(4):** 808460.
6. Takaishi M, Uchida K, Fujita F, Tominaga M. (2014) Inhibitory effects of monoterpenes on human TRPA1 and the structural basis of their activity. *J Physiol Sci* **64(1):** 47–57.
7. Zhou HH, Zhang L, Zhou QG, *et al.* (2016) (+)-borneol attenuates oxaliplatin-induced neuropathic hyperalgesia in mice. *Neuroreport* **27(3):** 160–165.

8. Jiang J, Shen YY, Li J, *et al.* (2015) (+)-borneol alleviates mechanical hyperalgesia in models of chronic inflammatory and neuropathic pain in mice. *Eur J Pharmacol* **757:** 53–58.
9. Sherkheli MA, Schreiner B, Haq R, *et al.* (2015) Borneol inhibits TRPA1, a proinflammatory and noxious pain-sensing cation channel. *Pak J Pharm Sci* **28(4):** 1357–1363.
10. Ohtsubo S, Fujita T, Matsushita A, Kumamoto E. (2015) Inhibition of the compound action potentials of frog sciatic nerves by aroma oil compounds having various chemical structures. *Pharmacol Res Perspect* **3(2):** e00127.
11. Pergolizzi JV, Jr., Taylor R, Jr., LeQuang JA, *et al.* (2018) The role and mechanism of action of menthol in topical analgesic products. *J Clin Pharm Ther* **43(3):** 313–319.
12. Wang S, Zhang D, Hu J, *et al.* (2017) A clinical and mechanistic study of topical borneol-induced analgesia. *EMBO Mol Med* **9(6):** 802–815.
13. Wang R, Wu ZM, Yang SF, *et al.* (2017) A molecular interpretation on the different penetration enhancement effect of borneol and menthol towards 5-fluorouracil. *Int J Mol Sci* **18(12):** 2747.
14. Dai X, Yin Q, Wan G, *et al.* (2016) Effects of concentrations on the transdermal permeation enhancing mechanisms of borneol: A coarse-grained molecular dynamics simulation on mixed-bilayer membranes. *Int J Mol Sci* **17(8):** 1349.
15. Yin QQ, Wang R, Yang SF, *et al.* (2017) Influence of temperature on transdermal penetration enhancing mechanism of borneol: A multi-scale study. *Int J Mol Sci* **18(1):** 195.
16. Dai X, Wang R, Wu Z, *et al.* (2018) Permeation-enhancing effects and mechanisms of borneol and menthol on ligustrazine: A multiscale study using in vitro and coarse-grained molecular dynamics simulation methods. *Chem Biol Drug Des* **92(5):** 1830–1837.
17. Yi QF, Yan J, Tang SY, *et al.* (2016) Effect of borneol on the transdermal permeation of drugs with differing lipophilicity and molecular organization of stratum corneum lipids. *Drug Dev Ind Pharm* **42(7):** 1086–1093.
18. Zhang QL, Fu BMM, Zhang ZJ. (2017) Borneol, a novel agent that improves central nervous system drug delivery by enhancing blood-brain barrier permeability. *Drug Deliv* **24(1):** 1037–1044.
19. Wu JY, Li YJ, Yang L, *et al.* (2018) Borneol and alpha-asarone as adjuvant agents for improving blood-brain barrier permeability of puerarin and tetramethylpyrazine by activating adenosine receptors. *Drug Deliv* **25(1):** 1858–1864.

20. Wu T, Zhang AQ, Lu HY, Cheng QY. (2018) The role and mechanism of borneol to open the blood-brain barrier. *Integr Cancer Ther* **17(3):** 806–812.
21. Zheng Q, Chen ZX, Xu MB, *et al.* (2018) Borneol, a messenger agent, improves central nervous system drug delivery through enhancing blood-brain barrier permeability: A preclinical systematic review and meta-analysis. *Drug Deliv* **25(1):** 1617–1633.
22. Jiangsu New Medical Academy, ed. (1986) *Zhong Yao Da Ci Dian* [*Great Compendium Of Chinese Medicines*]. Shanghai Scientific and Technical Publishers, Shanghai.
23. Li YL, Tian M, Yu J, *et al.* (2010) Studies on morphology and aristolochic acid analogue constituents of asarum campaniflorum and a comparison with two official species of Asari Radix et Rhizoma. *J Nat Med* **64(4):** 442–451.
24. Zhao ZZ, Liang ZT, Jiang ZH, *et al.* (2008) Comparative study on the aristolochic acid I content of Herba Asari for safe use. *Phytomedicine* **15(9):** 741–748.
25. Li C, Xu F, Cao C, *et al.* (2013) Comparative analysis of two species of Asari Radix et Rhizoma by electronic nose, headspace GC-MS and chemometrics. *J Pharm Biomed Anal* **85:** 231–238.
26. Kim SJ, Gao ZC, Taek LJ. (2003) Mechanism of anti-nociceptive effects of Asarum sieboldii Miq. radix: Potential role of bradykinin, histamine and opioid receptor-mediated pathways. *J Ethnopharmacol* **88(1):** 5–9.
27. Suzuki Y, Yuzurihara M, Hibino T, *et al.* (2009) Aqueous extract of Asiasari radix inhibits formalin-induced hyperalgesia via NMDA receptors. *J Ethnopharmacol* **123(1):** 128–133.
28. Yano S, Suzuki Y, Yuzurihara M, *et al.* (2006) Antinociceptive effect of methyleugenol on formalin-induced hyperalgesia in mice. *Eur J Pharmacol* **553(1–3):** 99–103.
29. Wang ZJ, Tabakoff B, Levinson SR, Heinbockel T. (2015) Inhibition of NAV1.7 channels by methyl eugenol as a mechanism underlying its antinociceptive and anesthetic actions. *Acta Pharmacol Sin* **36(7):** 791–799.
30. Wang C, Wang S, Fan G, Zou H. (2010) Screening of antinociceptive components in Corydalis yanhusuo W.T. Wang by comprehensive two-dimensional liquid chromatography/tandem mass spectrometry. *Anal Bioanal Chem* **396(5):** 1731–1740.
31. Wu H, Waldbauer K, Tang L, *et al.* (2014) Influence of vinegar and wine processing on the alkaloid content and composition of the tradi-

tional Chinese medicine Corydalis Rhizoma (Yanhusuo). *Molecules* **19(8):** 11487–11504.
32. Yan J, He X, Feng S, *et al.* (2014) Up-regulation on cytochromes P450 in rat mediated by total alkaloid extract from Corydalis yanhusuo. *BMC Complement Altern Med* **14:** 306.
33. Du W, Jin L, Li L, *et al.* (2018) Development and validation of a HPLC-ESI-MS/MS method for simultaneous quantification of fourteen alkaloids in mouse plasma after oral administration of the extract of Corydalis yanhusuo tuber: Application to pharmacokinetic study. *Molecules* **23(4):** 714
34. Yuan CS, Mehendale SR, Wang CZ, *et al.* (2004) Effects of Corydalis yanhusuo and Angelicae dahuricae on cold pressor-induced pain in humans: A controlled trial. *J Clin Pharmacol* **44(11):** 1323–1327.
35. Chu H, Jin G, Friedman E, Zhen X. (2008) Recent development in studies of tetrahydroprotoberberines: Mechanism in antinociception and drug addiction. *Cell Mol Neurobiol* **28(4):** 491–499.
36. Wang JB, Mantsch JR. (2012) L-tetrahydropalamatine: A potential new medication for the treatment of cocaine addiction. *Future Med Chem* **4(2):** 177–186.
37. Wang L, Zhang Y, Wang ZW, *et al.* (2016) The antinociceptive properties of the Corydalis yanhusuo extract. *PloS One* **11(9):** e0162875.
38. Guo ZG, Man YY, Wang XY, *et al.* (2014) Levo-tetrahydropalmatine attenuates oxaliplatin-induced mechanical hyperalgesia in mice. *Sci Rep* **4:** 3905.
39. Zhou HH, Wu DL, Gao LY, *et al.* (2016) L-tetrahydropalmatine alleviates mechanical hyperalgesia in models of chronic inflammatory and neuropathic pain in mice. *Neuroreport* **27(7):** 476–480.
40. Kang DW, Moon JY, Choi JG, *et al.* (2016) Antinociceptive profile of levo-tetrahydropalmatine in acute and chronic pain mice models: Role of spinal sigma-1 receptor. *Sci Rep* **6:** 37850.
41. Liu TT, Qu ZW, Qiu CY, *et al.* (2015) Inhibition of acid-sensing ion channels by levo-tetrahydropalmatine in rat dorsal root ganglion neurons. *J Neurosci Res* **93(2):** 333–339.
42. Zhang MY, Liu YP, Zhang LY, *et al.* (2015) Levo-tetrahydropalmatine attenuates bone cancer pain by inhibiting microglial cells activation. *Mediators of Inflamm* **2015:** 752512.
43. Zhang Y, Wang C, Wang L, *et al.* (2014) A novel analgesic isolated from a traditional Chinese medicine. *Curr Biol* **24(2):** 117–123.

44. Dai WL, Yan B, Jiang N, *et al.* (2017) Simultaneous inhibition of NMDA and MGLU1/5 receptors by levo-corydalmine in rat spinal cord attenuates bone cancer pain. *Int J Cancer* **141(4):** 805–815.
45. Hu Y, Kodithuwakku ND, Zhou L, *et al.* (2017) Levo-corydalmine alleviates neuropathic cancer pain induced by tumor compression via the CCL2/CCR2 pathway. *Molecules* **22(6):** 937.
46. Zhou L, Hu YH, Li CY, *et al.* (2018) Levo-corydalmine alleviates vincristine-induced neuropathic pain in mice by inhibiting an NF-KAPPA B-dependent CXCL1/CXCR2 signaling pathway. *Neuropharmacology* **135:** 34–47.
47. Yin ZY, Li L, Chu SS, *et al.* (2016) Antinociceptive effects of dehydrocorydaline in mouse models of inflammatory pain involve the opioid receptor and inflammatory cytokines. *Sci Rep* **6:** 27129.
48. Huo WW, Zhang Y, Liu Y, *et al.* (2018) Dehydrocorydaline attenuates bone cancer pain by shifting microglial M1/M2 polarization toward the M2 phenotype. *Mol Pain* **14:** 1744806918781733.
49. Wang XM, Feng L, Zhou T, *et al.* (2018) Genetic and chemical differentiation characterizes top-geoherb and non-top-geoherb areas in the TCM herb rhubarb. *Sci Rep* **8:** 9424.
50. Sui F, Huo HR, Zhang CB, *et al.* (2010) Emodin down-regulates expression of TRPV1 mRNA and its function in DRG neurons in vitro. *Am J Chin Med* **38(4):** 789–800.
51. Gao Y, Liu H, Deng L, *et al.* (2011) Effect of emodin on neuropathic pain transmission mediated by P2X2/3 receptor of primary sensory neurons. *Brain Res Bull* **84(6):** 406–413.
52. Li L, Sheng X, Zhao S, *et al.* (2017) Nanoparticle-encapsulated emodin decreases diabetic neuropathic pain probably via a mechanism involving P2X3 receptor in the dorsal root ganglia. *Purinergic Signal* **13(4):** 559–568.
53. Gadotti VM, Martins DF, Pinto HF, *et al.* (2012) Diacerein decreases visceral pain through inhibition of glutamatergic neurotransmission and cytokine signaling in mice. *Pharmacol Biochem Behav* **102(4):** 549–554.
54. da Silva MD, Cidral FJ, Winkelmann-Duarte EC, *et al.* (2017) Diacerein reduces joint damage, pain behavior and inhibits transient receptor potential vanilloid 1, matrix metalloproteinase and glial cells in rat spinal cord. *Int J Rheum Dis* **20(10):** 1337–1349.
55. Sharma A, Rathod R, Baliga VP. (2008) An open prospective study on postmarketing evaluation of the efficacy and tolerability of diacerein

in osteo-arthritis of the knee (DOK). *J Indian Med Assoc* **106(1):** 54–56, 58.
56. Brahmachari B, Chatterjee S, Ghosh A. (2009) Efficacy and safety of diacerein in early knee osteoarthritis: A randomized placebo-controlled trial. *Clin Rheumatol* **28(10):** 1193–1198.
57. Pavelka K, Bruyere O, Cooper C, *et al.* (2016) Diacerein: Benefits, risks and place in the management of osteoarthritis. An opinion-based report from the ESCEO. *Drugs Aging* **33(2):** 75–85.
58. Krogh R, Yunes RA, Andricopulo AD. (2000) Structure-activity relationships for the analgesic activity of gallic acid derivatives. *Farmaco* **55(11–12):** 730–735.
59. Trevisan G, Rossato MF, Tonello R, *et al.* (2014) Gallic acid functions as a TRPA1 antagonist with relevant antinociceptive and antiedematogenic effects in mice. *Naunyn Schmiedebergs Arch Pharmacol* **387(7):** 679–689.
60. Tang LQ, Wei W, Wang XY. (2007) Effects and mechanisms of catechin for adjuvant arthritis in rats. *Adv Ther* **24(3):** 679–690.
61. Lopes LS, Marques RB, Pereira SS, *et al.* (2010) Antinociceptive effect on mice of the hydroalcoholic fraction and (–) epicatechin obtained from Combretum leprosum Mart & Eich. *Brazilian J Med Biol Res* **43(12):** 1184–1192.
62. Quinonez-Bastidas GN, Cervantes-Duran C, Rocha-Gonzalez HI, *et al.* (2013) Analysis of the mechanisms underlying the antinociceptive effect of epicatechin in diabetic rats. *Life Sci* **93(17):** 637–645.
63. Bimonte S, Cascella M, Schiavone V, *et al.* (2017) The roles of epigallocatechin-3-gallate in the treatment of neuropathic pain: An update on preclinical in vivo studies and future perspectives. *Drug Des Devel Ther* **11:** 2737–2742.
64. Azevedo MI, Pereira AF, Nogueira RB, *et al.* (2013) The antioxidant effects of the flavonoids rutin and quercetin inhibit oxaliplatin-induced chronic painful peripheral neuropathy. *Mol Pain* **9:** 53
65. Rylski M, Duriasz-Rowinska H, Rewerski W. (1979) The analgesic action of some flavonoids in the hot plate test. *Acta Physiol Pol* **30(3):** 385–388.
66. Selvaraj G, Kahamurthi S, Thirungnasambandam R, *et al.* (2014) Antinociceptive effect in mice of thillai flavonoid rutin. *Biomed Environ Sci* **27(4):** 295–299.
67. Lapa FD, Gadotti VM, Missau FC, *et al.* (2009) Antinociceptive properties of the hydroalcoholic extract and the flavonoid rutin obtained

from Polygala paniculata L. in mice. *Basic Clin Pharmacol Toxicol* **104(4):** 306–315.
68. Hernandez-Leon A, Fernandez-Guasti A, Gonzalez-Trujano ME. (2016) Rutin antinociception involves opioidergic mechanism and descending modulation of ventrolateral periaqueductal grey matter in rats. *Eur J Pain* **20(2):** 274–283.
69. Schwingel TE, Klein CP, Nicoletti NF, *et al.* (2014) Effects of the compounds resveratrol, rutin, quercetin, and quercetin nanoemulsion on oxaliplatin-induced hepatotoxicity and neurotoxicity in mice. *Naunyn Schmiedebergs Arch Pharmacol* **387(9):** 837–848.
70. Abreu FF, Souza ACA, Teixeira SA, *et al.* (2016) Elucidating the role of oxidative stress in the therapeutic effect of rutin on experimental acute pancreatitis. *Free Radic Res* **50(12):** 1350–1360.
71. Mittal R, Kumar A, Singh DP, *et al.* (2018) Ameliorative potential of rutin in combination with nimesulide in STZ model of diabetic neuropathy: Targeting Nrf2/HO-1/NF-kB and COX signalling pathway. *Inflammopharmacology* **26(3):** 755–768.
72. Hasanein P, Emamjomeh A, Chenarani N, Bohlooli M. (2018) Beneficial effects of rutin in diabetes-induced deficits in acquisition learning, retention memory and pain perception in rats. *Nutr Neurosci* **23(7):** 1–12.
73. Csupor D, Wenzig EM, Zupko I, *et al.* (2009) Qualitative and quantitative analysis of aconitine-type and lipo-alkaloids of Aconitum carmichaelii roots. *J Chromatogr A* **1216(11):** 2079–2086.
74. Sun H, Ni B, Zhang AH, *et al.* (2012) Metabolomics study on Fuzi and its processed products using ultra-performance liquid-chromatography/electrospray-ionization synapt high-definition mass spectrometry coupled with pattern recognition analysis. *Analyst* **137(1):** 170–185.
75. Tai CJ, El-Shazly M, Wu TY, *et al.* (2015) Clinical aspects of Aconitum preparations. *Planta Med* **81(12–13):** 1017–1028.
76. Nyirimigabo E, Xu YY, Li YB, *et al.* (2015) A review on phytochemistry, pharmacology and toxicology studies of Aconitum. *J Pharm Pharmacol* **67(1):** 1–19.
77. Liou SS, Liu IM, Lai MC, Cheng JT. (2005) Comparison of the antinociceptive action of crude Fuzei, the root of Aconitum, and its processed products. *J Ethnopharmacol* **99(3):** 379–383.
78. Xu H, Arita H, Hayashida M, *et al.* (2006) Pain-relieving effects of processed Aconiti tuber in CCI-neuropathic rats. *J Ethnopharmacol* **103(3):** 392–397.

79. Shibata K, Sugawara T, Fujishita K, *et al.* (2011) The astrocyte-targeted therapy by Bushi for the neuropathic pain in mice. *PloS One* **6(8):** e23510.
80. Wang C, Sun DN, Liu CF, *et al.* (2015) Mother root of Aconitum carmichaelii Debeaux exerts antinociceptive effect in complete Freund's adjuvant-induced mice: Roles of dynorpin/kappa-opioid system and transient receptor potential vanilloid type-1 ion channel. *J Transl Med* **13:** 284.
81. Suzuki T, Miyamoto K, Yokoyama N, *et al.* (2016) Processed aconite root and its active ingredient neoline may alleviate oxaliplatin-induced peripheral neuropathic pain. *J Ethnopharmacol* **186:** 44–52.
82. Nesterova YV, Povet'yeva TN, Suslov NI, *et al.* (2014) Analgesic activity of diterpene alkaloids from Aconitum baikalensis. *Bull Exp Biol Med* **157(4):** 488–491.
83. Nesterova YV, Povetieva TN, Suslov NI, *et al.* (2014) Anti-inflammatory activity of diterpene alkaloids from Aconitum baikalense. *Bull Exp Biol Med* **156(5):** 665–668.
84. Khan H, Nabavi SM, Sureda A, *et al.* (2018) Therapeutic potential of songorine, a diterpenoid alkaloid of the genus Aconitum. *Eur J Med Chem* **153:** 29–33.
85. Shu HH, Arita H, Hayashida M, *et al.* (2006) Effects of processed Aconiti tuber and its ingredient alkaloids on the development of antinociceptive tolerance to morphine. *J Ethnopharmacol* **103(3):** 398–405.
86. Shu H, Arita H, Hayashida M, *et al.* (2006) Inhibition of morphine tolerance by processed Aconiti tuber is mediated by kappa-opioid receptors. *J Ethnopharmacol* **106(2):** 263–271.
87. Shu HH, Hayashida M, Arita H, *et al.* (2008) High doses of processed Aconiti tuber inhibit the acute but potentiate the chronic antinociception of morphine. *J Ethnopharmacol* **119(2):** 276–283.
88. Dudai N, Shachter A, Satyal P, Setzer WN. (2017) Chemical composition and monoterpenoid enantiomeric distribution of the essential oils from Apharsemon (Commiphora gileadensis). *Medicines (Basel)* **4(3):** 66.
89. Hanus LO, Rezanka T, Dembitsky VM, Moussaieff A. (2005) Myrrh: Commiphora chemistry. *Biomed Pap Med Fac Univ Palacky Olomouc Czech Repub* **149(1):** 3–27.

90. Morteza-Semnani K, Saeedi M. (2003) Constituents of the essential oil of Commiphora myrrha (Nees) Engl. var. molmol. *J Essential Oil Res* **15(1):** 50–1.
91. Dolara P, Luceri C, Ghelardini C, *et al.* (1996) Analgesic effects of myrrh. *Nature* **379(6560):** 29.
92. Germano A, Occhipinti A, Barbero F, Maffei ME. (2017) A pilot study on bioactive constituents and analgesic effects of MyrLiq®, a Commiphora myrrha extract with a high furanodiene content. *Biomed Res Int* **2017:** 3804356.
93. Marongiu B, Piras A, Porcedda S, Scorciapino A. (2005) Chemical composition of the essential oil and supercritical CO2 extract of Commiphora myrrha (Nees) Engl. and of Acorus calamus L. *J Agri Food Chem* **53(20):** 7939–7943.
94. Tonkal AMD, Morsy TA. (2008) An update review on Commiphora molmol and related species. *J Egypt Soc Parasitol* **38(3):** 763–796.
95. Shen T, Li GH, Wang XN, Lou HX. (2012) The genus Commiphora: A review of its traditional uses, phytochemistry and pharmacology. *J Ethnopharmacol* **142(2):** 319–330.
96. Su SL, Wang TJ, Duan JA, *et al.* (2011) Anti-inflammatory and analgesic activity of different extracts of Commiphora myrrha. *J Ethnopharmacol* **134(2):** 251–258.
97. Su SL, Hua YQ, Wang YY, *et al.* (2012) Evaluation of the anti-inflammatory and analgesic properties of individual and combined extracts from Commiphora myrrha, and Boswellia carterii. *J Ethnopharmacol* **139(2):** 649–656.
98. Shalaby MA, Hammouda AA-E. (2014) Analgesic, anti-inflammatory and anti-hyperlipidemic activities of Commiphora molmol extract (Myrrh). *J Intercult ethnopharmacol* **3(2):** 56–62.
99. Ozaki Y. (1990) Antiinflammatory effect of Curcuma xanthorrhiza Roxb and its active principles. *Chem Pharm Bull* **38(4):** 1045–1048.
100. Hossain CF, Al-Amin M, Sayem ASM, *et al.* (2015) Antinociceptive principle from Curcuma aeruginosa. *BMC Complement Altern Med* **15(1)**.
101. Abdel-Tawab M, Werz O, Schubert-Zsilavecz M. (2011) Boswellia serrata: An overall assessment of in vitro, preclinical, pharmacokinetic and clinical data. *Clin Pharmacokinet* **50(6):** 349–369.

102. Moussaieff A, Shein NA, Tsenter J, *et al.* (2008) Incensole acetate: A novel neuroprotective agent isolated from Boswellia carterii. *J Cereb Blood Flow Metab* **28(7):** 1341–1352.
103. Mostafa DM, Ammar NM, Basha M, *et al.* (2015) Transdermal microemulsions of Boswellia carterii Bird: Formulation, characterization and in vivo evaluation of anti-inflammatory activity. *Drug Deliv* **22(6):** 748–756.
104. Hamm S, Bleton J, Connan J, Tchapla A. (2005) A chemical investigation by headspace SPME and GC-MS of volatile and semi-volatile terpenes in various olibanum samples. *Phytochemistry* **66(12):** 1499–1514.
105. Moussaieff A, Mechoulam R. (2009) Boswellia resin: From religious ceremonies to medical uses; a review of in-vitro, in-vivo and clinical trials. *J Pharm Pharmacol* **61(10):** 1281–1293.
106. Paul M, Bruning G, Bergmann J, Jauch J. (2012) A thin-layer chromatography method for the identification of three different olibanum resins (Boswellia serrata, Boswellia papyrifera and Boswellia carterii, respectively, Boswellia sacra). *Phytochem Anal* **23(2):** 184–189.
107. Hu DY, Wang CM, Li FX, *et al.* (2017) A combined water extract of frankincense and myrrh alleviates neuropathic pain in mice via modulation of TRPV1. *Neural Plast* **2017:** 3710821.
108. Banno N, Akihisa T, Yasukawa K, *et al.* (2006) Anti-inflammatory activities of the triterpene acids from the resin of Boswellia carteri. *J Ethnopharmacol* **107(2):** 249–253.
109. Fan AY, Lao LX, Zhang RX, *et al.* (2005) Effects of an acetone extract of Boswellia carterii Birdw. (Burseraceae) gum resin on rats with persistent inflammation. *J Altern Complement Med* **11(2):** 323–331.
110. Fan AY, Lao L, Zhang RX, *et al.* (2005) Effects of an acetone extract of Boswellia carterii Birdw. (Burseraceae) gum resin on adjuvant-induced arthritis in Lewis rats. *J Ethnopharmacol* **101(1-3):** 104–109.
111. Li XJ, Yang YJ, Li YS, *et al.* (2016) Alpha-pinene, linalool, and 1-octanol contribute to the topical anti-inflammatory and analgesic activities of frankincense by inhibiting Cox-2. *J Ethnopharmacol* **179:** 22–26.
112. Belcaro G, Dugall M, Luzzi R, *et al.* (2014) Flexiqule (Boswellia extract) in the supplementary management of osteoarthritis: A supplement registry. *Minerva Med* **105(6 Suppl 2):** 9–16.
113. Belcaro G, Dugall M, Luzzi R, *et al.* (2018) Phytoproflex: Supplementary management of osteoarthrosis: A supplement registry. *Minerva Med* **109(2):** 88–94.

114. Franceschi F, Togni S, Belcaro G, *et al.* (2016) A novel lecithin based delivery form of boswellic acids (Casperome®) for the management of osteo-muscular pain: A registry study in young rugby players. *Eur Rev Med Pharmacol Sci* **20(19):** 4156–4161.
115. Haroyan A, Mukuchyan V, Mkrtchyan N, *et al.* (2018) Efficacy and safety of curcumin and its combination with boswellic acid in osteoarthritis: A comparative, randomized, double-blind, placebo-controlled study. *BMC Complement Altern Med* **18(1):** 7.
116. Feragalli B, Ippolito E, Dugall M, *et al.* (2017) Effectiveness of a novel boswellic acids delivery form (Casperome®) in the management of grade II ankle sprains due to sport trauma: A registry study. *Eur Rev Med Pharmacol Sci* **21(20):** 4726–4732.
117. Bannuru RR, Osani MC, Al-Eid F, Wang C. (2018) Efficacy of curcumin and Boswellia for knee osteoarthritis: Systematic review and meta-analysis. *Semin Arthritis Rheum* **48(3):** 416–429.
118. Liu XQ, Machado GC, Eyles JP, *et al.* (2018) Dietary supplements for treating osteoarthritis: A systematic review and meta-analysis. *Br J Sports Med* **52(3):** 167–175.
119. Amelia B, Saepudin E, Cahyana AH, *et al.* (2017) GC-MS analysis of clove (Syzygium aromaticum) bud essential oil from Java and Manado. International Symposium on Current Progress in Mathematics and Sciences 2016.
120. Chaieb K, Hajlaoui H, Zmantar T, *et al.* (2007) The chemical composition and biological activity of clove essential oil, eugenia caryophyllata (Syzigium aromaticum L. Myrtaceae): A short review. *Phytother Res* **21(6):** 501–506.
121. Kamatou GP, Vermaak I, Viljoen AM. (2012) Eugenol from the remote Maluku Islands to the international market place: A review of a remarkable and versatile molecule. *Molecules* **17(6):** 6953–6981.
122. Alqareer A, Alyahya A, Andersson L. (2006) The effect of clove and benzocaine versus placebo as topical anesthetics. *J Dent* **34(10):** 747–750.
123. Halder S, Mehta AK, Mediratta PK, Sharma KK. (2012) Acute effect of essential oil of Eugenia caryophyllata on cognition and pain in mice. *Naunyn Schmiedebergs Arch Pharmacol* **385(6):** 587–593.
124. Taher YA, Samud AM, El-Taher FE, *et al.* (2015) Experimental evaluation of anti-inflammatory, antinociceptive and antipyretic activities of clove oil in mice. *Libyan J Med* **10:** 28685.
125. Tanko Y, Mohammed A, Okasha MA, *et al.* (2008) Anti-nociceptive and anti-inflammatory activities of ethanol extract of Syzygium aro-

maticum flower bud in Wistar rats and mice. *Afr J Tradit Complement Altern Med* **5(2):** 209–212.

126. Khalilzadeh E, Hazrati R, Saiah GV. (2016) Effects of topical and systemic administration of Eugenia caryophyllata buds essential oil on corneal anesthesia and analgesia. *Res Pharm Sci* **11(4):** 293–302.
127. Ferland CE, Beaudry F, Vachon P. (2012) Antinociceptive effects of eugenol evaluated in a monoiodoacetate-induced osteoarthritis rat model. *Phytother Res* **26(9):** 1278–1285.
128. Dal Bo W, Luiz AP, Martins DF, *et al.* (2013) Eugenol reduces acute pain in mice by modulating the glutamatergic and tumor necrosis factor alpha (TNF-alpha) pathways. *Fundam Clin Pharmacol* **27(5):** 517–525.
129. Park SH, Sim YB, Lee JK, *et al.* (2011) The analgesic effects and mechanisms of orally administered eugenol. *Arch Pharm Res* **34(3):** 501–507.
130. Guenette SA, Beaudry F, Marier JF, Vachon P. (2006) Pharmacokinetics and anesthetic activity of eugenol in male Sprague-Dawley rats. *J Vet Pharmacol Ther* **29(4):** 265–270.
131. Guenette SA, Ross A, Marier JF, *et al.* (2007) Pharmacokinetics of eugenol and its effects on thermal hypersensitivity in rats. *Eur J Pharmacol* **562(1–2):** 60–67.
132. Lionnet L, Beaudry F, Vachon P. (2010) Intrathecal eugenol administration alleviates neuropathic pain in male Sprague-Dawley rats. *Phytother Res* **24(11):** 1645–1653.
133. Lee SH, Moon JY, Jung SJ, *et al.* (2015) Eugenol inhibits the $GABA_A$ current in trigeminal ganglion neurons. *PloS One* **10(1):** e0117316.
134. Chung G, Im ST, Kim YH, *et al.* (2014) Activation of transient receptor potential ankyrin 1 by eugenol. *Neuroscience* **261:** 153–160.
135. Shen Q, Li W, Li W. (2007) The effect of clove oil on the transdermal delivery of ibuprofen in the rabbit by in vitro and in vivo methods. *Drug Dev Ind Pharm* **33(12):** 1369–1374.
136. Chen J, Jiang QD, Wu YM, *et al.* (2015) Potential of essential oils as penetration enhancers for transdermal administration of ibuprofen to treat dysmenorrhoea. *Molecules* **20(10):** 18219–18236.
137. Jiang QD, Wu YM, Zhang H, *et al.* (2017) Development of essential oils as skin permeation enhancers: Penetration enhancement effect and mechanism of action. *Pharm Biol* **55(1):** 1592–1600.
138. Cui Y, Guo GL, Ma L, *et al.* (2010) Structure and function relationship of toxin from Chinese scorpion Buthus martensii Karsch (BmKAGAP):

Gaining insight into related sites of analgesic activity. *Peptides* **31(6):** 995–1000.
139. Cui Y, Liu YF, Chen QQ, *et al.* (2010) Genomic cloning, characterization and statistical analysis of an antitumor-analgesic peptide from Chinese scorpion Buthus martensii Karsch. *Toxicon* **56(3):** 432–439.
140. Lai LL, Huang TT, Wang Y, *et al.* (2009) The expression of analgesic-antitumor peptide (AGAP) from Chinese Buthus martensii Karsch in transgenic tobacco and tomato. *Mol Biol Rep* **36(5):** 1033–1039.
141. Liu YF, Ma RL, Wang SL, *et al.* (2003) Expression of an antitumor-analgesic peptide from the venom of Chinese scorpion Buthus martensii Karsch in Escherichia coli. *Protein Expr Purif* **27(2):** 253–258.
142. Ma R, Cui Y, Zhou Y, *et al.* (2010) Location of the analgesic domain in scorpion toxin BMK AGAP by mutagenesis of disulfide bridges. *Biochem Biophys Res Commun* **394(2):** 330–334.
143. Mao QH, Ruan JP, Cai XT, *et al.* (2013) Antinociceptive effects of analgesic-antitumor peptide (AGAP), a neurotoxin from the scorpion Buthus martensii Karsch, on formalin-induced inflammatory pain through a mitogen-activated protein kinases-dependent mechanism in mice. *PloS One* **8(11):** e78239.
144. Ruan JP, Mao QH, Lu WG, *et al.* (2018) Inhibition of spinal MAPKS by scorpion venom peptide BMK AGAP produces a sensory-specific analgesic effect. *Mol Pain* **14:** 1744806918761238.
145. Shao JH, Cui Y, Zhao MY, *et al.* (2014) Purification, characterization, and bioactivity of a new analgesic-antitumor peptide from Chinese scorpion Buthus martensii Karsch. *Peptides* **53**: 89–96.
146. Wang Y, Wang L, Cui Y, *et al.* (2011) Purification, characterization and functional expression of a new peptide with an analgesic effect from Chinese scorpion Buthus martensii Karsch (BMK AGP-SYPU1). *Biomed Chromatogr* **25(7):** 801–807.
147. Song YB, Liu ZY, Zhang Q, *et al.* (2017) Investigation of binding modes and functional surface of scorpion toxins ANEP to sodium channels 1.7. *Toxins (Basel)* **9(12):** 387.
148. Shao JH, Kang N, Liu YF, *et al.* (2007) Purification and characterization of an analgesic peptide from Buthus martensii Karsch. *Biomed Chromatogr* **21(12):** 1266–1271.
149. Liu T, Pang XY, Jiang F, *et al.* (2008) Anti-nociceptive effects induced by intrathecal injection of BMK as a polypeptide from the venom of

Chinese scorpion Buthus martensii Karsch, in rat formalin test. *J Ethnopharmacol* **117(2):** 332–338.
150. Wang YQ, Hao ZH, Shao JH, *et al.* (2011) The role of Ser54 in the antinociceptive activity of BMK9, a neurotoxin from the scorpion Buthus martensii Karsch. *Toxicon* **58(6–7):** 527–532.
151. Cao Z, Wang W, Mao X, *et al.* (2007) High-level expression and purification of an analgesic peptide from Buthus martensii Karsch. *Protein Pept Lett* **14(3):** 247–251.
152. Cao ZY, Mi ZM, Cheng GF, *et al.* (2004) Purification and characterization of a new peptide with analgesic effect from the scorpion Buthus martensii Karsch. *J Pept Res* **64(1):** 33–41.
153. Zhang XY, Bai ZT, Chai ZF, *et al.* (2003) Suppressive effects of BmK IT2 on nociceptive behavior and c-Fos expression in spinal cord induced by formalin. *J Neurosci Res* **74(1):** 167–173.
154. Bai ZT, Liu T, Pang XY, *et al.* (2007) Suppression by intrathecal BmK IT2 on rat spontaneous pain behaviors and spinal c-Fos expression induced by formalin. *Brain Res Bull* **73(4–6):** 248–253.
155. Li C, Guan RJ, Xiang Y, *et al.* (2005) Structure of an excitatory insect-specific toxin with an analgesic effect on mammals from the scorpion Buthus martensii Karsch. *Acta Crystallogr D Struct Biol* **61:** 14–21.
156. Xiong YM, Lan ZD, Wang M, *et al.* (1999) Molecular characterization of a new excitatory insect neurotoxin with an analgesic effect on mice from the scorpion Buthus martensii Karsch. *Toxicon* **37(8):** 1165–1180.
157. Guan RJ, Wang CG, Wang M, Wang DC. (2001) A depressant insect toxin with a novel analgesic effect from scorpion Buthus martensii Karsch. *Biochim Biophys Acta Protein Struct Mol Enzymol* **1549(1):** 9–18.
158. Guan RJ, Wang M, Wang D, Wang DC. (2001) A new insect neurotoxin ANGP1 with analgesic effect from the scorpion Buthus martensii Karsch: Purification and characterization. *J Pept Res* **58(1):** 27–35.
159. Uzair B, Bint-E-Irshad S, Khan BA, *et al.* (2018) Scorpion venom peptides as a potential source for human drug candidates. *Protein Pept Lett* **25(7):** 702–708.
160. Jura-Morawiec J, Tulik M. (2016) Dragon's blood secretion and its ecological significance. *Chemoecology* **26:** 101–105.
161. Gupta D, Bleakley B, Gupta RK. (2008) Dragon's blood: Botany, chemistry and therapeutic uses. *J Ethnopharmacol* **115(3):** 361–380.
162. State Administration of Traditional Chinese Medicine, Chinese Materia Medica Committee, ed. (1998) *Zhong Hua Ben Cao: Jing Xuan Ben*

[*Chinese Materia Medica: Abridged Version*]. Shanghai Scientific and Technical Publishers, Shanghai.

163. Shi J, Hu R, Lu Y, *et al.* (2009) Single-step purification of dracorhodin from dragon's blood resin of Daemonorops draco using high-speed counter-current chromatography combined with pH modulation. *J Sep Sci* **32(23–24):** 4040–4047.
164. Wan Y, Yu Y, Pan X, *et al.* (2019) Inhibition on acid-sensing ion channels and analgesic activities of flavonoids isolated from dragon's blood resin. *Phytother Res* **33(3):** 718–727.
165. Yi T, Chen HB, Zhao ZZ, *et al.* (2011) Comparison of the chemical profiles and anti-platelet aggregation effects of two "dragon's blood" drugs used in traditional Chinese medicine. *J Ethnopharmacol* **133(2):** 796–802.
166. Fan JY, Yi T, Sze-To CM, *et al.* (2014) A systematic review of the botanical, phytochemical and pharmacological profile of Dracaena cochinchinensis, a plant source of the ethnomedicine "dragon's blood". *Molecules* **19(7):** 10650–10669.
167. Zhao H, Chen Z. (2013) An HPLC-ESI-MS method for analysis of loureirin A and B in dragon's blood and application in pharmacokinetics and tissue distribution in rats. *Fitoterapia* **86:** 149–158.
168. Liu X, Chen S, Yin S, Mei Z. (2004) Effects of dragon's blood resin and its component loureirin B on tetrodotoxin-sensitive voltage-gated sodium currents in rat dorsal root ganglion neurons. *Sci China C Life Sci* **47(4):** 340–348.
169. Liu X, Chen S, Zhang Y, Zhang F. (2006) Modulation of dragon's blood on tetrodotoxin-resistant sodium currents in dorsal root ganglion neurons and identification of its material basis for efficacy. *Sci China C Life Sci* **49(3):** 274–285.
170. Liu X, Yin S, Chen S, Ma Q. (2005) Loureirin b: An effective component in dragon's blood modulating sodium currents in TG neurons. Conference proceedings: Annual International Conference of the IEEE Engineering in Medicine and Biology Society **5:** 4962–4965.
171. Guo M, Chen S, Liu X. (2008) Material basis for inhibition of dragon's blood on evoked discharges of wide dynamic range neurons in spinal dorsal horn of rats. *Sci China C Life Sci* **51(11):** 1025–1038.
172. Wang ST, Chen S, Guo M, Liu XM. (2008) Inhibitory effect of cochinchinenin B on capsaicin-activated responses in rat dorsal root ganglion neurons. *Brain Res* **1201:** 34–40.

173. Yang YN, Chen JX, Pang XY, *et al.* (2009) Slow rise of intracellular ca(2+) concentration in rat primary sensory neurons triggered by loureirin B. *Sheng Li Xue Bao* [*Acta Physiologica Sinica*] **61(2):** 115–120.
174. Wei LS, Chen S, Huang XJ, *et al.* (2013) Material basis for inhibition of dragon's blood on capsaicin-induced TRPV1 receptor currents in rat dorsal root ganglion neurons. *Eur J Pharmacol* **702(1–3):** 275–284.
175. Li YS, Wang JX, Jia MM, *et al.* (2012) Dragon's blood inhibits chronic inflammatory and neuropathic pain responses by blocking the synthesis and release of substance P in rats. *J Pharmacol Sci* **118(1):** 43–54.
176. Chen FF, Huo FQ, Xiong H, *et al.* (2015) Analgesic effect of total flavonoids from Sanguis draxonis on spared nerve injury rat model of neuropathic pain. *Phytomedicine* **22(12):** 1125–1132.
177. Tan KH, Nishida R. (2012) Methyl eugenol: Its occurrence, distribution, and role in nature, especially in relation to insect behavior and pollination. *J Insect Sci* **12:** 1–74.
178. Brookes ME, Eldabe S, Batterham A. (2017) Ziconotide monotherapy: A systematic review of randomised controlled trials. *Curr Neuropharmacol* **15(2):** 217–231.
179. Pope JE, Deer TR. (2013) Ziconotide: A clinical update and pharmacologic review. *Expert Opin Pharmacother* **14(7):** 957–966.

7

Clinical Evidence for Acupuncture and Related Therapies

OVERVIEW

The searches identified 21 randomised controlled trials, one non-randomised controlled study and ten non-controlled studies. The main interventions were acupuncture or electroacupuncture on traditional points, ear acupuncture and ear acupressure, moxibustion, and combinations of traditional acupuncture plus ear acupuncture/ acupressure. Control groups included sham acupuncture, no acupuncture and conventional analgesic medications. The main outcomes that provided data suitable for meta-analysis were pain intensity and quality of life.

Introduction

Acupuncture is a family of techniques which stimulate acupuncture points to correct imbalances of energy (*qi* 气) and restore health to the body. Methods of stimulating acupuncture points include:

- Manual acupuncture: insertion of an acupuncture needle into acupuncture points;
- Electroacupuncture: application of electrical stimulation to acupuncture points;
- Ear acupuncture: insertion of small needles into points or zones located on the ear;
- Ear acupressure: application of pressure to points or zones located on the ear;

- Scalp acupuncture: insertion of needles (usually at an oblique angle) into the scalp along zones that correspond to areas of the body and/or physiological functions;
- Moxibustion: burning of a herb (usually *ai ye* 艾叶 *Artemesia vulgaris* L.) close to or on the skin to induce a warming sensation.

Whilst many of these therapies have ancient roots, several have emerged as new techniques in the last century, including electroacupuncture, ear acupuncture and scalp acupuncture.

Previous Systematic Reviews

There were 23 previous systematic reviews involving acupuncture and related therapies for pain symptoms of cancer patients. Ten systematic reviews investigated acupuncture,[1–9] or complementary and alternative medicine (CAM)[10] therapies for reducing general cancer pain, and eight systematic reviews focused on the management of therapy-related adverse events in patients with breast cancer.[11–18] The remaining five systematic reviews were for palliative cancer care including pain relief with acupuncture and related therapies.[19–23] These systematic reviews included 41 primary studies (following removal of duplicates). Most of the systematic reviews only included randomised controlled trials (RCTs) as the primary studies and four systematic reviews also included non-randomised controlled clinical trials (CCTs) and non-controlled clinical trials such as one-arm studies, case series and case reports.[9,12,18,23]

The findings favoured the effectiveness of acupuncture and related therapies for cancer pain in 14 of the included systematic reviews,[1–3,5,8,12–14,16,17,19–21,23] eight of which conducted meta-analyses of RCTs.[1–3,12–14,19,20] However, concerns about the considerable heterogeneity among primary studies were raised in all systematic reviews. In some, this precluded evidence synthesis or downgraded the strength of clinical recommendations. Heterogeneity existed in the studies' scope (e.g., tumour compression pain, chemotherapy-induced pain, surgery-induced pain), interventions (e.g. type of acupuncture and related therapy, acupuncture protocol including point selection, treatment frequency, number of sessions, duration of each session, point stimulation/manipulation method) and outcome measurements (e.g. patient-reported pain intensity or pain relief, quality of life measured by various scales, typical scales for specific conditions).

Identification of Clinical Studies

Thirty-two clinical trials of acupuncture and related therapies met the inclusion criteria, including 21 RCTs (A1–A21), one CCT (A22) and ten non-controlled studies (A23–A32) (Fig. 7.1). Among the included studies, three were three-arm RCTs (A1, A11, A21) involving a sham-control group, seven were sham-controlled two-arm RCTs (A2, A3, A10, A12, A13, A14, A18), ten were open-label two-arm RCTs (A4–A9, A15–A17, A19) and one was a randomised, crossover study (A20). For the included non-controlled studies, there were six case series (A25–A28, A30, A32), one retrospective study (A23), and three case reports (A24, A29, A31).

For the RCTs, ten studies (A2, A4, A5, A7, A8, A11–A15) investigated manual or electroacupuncture on traditional acupuncture points based on the theory of Meridians and Collaterals in Traditional Chinese Medicine. There were four RCTs (A3, A9, A16, A21) on ear acupuncture/acupressure and two (A6, A10) on moxibustion. Five RCTs (A1, A17–A20) used acupuncture on traditional points combined with ear acupuncture or acupressure and one of these (A19) also included scalp acupuncture zones.

The CCT (A22) investigated electroacupuncture. Of the non-controlled studies, seven studies (A23, A24, A27–A31) used manual or electroacupuncture, while two studies (A25, A32) applied ear acupuncture or acupressure. In addition, one study (A26) used acupuncture on both traditional and ear acupuncture points. No studies that used acupressure on traditional points to treat cancer pain were identified.

Nine included RCTs (A4, A6–A9, A13, A15–A17) were conducted in mainland China; while there were six studies (A1, A11, A12, A18–A20) in the United States, two (A3, A5) in Brazil, two (A2, A10) in Korea, one (A14) in Australia and one (A21) in France. The CCT was

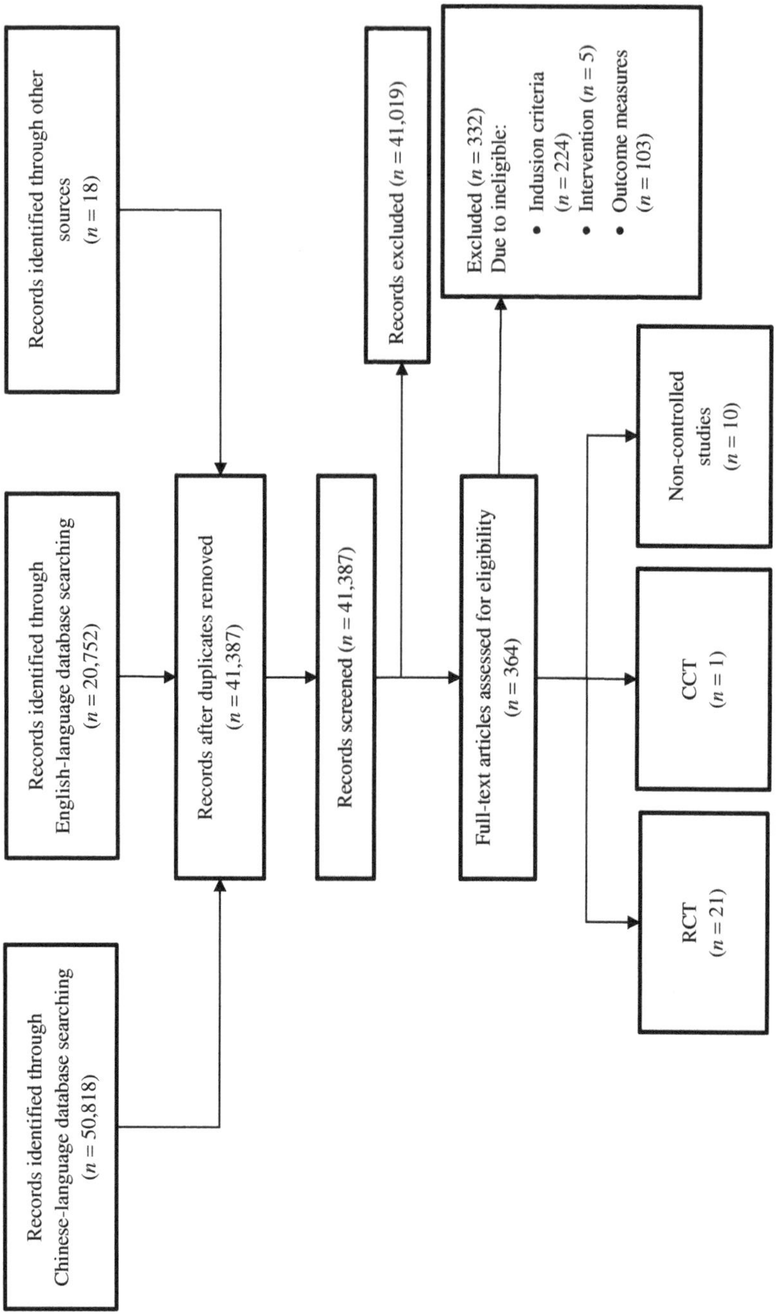

Fig. 7.1 Flowchart of study selection process: Acupuncture and related therapies

conducted in mainland China while all the non-controlled studies were not in mainland China. The majority of the non-controlled studies (A23, A25–A27, A30) took place in the United States, plus three (A28, A29, A31) in the United Kingdom, one (A32) in France and one (A24) in Taiwan.

Aromatase inhibitor-associated musculoskeletal symptoms (AIMSS) was the most commonly researched type of cancer pain, with six RCTs (A1, A11, A12, A14, A18, A20) and one non-controlled study (A30). Metastatic disease was the main cause of pain in three RCTs (A9, A10, A16) and three non-controlled studies (A24, A28, A29).

Outline of the Data Analyses

Studies are grouped by the type of study (RCT, non-controlled study) and by the type of acupuncture and related therapies as follows:

- Manual acupuncture and/or electroacupuncture (ten RCTs, one CCT, seven non-controlled studies),
- Ear acupuncture or acupressure (four RCTs, two non-controlled studies),
- Ear acupuncture or ear acupressure plus manual acupuncture (five RCTs, one non-controlled study),
- Moxibustion (two RCTs).

Meta-analysis results of RCTs are presented for each type of acupuncture and related therapies for the following outcomes (if available):

- Pain intensity
  - Numerical rating scale (NRS);
  - Visual analogue scale (VAS);
  - Brief pain inventory (BPI);
- Analgesic onset time;
- Frequency of breakthrough pain;
- Duration of analgesia;

- Analgesic dose;
- Quality of life;
- Karnofsky Performance Status; and
- Adverse events.

Studies of Acupuncture and Electroacupuncture

Ten RCTs, one CCT, and seven non-controlled studies used manual acupuncture or electroacupuncture at traditional points. In addition, five RCTs combined ear acupressure or ear acupuncture with acupuncture at traditional points (A1, A17–A20). These five RCTs are included in the acupuncture point calculations for RCTs in this section but the outcome results are reported separately in the section on ear acupuncture or ear acupressure plus manual acupuncture.

Randomised Controlled Trials of Acupuncture and Electroacupuncture

In the ten RCTs (A2, A4, A5, A7, A8, A11–A15) using acupuncture on traditional acupuncture points, there were 574 participants with a confirmed diagnosis of cancer. The average age of participants ranged from 53 to 65 years; but one study (A14) reported the numbers of participants aged less than 45 years and not less than 45 years rather than the average age. Based on the reported means and standard deviations for ages, most participants were aged between 50 and 70 years. Following drop-outs, 549 participants completed the studies.

Test interventions were acupuncture using needles with skin penetration at specific points of the body in all ten RCTs. Of these, six RCTs (A4, A7, A11, A13–A15) added electrical stimulation to the needles.

One RCT (A11) included three groups comparing real electroacupuncture to sham electroacupuncture or no acupuncture (waitlist), so these were separated for analysis (A11.1, A11.2).

Ten RCTs were included in the comparisons below:

- Two RCTs for acupuncture versus sham acupuncture (A2, A12);

- Three RCTs of electroacupuncture versus sham electroacupuncture (A11.1, A13, A14);
- One RCT for acupuncture plus conventional analgesic versus conventional analgesic (A8);
- Three RCTs of electroacupuncture plus conventional analgesic versus conventional analgesic (A4, A11.2, A15);
- One RCT of electroacupuncture plus conventional analgesic plus zolpidem versus conventional analgesic plus zolpidem (A7);
- One RCT of acupuncture plus kinesiotherapy versus kinesiotherapy alone (A5).

The groups that combined acupuncture with conventional analgesics are referred to as 'integrative medicine' groups.

Syndromes

One study (A11) developed the acupuncture protocol based on *bi* syndrome (*bi zheng* 痹症) in Traditional Chinese Medicine theory. Another study (A12) stated selection of *qi* enhancing (*bu qi* 补气) acupuncture points due to *qi* deficiency (*qi xu* 气虚) syndrome of the patients.

Frequently Used Points for Acupuncture

The acupuncture points used most frequently in the 15 RCTs that used acupuncture at traditional points, including the five studies that combined traditional points and ear points, were: LI4 *Hegu* 合谷, ST36 *Zusanli* 足三里, LR3 *Taichong* 太冲, GB34 *Yanglingquan* 阳陵泉, PC6 *Neiguan* 内关, SP6 *Sanyinjiao* 三阴交, and KI3 *Taixi* 太溪 (Table 7.1).

Risk of Bias for Acupuncture

Ten RCTs of acupuncture or electroacupuncture are included in this risk of bias assessment. One RCT (A11) included comparisons with a sham control and no acupuncture (waitlist), so there were 11

Table 7.1 Frequently, Used Acupuncture Points in the Randomised Controlled Trials

Point Name	N. studies
LI4 *Hegu* 合谷	12
ST36 *Zusanli* 足三里	7
LR3 *Taichong* 太冲	6
GB34 *Yanglingquan* 阳陵泉	6
PC6 *Neiguan* 内关	5
SP6 *Sanyinjiao* 三阴交	5
KI3 *Taixi* 太溪	5
TE5 *Waiguan* 外关	4
GB41 *Zulinqi* 足临泣	4
GV20 *Baihui* 百会	3
ST41 *Jiexi* 解溪	3
LI11 *Quchi* 曲池	3

Note: Analysis is based on the main points and does not include extra points added for certain symptoms.

comparisons for blinding. For sequence generation, all studies were described as 'randomised'; but one study (A4) did not provide details of sequence generation, so nine studies were judged 'low risk' for use of a correct method of sequence generation (Table 7.2). Five studies described a reliable method of allocation concealment and were judged 'low risk', while the others were judged 'unclear risk' due to the lack of a relevant statement. Five comparisons involving sham acupuncture were judged 'low risk' for blinding the participants and outcome assessors, while the open-label studies as well as the no-acupuncture arm in the three-arm study were 'high risk' for blinding of participants. Blinding of study personnel was not described in any study, so all were judged as 'high risk' of bias since it is not practical to blind the people who perform acupuncture. As the measurements for pain are subjective outcomes reported by participants, blinding of outcome assessors were judged as 'high risk' of bias if participants were not blinded to the treatments. There were no drop-outs or few

Table 7.2 Risk of Bias of Randomised Controlled Trials of Acupuncture

Risk of Bias Domain	Low Risk *n* (%)	Unclear Risk *n* (%)	High Risk *n* (%)
Sequence generation	9 (90)	1 (10)	0 (0)
Allocation concealment	5 (50)	5 (50)	0 (0)
Blinding of participants*	5 (45.45)	0 (0)	6 (54.55)
Blinding of personnel*	0 (0)	0 (0)	11 (100)
Blinding of outcome assessors*	5 (45.45)	0 (0)	6 (54.55)
Incomplete outcome data	10 (100)	0 (0)	0 (0)
Selective reporting	0	10 (100)	0 (0)

*Based on 11 comparisons.

drop-outs, so all were assessed as 'low risk' of bias for incomplete outcome data. Trial protocols were unavailable for all the studies. All studies were judged 'unclear risk' for selective reporting as their protocols were unavailable.

Acupuncture or Electroacupuncture versus Sham Controls

Five RCTs used sham controls. Two compared acupuncture to sham acupuncture (A2, A12), and three compared electroacupuncture to sham electroacupuncture (A11.1, A13, A14).

In the study on intradermal acupuncture combined with analgesics for pain control in advanced cancer (A2), patients were randomly assigned to receive acupuncture or sham acupuncture for three weeks on CV12 *Zhongwan* 中脘, ST25 *Tianshu* 天枢, LI4 *Hegu* 合谷, LR3 *Taichong* 太冲, PC6 *Neiguan* 内关, and on from zero to three *ashi* 阿是 points. Each intradermal acupuncture needle was kept attached in the skin for 48 to 72 hours, and all patients were instructed to press all the needle sites with their hands twice a day. Every week, the attached skin sites were sterilised and checked by the clinicians. In the sham group, all interventions were the same as those of the experimental group, including the issuance of the same instructions. However, the tip of the needle was bent to cause a pricking sensation mimicking real acupuncture without actually puncturing the skin. Follow-up evaluations were conducted three weeks after the end of treatment. One participant in the real acupuncture group and two in the sham acupuncture group withdrew consent after enrolment but no dropouts occurred during the treatment.

A two-arm sham-controlled study on acupuncture for AIMSS (A12) enrolled 51 participants who were randomised into two groups to receive acupuncture (n = 25) or sham acupuncture (n = 26). The real acupuncture points were: CV4 *Guanyuan* 关元, CV6 *Qihai* 气海, CV12 *Zhongwan* 中脘, LI4 *Hegu* 合谷, PC6 *Neiguan* 内关, GB34 *Yanglingquan* 阳陵泉, ST36 *Zusanli* 足三里, KI3 *Taixi* 太溪, and BL65 *Shugu* 束骨. In the sham acupuncture group, 14 sham acupuncture points, which were located at the midpoint of the line connecting two real acupuncture points, were used. Needles remained in the body for 20 minutes and acupuncture treatments were delivered weekly for eight weeks. Four participants were excluded from the analysis due to failure to receive the intervention (one in the acupuncture and two in the sham acupuncture group) or early withdrawal from the study (one in the acupuncture group).

The three-arm trial investigating electroacupuncture for AIMSS (A11) enrolled 67 participants who were randomised equally into three groups: 22 in the electroacupuncture group, 22 in the sham electroacupuncture group and 23 in the no acupuncture (waitlist) group. At least four acupuncture points were chosen around the joint with the most pain and at least four more distal points were used to address constitutional symptoms. The needles were inserted until *de qi* 得气 (sensation of soreness, tingling, etc.) and then left in place for 30 minutes with brief manipulation at the beginning and the end of therapy. As for sham electroacupuncture, between eight and 12 non-acupuncture, non-trigger points at least 5 cm from the joint with the most pain were selected by the acupuncturist. Instead of eliciting *de qi* 得气, the needles were minimally manipulated to avoid eliciting sensations other than initial contact with skin. The real or sham acupuncture treatments were delivered twice a week for two weeks, then weekly for six more weeks, for a total of 10 treatments over eight weeks. Eight participants were lost to follow-up, three in the electroacupuncture group, three in the sham electroacupuncture group, and two in the no-acupuncture control group.

The other two-arm study for AIMSS (A14) enrolled 32 participants whose baseline worst pain score on the BPI-SF was ≥3. They were randomly divided into electroacupuncture or sham electroacupuncture groups. The acupuncture points for the electroacupuncture group were: LI4 *Hegu* 合谷, LI11 *Quchi* 曲池, GB34 *Yanglingquan* 阳陵泉, ST40 *Fenglong* 丰隆, LR3 *Taichong* 太冲, GV20 *Baihui* 百会, *Sishencong* 四神聪, and EX-UE9 *Baxie* 八邪 on day 1; and GB21 *Jianjing* 肩井, TE5 *Waiguan* 外关, ST36 *Zusanli* 足三里, SP6 *Sanyinjiao* 三阴交, LR3 *Taichong* 太冲, GV20 *Baihui* 百会, EX-HN3 *Sishencong* 四神聪, and EX-UE9 *Baxie* 八邪 on day 2. Six of the above acupuncture points (GB21 *Jianjing* 肩井, TE5 *Waiguan* 外关, LI11 *Quchi* 曲池, LI4 *Hegu* 合谷, ST36 *Zusanli* 足三里, and LR3 *Taichong* 太冲) were used for the sham group with a Streitberger placebo needle. The *de qi* 得气 sensation was achieved in the electroacupuncture group but avoided in the sham group. Participants received treatment twice weekly for six weeks and each treatment session took approximately 30 minutes, comprising 10 minutes of consultation and 20 minutes in which the acupuncture needles were stimulated. There were two dropouts in the electroacupuncture group and one in the sham group due to the complaints of ineffectiveness ($n = 1$) and conflict with work hours ($n = 2$).

The study on electroacupuncture for stage III–IV pancreatic cancer with pain intensity 3–6 on NRS (A13) enrolled 60 participants, who received electroacupuncture or sham electroacupuncture bilaterally at EX-B2 *Jiaji* points 夹脊穴 from T8 to T12 for 30 minutes once a day for three days. The Park Sham Device was used for the application of sham electroacupuncture. All patients were requested to maintain the same analgesic drug treatment after randomization. One patient in the control group dropped out because the analgesic medication was modified due to breakthrough pain before the third treatment but has been included in the intent to treat (ITT) analysis.

Pain Intensity

All the studies reported the change in pain intensity from baseline. Two studies used NRS (A2, A13), two studies used BPI (A11, A14) and one study used VAS (A12). Only the data from three RCTs (A2, A11.1, A13) could be pooled due to the different reporting methods.

The study on electroacupuncture for pancreatic cancer pain (A13) found that, compared to sham electroacupuncture, there was a significant reduction in NRS in the electroacupuncture group (MD −1.51 [−1.80, −1.22]) at the end of treatment. There were no significant differences between groups for the other studies. The pooled result for the three studies showed no difference between the groups (MD −0.73 [−1.82, 0.36] I^2 = 78%) with substantial heterogeneity. The heterogeneity was likely due to the study that enrolled AIMSS participants and used BPI (A11.1). When this study was removed, there was a significant reduction in pain intensity on NRS for acupuncture or electroacupuncture, compared with sham controls (MD −1.09 [−2.15, −0.03] I^2 = 71%) with reduced but substantial heterogeneity (Table 7.3).

One study (A12) reported results as median with a range and did not observe a statistically significant difference in VAS between the two groups. Another study (A14) presented results in figures and reported that there were no significant differences in pain severity and interference measured on the Brief Pain Inventory-Short Form (BPI-SF).

Quality of Life

Two studies (A2, A14) reported data on quality of life (QOL).

One study reported on Functional Assessment of Cancer Therapy-General (FACT-G) (A14). The FACT-G is a 27 item self-report questionnaire that has versions in multiple languages including Chinese.[24,25] To obtain total scores, some subscales are reverse-scored so that higher total scores indicate better QOL. At the end of treatment there was no significant difference between groups (detailed data unavailable for analysis).

Table 7.3 Acupuncture or Electroacupuncture versus Sham Acupuncture: Change in Pain Intensity

Outcome	Cancer, Pain Intensity, Intervention (N. Participants)	Effect Size MD [95% CI] I^2	Included Studies
NRS	Advanced cancer, AC (27)	−0.39 [−1.53, 0.75]	A2
BPI-pain severity	AIMSS, BPI-worst pain ≥ 4, EA (44)	0.10 [−1.16, 1.36]	A11.1
NRS	Stage III-IV pancreatic cancer, NRS 3-6, EA (60)	−1.51 [−1.80, −1.22]*	A13
Pooled result (all)	3 studies (131)	−0.73 [−1.82, 0.36] 78%	A2, A11.1, A13
Pooled result (NRS)	2 studies (87)	−1.09 [−2.15, −0.03]*, 71%	A2, A13

*Statistically significant. Abbreviations: AIMSS, aromatase inhibitor-associated musculoskeletal symptoms; NRS, Numerical rating scale; BPI, Brief Pain Inventory; CI, confidence interval; AC, acupuncture; EA, electroacupuncture; N., number; MD, mean difference.

Another study (A2) used European Organisation for Research and Treatment of Cancer Quality of Life Questionnaire (EORTC QLQ-C30). The EORTC QLQ-C30 is a thirty-item questionnaire available in multiple languages that includes five functional scales, a scale for global health status/QOL and scales for multiple symptoms.[25,26] Scoring is normed at 100 with higher scores indicating better QOL for the first six scales with the reverse for the symptoms. In the following analysis, only the global health status/QOL scale was used. On the global health status, there was no significant difference between groups at the end of treatment (MD 1.48 [−6.73, 9.69], $n = 27$).

Acupuncture or Electroacupuncture plus Conventional Analgesic versus Conventional Analgesic

Four RCTs compared acupuncture or electroacupuncture plus conventional analgesic(s) to the same conventional analgesic(s) without the use of sham controls. There was one comparison for acupuncture (A8), and three comparisons for electroacupuncture (A4, A11.2, A15).

One study (A8) enrolled 64 patients with advanced gastric cancer and cancer pain. All participants received World Health Organization (WHO) three-step analgesic ladder treatment. The acupuncture points for the acupuncture group were: ST36 *Zusanli* 足三里, SP6 *Sanyinjiao* 三阴交, LI4 *Hegu* 合谷 and PC6 *Neiguan* 内关. After achieving the sensation of *de qi* 得气, needles were left in place for 30 minutes, once a day, with five acupuncture treatments per week for eight weeks. There were no dropouts.

In one study (A4), all 60 participants had non-small cell lung cancer (NSCLC) with cancer pain and were receiving oxycodone hydrochloride prolonged-release tablets orally with the dose adjusted according to the patient's pain relief. In the electroacupuncture group, patients received electroacupuncture at LI4 *Hegu* 合谷, PC6 *Neiguan* 内关, ST36 *Zusanli* 足三里, and SP6 *Sanyinjiao* 三阴交. Treatment was once a day with needle retention for 30 minutes, for 14 days. There were no dropouts. In another study (A15), 60 patients with liver cancer and cancer pain were receiving Fentanyl Transdermal System (starting with 2.5 mg for moderate pain and 5 mg for severe pain), once every 72 hours, with dose adjustment according to the patient's pain relief. The integrative group was also treated with acupuncture at GV20 *Baihui* 百会, LI11 *Quchi* 曲池, PC6 *Neiguan* 内关, SP10 *Xuehai* 血海, ST36 *Zusanli* 足三里, SP6 *Sanyinjiao* 三阴交, KI3 *Taixi* 太溪, LR3 *Taichong* 太冲, and GB41 *Zulinqi* 足临泣. After achieving the sensation of *de qi* 得气, electroacupuncture was added at LI11 *Quchi* 曲池, PC6 *Neiguan* 内关, SP10 *Xuehai* 血海 and ST36 *Zusanli* 足三里 for 30 minutes, once a day for 14 days. Four people dropped out, three in the integrative group due to distrust of the clinical effect and one in the control group due to severe rash. The fourth study (A11.2) was a three-armed study and the characteristics have been described above.

Pain Intensity

All the studies reported data on pain intensity. Three studies (A8, A4, A15) that reported pain intensity after treatment could be pooled together. Another study (A11.2) that reported the change in pain from baseline on BPI, was separated for analysis.

One study (A8) found that, compared to oxycodone HCl extended-release tablets, there was a significant reduction in NRS in the integrative therapy group (MD −0.83 [−1.36, −0.30], *n* = 64), while there was a marginally significant reduction in NRS (MD −0.43 [−0.77, −0.09], *n* = 60) in the integrative therapy group compared to the WHO three-step analgesic ladder in another study (A4). One study (A15) used VAS and found there was no significant difference between groups (MD 0.13 [−0.65, 0.91], *n* = 56) for electroacupuncture plus Fentanyl Transdermal System versus Fentanyl Transdermal System. The pooled result for all three studies showed a significant difference between groups (MD −0.45 [−0.87, −0.02] I^2 = 51%) with moderate heterogeneity (Table 7.4). In the sensitivity analysis, for the two studies using electroacupuncture, the pooled result was not sig-

Table 7.4 Acupuncture plus Conventional Analgesic versus Conventional Analgesic: Pain Intensity

Outcome	Cancer, Comparator[1], Intervention (N. Participants)	Effect Size MD [95% CI] I^2	Included Studies
NRS	Advanced gastric cancer, WHO 3-step analgesic ladder, AC (64)	−0.83 [−1.36, −0.30]*	A8
NRS	NSCLC, Oxycodone HCl extended-release tablets, EA (60)	−0.43 [−0.77, −0.09]*	A4
VAS[2]	Liver cancer, Fentanyl Transdermal System, EA (56)	0.13 [−0.65, 0.91]	A15
Pooled result	3 studies (180)	−0.45 [−0.87, -0.02]* 51%	All above
Sensitivity analysis	EA, 2 studies (116)	−0.27 [−0.77, 0.23] 40%	A4, A15

*Statistically significant. Note: 1) The same analgesic was used in both groups; 2) One point on NRS is equivalent to 1 cm on VAS. Abbreviations: AC, acupuncture; EA, electroacupuncture; CI, confidence interval; MD, mean difference; N., number; NRS, numerical rating scale; NSCLC, non-small cell lung cancer; oxycodone HCl: oxycodone hydrochloride; VAS, visual analogue scale; WHO, World Health Organization.

nificant with slightly reduced heterogeneity (MD –0.27 [–0.77, 0.23] $I^2 = 40\%$).

In the study (A11.2) that reported the change in BPI pain severity from baseline, there was a significant difference between groups at the end of treatment (MD –2.00 [–3.11, –0.89], *n* = 45) in favour of the electroacupuncture group.

Analgesic Onset Time and Duration of Analgesia

One study (A4) reported on analgesic onset time and the results showed a significant difference between groups (MD –11.30 [–17.53, –5.07] minutes, *n* = 60) in favour of the integrative electroacupuncture group. This study also reported data for duration of analgesia, which showed a significant improvement in the integrative group (MD 11.90 [4.26, 19.54] hours, *n* = 60) versus the conventional analgesic group.

Frequency of Breakthrough Pain and Analgesic Dose

The same study (A4) reported data for breakthrough pain and analgesic dose. The results showed a significant reduction in the average frequency of breakthrough pain during the 14 days of treatment in the integrative medicine group (MD –2.30 [–4.27, –0.33] times per person, *n* = 60). This study also reported a significant reduction in the maintenance dose of analgesics in the integrative medicine group (MD –22.68 [–41.70, –3.66] mg/d, *n* = 60) compared to the group that only received conventional analgesics.

Quality of Life

Two studies reported on QLQ-C30 (A4, A8). There was a significant improvement for acupuncture or electroacupuncture combined with conventional analgesics in each study, and the pooled result of these two studies showed a significant improvement in global health status (MD 10.86 [5.01, 16.70], $I^2 = 0\%$) without heterogeneity (Table 7.5).

Table 7.5 Acupuncture plus Conventional Analgesic versus Conventional Analgesic: Quality of Life (QLQ-C30)

Comparator[1]	Cancer, Intervention (N. Participants)	Effect Size MD [95% CI], I^2	Included Studies
Oxycodone HCl extended-release tablets	NSCLC, EA (60)	11.05 [2.12, 19.98]*	A4
WHO three-step analgesic ladder	Advanced gastric cancer, AC (64)	10.71 [2.98, 18.44]*	A8
Total pool	2 studies (124)	10.86 [5.01, 16.70]* 0%	All above

*Statistically significant. Note: 1) The same analgesic was used in both groups. Abbreviations: AC, acupuncture; EA, electroacupuncture; CI, confidence interval; MD, mean difference; N., number; NSCLC, non-small cell lung cancer; oxycodone HCl: oxycodone hydrochloride; WHO, World Health Organization.

Adverse Reactions

Two studies (A4, A15) reported on adverse events and/or adverse reactions but did not specify the criteria used. One study (A15) reported adverse reactions and adverse events (AEs) together, so the data are presented in the section on safety. Therefore, only one study (A4) was analysed.

There were higher incidences of adverse reactions associated with analgesics in the control group (C) compared to the integrative electroacupuncture test group (T) as follows: constipation (T/C: 5/20), nausea and vomiting (8/17), dizziness (1/1), and itchy skin (0/1). The differences between groups were significant for constipation and nausea and vomiting (Table 7.6).

Acupuncture plus Conventional Analgesic plus Zolpidem versus Conventional Analgesic plus Zolpidem

In one RCT (A7), all participants had advanced lung cancer (n = 100) with moderate or severe pain (NRS ≥ 4). All were treated with conventional analgesics (based on WHO three-step analgesic ladder)

Table 7.6 Electroacupuncture plus Conventional Analgesic versus Conventional Analgesic: Adverse Reactions

Adverse reactions	Effect Size MD [95% CI] I^2	Included Study (N. Participants)
Constipation	0.25 [0.11, 0.58]*	A4 (60)
Nausea & vomiting	0.47 [0.24, 0.92]*	
Dizziness	1.00 [0.07, 15.26]	
Itchy skin	0.33 [0.01, 7.87]	

*Statistically significant. Abbreviations: CI, confidence interval; N., number; RR, risk ratio.

plus zolpidem (a non-benzodiazepine and hypnotic used for the short-term treatment of sleeping problems), 10 mg daily before sleep. Patients in one group also received a 30-minute electroacupuncture treatment daily for four weeks. The acupuncture points included KI6 *Zhaohai* 照海, BL62 *Shenmai* 申脉, HT7 *Shenmen* 神门, EX-HN3 *Yintang* 印堂, EX-HN3 *Sishencong* 四神聪 and *Anmian* 安眠 as main points; LI4 *Hegu* 合谷, LR3 *Taichong* 太冲, ST36 *Zusanli* 足三里, CV6 *Qihai* 气海 and LI11 *Quchi* 曲池 as auxiliary points. Additionally, some acupuncture points were selected according to the location and cause of the cancer pain. There was no drop-out in the study and the result showed a significant reduction in NRS scores (MD –2.12 [–2.55, –1.69], *n* = 100) in the integrative therapy group.

Acupuncture plus Kinesiotherapy versus Kinesiotherapy

One study (A5) evaluated the effectiveness of acupuncture plus kinesiotherapy (a therapeutic treatment of disease by passive and active muscular movements) in the rehabilitation of physical and functional disorders of women undergoing breast cancer surgery. Participants (*n* = 50) included in the study received weekly treatment for ten weeks. The acupuncture protocol consisted of CV3 *Zhongji* 中极, GB34 *Yanglingquan* 阳陵泉, ST36 *Zusanli* 足三里, KI7 *Fuliu* 复溜, LR3 *Taichong* 太冲, GB21 *Jianjing* 肩井, LI15 *Jianyu* 肩髃, HT14 *Lingdao* 灵道, LU5 *Chize* 尺泽, LI4 *Hegu* 合谷, ST38 *Tiaokou* 条口 and BL60

Kunlun 昆仑. The depth of needle insertion was determined according to the application site, patient age, body composition and intensity of reaction to the needle. The two drop-outs (one in each group) were the result of disease progression that made the presence of patients at the clinic for treatment impossible. There was a significant reduction in the integrative group for VAS at the end of the treatment compared to the control group (MD –1.60 [–2.93, –0.27], *n* = 48).

GRADE for Acupuncture and Electroacupuncture

GRADE assessments were conducted for the pooled results for pain intensity. The following two comparisons were assessed: (1) Real acupuncture or electroacupuncture versus sham acupuncture (see Table 7.3); (2) Acupuncture plus conventional analgesic versus conventional analgesic (see Table 7.4).

For the first comparison, two sham-controlled RCTs (A2, A13) of acupuncture were available. The pooled result showed a significant difference between groups with substantial heterogeneity (I^2 = 71%). The GRADE assessment was rated down by two categories to 'low' due to the inconsistency and small sample size (Table 7.7).

Table 7.7 GRADE for Change in Pain Intensity: Real Acupuncture versus Sham Acupuncture

Outcome	Absolute Effect: With Acupuncture	Absolute Effect: With Sham Acupuncture	Relative Effect (95% CI) *n* Studies (*n* Participants)	Certainty of the Evidence GRADE
NRS	**–1.55** points Average difference: 1.09 points lower (95% CI: 0.03 to 2.15 points lower)	**–0.46** points	**MD –1.09*** (–2.15 to –0.03 points) 2 (87)	⊕⊕○○ LOW[1,2]

*Statistically significant result. See Table 7.3 for included studies.

[1]Statistical heterogeneity was substantial.

[2]All RCTs had small sample sizes.

Abbreviations: CI, confidence interval; MD, mean difference; *n*, number; NRS, numeric rating scale.

Table 7.8 GRADE for Reduction of Pain Intensity: Acupuncture plus Conventional Analgesic versus Conventional Analgesic

Outcome	Absolute Effect: With Acupuncture	Absolute Effect: Without Acupuncture	Relative Effect (95% CI) *n* Studies (*n* Participants)	Certainty of the Evidence GRADE
NRS/VAS	**1.95** points	**2.40** points	**MD –0.45*** (–0.87 to –0.02 points) 3 (180)	⊕◯◯◯ VERY LOW[1,2,3]
	Average difference: 0.45 points lower (95% CI: 0.02 to 0.87 points lower)			

*Statistically significant result. See Table 7.4 for included studies.
[1]No blinding.
[2]Statistical heterogeneity was substantial.
[3]All RCTs had small sample sizes.
Abbreviations: CI, confidence interval; MD, mean difference; *n*, number; NRS, numeric rating scale; VAS, visual analogue scale.

For the open-label studies evaluating acupuncture adjunctive to conventional analgesics, three RCTs (A4, A8, A15) were available. The pooled result showed a significant decrease in NRS/VAS scores at the end of treatment with substantial heterogeneity (I^2 = 51%). The GRADE of evidence was rated down by three categories to 'very low' due to lack of blinding, heterogeneity and small sample size (Table 7.8).

Frequently Reported Acupuncture Points in Meta-analyses

Among the ten RCTs that assessed acupuncture or electroacupuncture, the most commonly used outcome in the meta-analyses was pain intensity (five RCTs).

The acupuncture points most frequently included in the two meta-analyses showing a favourable effect for pain intensity were PC6 *Neiguan* 内关 that was included in four RCTs; and LI4 *Hegu* 合谷, SP6 *Sanyinjiao* 三阴交 and ST36 *Zusanli* 足三里 which were each used in three RCTs (Table 7.9).

Table 7.9 Frequently Reported Acupuncture Points in Meta-analyses Showing a Favourable Effect for Pain Intensity

No. of Meta-analyses (Studies)	Acupuncture Points	Frequency of Use
2* (5)	PC6 *Neiguan* 内关	4
	LI4 *Hegu* 合谷	3
	SP6 *Sanyinjiao* 三阴交	3
	ST36 *Zusanli* 足三里	3
	LR3 *Taichong* 太冲	2

*Pain intensity.
For results see Table 7.3 and 7.4.

Controlled Clinical Trial of Electroacupuncture

One non-randomised controlled clinical trial (A22) divided 65 participants with advanced hepatocellular carcinoma with cancer pain into an electroacupuncture group (n = 32) or a fentanyl transdermal patch analgesia group (n = 33). In the electroacupuncture group, treatment was administered at acupuncture points, including GV20 *Baihui* 百会, LI11 *Quchi* 曲池, PC6 *Neiguan* 内关, SP10 *Xuchai* 血海, ST36 *Zusanli* 足三里, and SP6 *Sanyinjiao* 三阴交 once a day for seven days, while in the control group, a fentanyl transdermal patch was placed on the upper left arm and replaced once every three days. No dropout was reported. The VAS pain score of the electroacupuncture group was not significantly different from the control group at the end of the seven days of treatment (MD 0.20 [–0.94, 1.34], n = 65).

Non-controlled Clinical Trials of Acupuncture

Seven non-controlled studies of acupuncture including three case-series (A27, A28, A30), one retrospective case-series (A23), and three case reports (A24, A29, A31) were included. Four studies (A23, A27, A28, A30) used individualised or semi-individualised acupuncture protocols. The points used in multiple studies were ST36 *Zusanli* 足三里 (*n* = 3), SP6 *Sanyinjiao* 三阴交 (*n* = 2) and LI4 *Hegu* 合谷 (*n* = 2).

In a preliminary case series study (A27), two males and five females were provided a semi-standardised manual acupuncture treatment comprising one to three treatment sessions (20–30 minutes per session) per week for eight weeks. The acupuncture treatment was semi-standardised for all patients and based on the type of cancer and the patient's condition. However, the points ST36 *Zusanli* 足三里 and SP6 *Sanyinjiao* 三阴交 were used for all patients, because *qi* and *yin* will be deficient in all cancer patients, regardless of the type of cancer, according to the authors. The mean VAS scores decreased from 51±29.5 mm at the baseline to 36±28.8 mm at the end of week eight. The scores for overall QOL (EORTC QLQ-C30) increased from 55±22 to 69±22.9 at the end of treatment.

The pilot study on acupuncture for cancer-induced bone pain (A28) recruited patients experiencing significant pain from bony metastases (NRS ≥3). One treatment of acupuncture was given, using a minimum of four points and lasting approximately 20 minutes. Decisions on point selection were made according to the site of the painful bony metastases, the segmental distribution of the pain, and the presence of myofascial trigger points. The NRS for resting pain and scores on the Treatment Satisfaction Questionnaire (TSQ) were collected at 10 minutes after needle insertion, when needles were removed, and 48 hours after the treatment. Five patients (three males and two females) completed the study. All five patients responded that they were either 'very satisfied' or 'satisfied' to all questions on the TSQ, both during and after treatment. No adverse events were reported. Mean resting pain intensity immediately before treatment was 4.3 and this reduced to 0.8 during and post-treatment. When resting pain intensity was recorded 48 hours following treatment the mean intensity was 3.2.

The prospective case-series study on electroacupuncture for AIMSS (A30, *n* = 12) was the pilot trial for the three-arm RCT (A11), establishing the feasibility of recruitment and acceptance, as well as providing preliminary data on safety and effectiveness. The protocol for electroacupuncture treatment was the same as the final RCT (A11). The results showed significant reductions in pain severity

(5.3 to 1.9), stiffness (6.9 to 2.4), and joint symptom interference (4.7 to 0.8) from baseline to the end of treatment. No infection, or development / worsening of lymphedema was observed.

A retrospective case-series (A23) included cancer patients who were referred to palliative medicine and received acupuncture for pain management. One hundred and seventy acupuncture treatments from 68 individual patients were studied. All treatments were administered by a single palliative medicine physician while patients continuing standard medical and supportive care, including medication management and psychosocial support. The frequency and number of treatments were determined by both the provider and the patient. Point selection was individualised for each patient based upon their specific conditions and symptoms. Local points were selected based on Western medical acupuncture and myofascial trigger points. Distant points were selected based on the channel theory of traditional CM. The mean number of points per treatment was 13, with the most common being GV24 *Shenting* 神庭 and the bilateral points LR3 *Taichong* 太冲, LI4 *Hegu* 合谷, SP6 *Sanyinjiao* 三阴交, KI3 *Taixi* 太溪, ST36 *Zusanli* 足三里, and BL60 *Kunlun* 昆仑. The Edmonton Symptom Assessment System (ESAS), a validated numerical rating scale for the presence and severity of nine common cancer symptoms, was used for assessment.[27] Scores range from zero to 10; zero indicates no symptoms and 10 severe symptoms. Significant reductions in mean pain scores were observed after the first treatment (−1.9±1.8) and across all treatments (−1.7±1.9). The percentage of pain reduction was greatest in people with stage III/IV disease, and there were higher rates of clinically meaningful pain improvement in people with higher baseline pain scores. There were significant improvements in anxiety, depression, drowsiness, dyspnea, fatigue, nausea, and well-being after the first treatment and across all treatments.

There were three case reports on acupuncture for treating cancer-related pain. One (A24) reported that weekly acupuncture on GB29 *Juliao* 巨髎, GB30 *Huantiao* 环跳, GB34 *Yanglingquan* 阳陵泉, GB40 *Qiuxu* 丘墟, BL40 *Weizhong* 委中, and ST36 *Zusanli* 足三里 reduced breakthrough pain, improved symptoms and increased QOL in a patient with advanced liver cancer with neuropathic pain induced by bone metastasis. Another case report (A29) used two 30-minute acupuncture treatments per week for two weeks to manage the symptom of degenerative lower back pain for a 54-year-old woman with metastatic breast cancer. After treatment, the cancer pain was relieved. In the other case report (A31), a 41-year-old woman with advanced breast cancer was treated with a standard course of acupuncture for cancer pain, using paravertebral segmental points, trigger points, plus contralateral LI4 *Hegu* 合谷 on the non-lymphoedematous arm. She experienced an episode of galactorrhoea six days following the first treatment and during the second treatment. She had not previously lactated for four years. Computed tomography (CT) and magnetic resonance imaging (MRI) of the brain revealed no focal abnormality but recurrent malignant disease was found. There was short-term relief of lymphoedema but pain relief was not adequate and acupuncture was discontinued.

Safety of Acupuncture and Electroacupuncture

Six of the RCTs reported on AEs. Two of these mentioned there were no AEs associated with acupuncture and electroacupuncture (A12, A13). In the three-arm study on AIMSS (A11), eight participants reported AEs, but all were mild in severity and spontaneously resolved without additional medical interventions. The electroacupuncture group had more AEs reported (n = 16) than the sham control group (n = 4). A major category of AEs reported in the electroacupuncture group was related to the *de qi* 得气 sensation (n = 6) such as tingling, or numbness during the acupuncture process. There were similar rates of pain at the needling site in the electroacupuncture (n = 5) and sham control (n = 4) groups. In one study (A2), only one participant suffered from an acupuncture-related adverse event, fatigue, which resolved quickly. Minor bruising on acupuncture points (n = 5) was reported in another study (A14) but no participants experienced serious AEs due to the acupuncture treatment. In another study (A15), three participants in the integrative group suffered from bruising after acupuncture treatment that disappeared after hot topical treatment.

For treatment-related AEs in the CCT (A22), there were three cases of subcutaneous haemorrhage in the electroacupuncture group.

In the non-controlled studies, three studies reported on AEs. One study (A28) reported no AEs due to the acupuncture treatment. In one case series (A27), one participant reported aggravation of pain, burning, and dizziness after the first treatment and during the second visit. These symptoms subsided on their own within 24 hours and did not recur. One case report discussed galactorrhoea following acupuncture (A31).

Studies of Ear Acupuncture and Ear Acupressure

Four RCTs and two non-controlled studies used ear acupuncture or ear acupressure, excluding studies that combined ear points with traditional points.

Randomised Controlled Trials of Ear Acupuncture or Ear Acupressure

In the four RCTs on ear acupuncture or ear acupressure (A3, A9, A16, A21), 227 participants were enrolled and 208 completed the studies. The mean age of participants ranged from 52 to 62 years.

One RCT (A21) included three groups that compared ear acupuncture, sham ear acupuncture and sham ear acupressure but we have only included the comparison for ear acupuncture versus sham ear acupuncture.

Four RCTs were included the comparisons below:

- Two RCTs for ear acupuncture versus sham ear acupuncture (A3, A21);
- Two RCTs of ear acupressure plus conventional analgesic versus conventional analgesic (A9, A16).

Syndromes

None of the included studies referred to syndrome differentiation.

Frequently Used points in Randomised Controlled Trials of Ear Acupuncture or Ear Acupressure

The most frequently used ear points were TF4 *Shenmen* 神门 (*n* = 3) and AH6a *Jiaogan* 交感 (sympathetic nervous system) (*n* = 3).

Risk of Bias for Ear Acupuncture or Ear Acupressure

All studies were judged 'low risk' for sequence generation since they used random number tables, but three of them (A3, A9, A16) were judged 'unclear risk' for allocation concealment because none provided related information. One study (A21) used a centralised computerised randomisation system that enabled allocation concealment. For the sham-controlled studies (A3, A21), they were judged 'low risk' for blinding the participants and outcome assessors, while the open-label studies without sham controls were 'high risk' for these items. Incomplete outcome data were judged 'low risk' since the studies had no drop-outs (A9, A16) or missing outcome data were balanced in numbers between groups with similar reasons (A3). However, one study was judged 'high risk' for incomplete outcome data (A21) because it reported imbalanced drop-out numbers across intervention groups and did not perform intention to treat (ITT) analyses. No protocol or registration information was available for any study so they were judged as 'unclear risk' for selective reporting (Table 7.10).

Ear Acupuncture versus Sham Ear Acupuncture

Two RCTs used sham controls. In a two-arm sham-controlled study on ear acupuncture for cancer pain (A3), 31 participants who were receiving chemotherapy and had moderate or severe pain (NRS ≥4) were randomised to the real ear acupuncture group or to the sham control group. Patients in the study received ear acupuncture treatments weekly for eight weeks. In the real ear acupuncture group the mean time per session was 40 minutes, while in the sham group it

Table 7.10 Risk of Bias of Randomised Controlled Trials of Ear Acupuncture or Acupressure

Risk of Bias Domain	Low Risk *n* (%)	Unclear Risk *n* (%)	High Risk *n* (%)
Sequence generation	4 (100)	0 (0)	0 (0)
Allocation concealment	1 (25)	3 (75)	0 (0)
Blinding of participants	2 (50)	0 (0)	2 (50)
Blinding of personnel	0 (0)	0 (0)	4 (100)
Blinding of outcome assessors	2 (50)	0 (0)	2 (50)
Incomplete outcome data	3 (75)	0 (0)	1 (25)
Selective reporting	0	4 (100)	0 (0)

was 20 minutes. The ear points for the real ear acupuncture group were TF4 *Shenmen* 神门, CO10 *Shen* 肾 (kidney), AH6 *Jiaogan* 交感, muscle relaxation, and energy balance points, based on the five elements theory. The points LO5 *Yan* 眼 (eye) and CO16 *Qiguan* 气管 (trachea) were applied in the sham group. Eleven people dropped out (five in the real ear acupuncture group and three in the sham group), but the article did not report the reasons. Twenty-three participants were analysed at the end of the treatment.

In the other study (A21), all patients had chronic peripheral or central neuropathic pain (VAS ≥3 cm) arising after treatment of a cancer. They were randomly divided into the ear acupuncture group (n = 29) that received ear acupuncture at points where an electrodermal signal had been detected, a sham ear acupuncture group (n = 30) that received ear acupuncture at placebo points without any electrodermal signal, or a sham ear acupressure group (n = 30) that used Vaccaria seeds at placebo points. The treatments were delivered once a month for two months. There were two withdrawals from the sham group during the first treatment. One participant in the ear acupuncture group and four in the sham group refused to receive the second treatment, while one in the sham group changed analgesic before the second treatment.

Table 7.11 Ear Acupuncture versus Sham Ear Acupuncture: Pain Intensity

Outcome	Condition, Pain Intensity (N. Participants)	Effect Size MD [95% CI] I^2	Included Studies
NRS	Receiving chemotherapy, NRS ≥ 4 (23)	−4.24 [−5.72, −2.76]*	A3
VAS[1]	Chronic peripheral or central neuropathic pain arising after treatment of a cancer, VAS ≥ 3 cm (57)	−1.80 [−2.93, −0.67]*	A21
Pooled result	2 studies (80)	−2.97 [−5.36, −0.58]* 85%	A3, A21

*Statistically significant. Note: 1) One point on NRS is equivalent to 1 cm on VAS.
Abbreviations: CI, confidence interval; MD, mean difference; N., number; NRS, Numeric Rating Scale; VAS, Visual Analogue Scale.

Pain Intensity

Both studies reported data on pain intensity. One study used NRS scores (A3) and one study used VAS scores (A21) that have been converted from millimetres to centimetres for this analysis. In each of the RCTs, there were significantly greater reductions in pain intensity in the ear acupuncture groups compared to the sham control groups. In one study (A21), there was also a greater reduction in the comparison with sham ear acupressure (MD −2.10 [−3.11, −1.09] cm). The pooled result showed a significantly greater reduction in pain in the ear acupuncture groups (MD −2.97 [−5.36, −0.58] I^2 = 85%) compared with sham ear acupuncture, but with substantial heterogeneity (Table 7.11).

Analgesic Dose

Only one study (A3) reported the use of analgesics during the study. There were significantly fewer daily analgesic doses (MD −1.05 [−1.68, −0.42] doses/d, *n* = 23) in the real ear acupuncture group at the end of treatment compared to the sham control group.

Ear Acupressure plus Conventional Analgesic versus Conventional Analgesic

Two RCTs (A9, A16) were included. All participants completed the studies as no drop-out was reported.

In one RCT (A9), all participants had bone metastases (*n* = 60) and had their moderate to severe pain (NRS ≥4) treated with oxycodone and acetaminophen tablets. Thirty people in the integrative therapy group also received ear acupressure with *Vaccaria* seeds (*wang bu liu xing* 王不留行) once a day for seven days. The ear acupressure points were selected according to symptoms as follows: CO4 *Wei* 胃, CO12 *Gan* 肝, CO13 *Pi* 脾, CO3 *Benmen* 贲门, AH6a *Jiaogan* 交感, TF4 *Shenmen* 神门 and AT4 *Pizhixia* 皮质下 for alleviating pain, nausea and vomiting; HX2 *Zhichang* 直肠, CO7 *Dachang* 大肠, AH8 *Fu* 腹, CO17 *Sanjiao* 三焦, and TF3 *Bianmidian* 便秘点 for preventing constipation; and the point corresponding to the location of tumour invasion, for example, CO12 *Gan* 肝 for hepatoma, CO14 *Fei* 肺 for lung cancer (one point for each patient at most).

Another RCT (A16) required all the participants (*n* = 46) have malignant neuropathic pain graded moderate to severe (VAS ≥4). All received oxycodone HCl extended-release tablets (starting with 10 mg, once every 12 hours, with dose adjustment according to the patient's pain relief). Participants in the integrative therapy group (*n* = 23) also received ear acupressure using magnetic beads applied to specific points and maintained for five days. The whole treatment course was four weeks. The main ear acupressure points included TF4 *Shenmen* 神门, AT4 *Pizhixia* 皮质下, AH6a *Jiaogan* 交感, CO12 *Gan* 肝, CO13 *Pi* 脾, CO4 *Wei* 胃, TF2 *Zigong* 子宫 and CO18 *Neifenmi* 内分泌.

Pain Intensity

Both studies reported data on pain intensity. In each RCT, there was a significantly greater reduction in pain in the integrative therapy

Table 7.12 Ear Acupressure plus Conventional Analgesic versus Conventional Analgesic: Pain Intensity

Outcome	Cancer, Comparator[1] (N. Participants)	Effect Size MD [95% CI], I^2	Included Studies
NRS	Bone metastases, NRS ≥ 4, oxycodone & acetaminophen tablets (60)	−1.93 [−2.24, −1.62]*	A9
VAS[2]	Malignant neuropathic pain, VAS[2] ≥ 4 (46)	−1.60 [−1.84, −1.36]*	A16
Pooled result	2 studies (106)	−1.75 [−2.07, −1.43]* 64%	All above

*Statistically significant; *Note*: 1) The same analgesic was used in both groups; 2) One point on NRS is equivalent to 1 cm on VAS. Abbreviations: CI, confidence interval; MD, mean difference; N., number; NRS, Numeric Rating Scale; VAS, Visual Analogue Scale.

group compared to the control group. The pooled result showed a significantly greater pain reduction in the groups that received ear acupressure combined with conventional analgesics (MD −1.75 [−2.07, −1.43] I^2 = 64%), with substantial heterogeneity (Table 7.12).

Analgesic Dose

One study (A16) reported the dose of analgesics used during the treatment. There was a significantly lower analgesic consumption (MD −19.80 [−24.95, −14.65] mg/d of oxycodone HCl, *n* = 46) in the ear acupressure plus conventional analgesic group compared to the control group.

Karnofsky Performance Status

The study of ear acupressure for moderate and severe cancer pain due to bone metastasis (A9) reported Karnofsky Performance Status (KPS) scores. The authors reported a greater improvement in KPS after treatment in the ear acupressure plus analgesic but the analysis showed no statistical difference between the two groups (MD 4.33 [−2.39, 11.05], *n* = 60).

GRADE for Ear Acupuncture or Ear Acupressure

Assessments of ear acupuncture or ear acupressure for reduction of pain intensity were conducted using the GRADE approach. The following two comparisons were assessed: 1) Ear acupuncture versus sham ear acupuncture (Table 7.11); 2) Ear acupressure plus conventional analgesic versus conventional analgesic (Table 7.12).

For the first comparison, there was a difference of −2.97 points. This was a significant difference in favour of ear acupuncture but there was substantial heterogeneity (I^2 = 85%). The certainty of the evidence was reduced by two categories to 'low' due to the inconsistency and small sample size (Table 7.13).

For the second comparison, there was a significantly greater reduction in pain intensity in the groups that received ear acupressure compared to the groups without acupressure (MD −1.75 points) with substantial heterogeneity (I^2 = 64%). The certainty of this evidence was rated down by three categories to 'very low' due to lack of blinding, heterogeneity, and small sample size (Table 7.14).

Table 7.13 GRADE for Pain Intensity: Ear Acupuncture versus Sham Ear Acupuncture

	Absolute Effect			
Outcome	**With Ear Acupuncture**	**With Sham Ear Acupuncture**	**Relative Effect (95% CI) N. Studies (Participants)**	**Certainty of the Evidence GRADE**
NRS/VAS scores	**2.78** points	**5.75** points	**MD −2.97*** (−5.36 to −0.58 points) 2 (80)	⊕⊕◯◯ LOW[1,2]
	Average difference: 2.97 points lower (95% CI: 0.58 to 5.38 lower)			

*Statistically significant result, random effect model. Note: 1) Statistical heterogeneity was substantial; 2) Both RCTs had small sample sizes. Abbreviations: CI, confidence interval; GRADE, Grading of Recommendations Assessment, Development and Evaluation; MD, mean difference; N., number; NRS, numeric rating scale; VAS, visual analogue scale. See Table 7.11 for included studies.

Table 7.14 GRADE for Pain Intensity: Ear Acupressure plus Conventional Analgesic versus Conventional Analgesic

	Absolute Effect			
Outcome	**With Ear Acupuncture**	**Without Ear Acupressure**	**Relative Effect (95% CI) N. Studies (Participants)**	**Certainty of the Evidence GRADE**
NRS/VAS scores	**1.13** points	**2.88** points	**MD –1.75*** (–2.07 to –1.43 points) 2 (106)	⊕○○○ VERY LOW[1,2,3]
	Average difference: 1.75 points lower (95% CI: 1.43 to 2.07 lower)			

*Statistically significant result, random effect model. Note: 1) No blinding; 2) Statistical heterogeneity was substantial; 3) Both randomised controlled trials had small sample sizes. Abbreviations: CI, confidence interval; GRADE, Grading of Recommendations Assessment, Development and Evaluation; MD, mean difference; N., number; NRS, numeric rating scale; VAS, visual analogue scale. See Table 7.12 for included studies

Non-controlled Clinical Trials of Ear Acupuncture or Ear Acupressure

No non-randomised CCT on ear acupuncture or ear acupressure to treat cancer pain was identified but two non-controlled studies were included (A25, A32).

A prospective case-series study (A25) enrolled 50 participants to investigate the effects of ear acupressure for cancer pain. The ear points selected for pain treatment were AH6a *Jiaogan* 交感 and AT4 *Pizhixia* 皮质下, plus ear points corresponding to the locations where patients had pain. Five to nine acupuncture points were selected for each participant and *Vaccaria* seeds held in place by tape were used to stimulate the ear points. The study found preliminary evidence for the analgesic effects of ear acupressure for cancer pain management with reductions of more than 55% for worst pain and about 57% for both average pain and pain intensity. Moreover, the use of pain medication was reduced during the ear acupressure with the authors reporting that 78% of patients took less pain medication than before the treatment.

One pilot study (A32) was reported in the form of a letter to the editor. This was a pilot study for the three-arm sham-controlled RCT

(A21) described previously. In this pilot study (A32), 20 patients with chronic pain syndrome with peripheral or central neuropathic pain were treated by auricular acupuncture. Initial pain, as measured on the VAS, attained 76 ± 16 mm on average. At day 0 (baseline) there was a correlation between pain intensity and the electrodermal response at the main auricular projection points on the ear corresponding to the location of the pain. Intradermal needles used for auricular acupuncture were applied at these points and left in place during the study (60 days). The needles fell out between 5 and 35 days after the auricular acupuncture commenced. Pain intensity decreased or remained stable after auricular acupuncture in all patients. The average pain intensity decreased by 33 ± 5 mm between day 0 and day 60. It is noteworthy that the improvement was not limited to diminution of the pain. Patients who experienced improvement after auricular acupuncture also said that they felt better and some felt well enough to propose interrupting their analgesic treatment.

Safety of Ear Acupuncture or Ear Acupressure

Two of the RCTs reported on AEs. One study on ear acupuncture (A21) reported there were no AEs. Another study (A3) stated there were no major AEs that required medical evaluations or any specific interventions during the study, although some participants reported pain or slightly intense sensation at the site of application of the needles for a maximum duration of three days.

The two non-controlled studies (A25, A32) did not report on AEs.

Studies of Ear Acupuncture or Ear Acupressure plus Acupuncture

Five RCTs and one non-controlled study used ear acupuncture or ear acupressure plus acupuncture on traditional points.

Randomised Controlled Trials of Ear Acupuncture or Ear Acupressure plus Acupuncture

Five RCTs of ear acupuncture or ear acupressure plus acupuncture on traditional points (A1, A17–A20) enrolled 420 participants, who ranged from 48 to 61 years old. Following dropouts, 381 participants completed the studies.

One three-arm RCT included three groups that compared a true intervention group to a sham control and a no acupuncture (waitlist) control (A1), so these groups were separated for analysis (A1.1, A1.2). Three were two-arm RCTs (A17–A18) and one was a cross-over RCT (A20).

The studies and comparisons included:

- Two RCTs for ear acupuncture plus acupuncture versus sham control (A1.1, A18);
- Three RCTs of ear acupuncture plus acupuncture versus no acupuncture (A1.2, A19, A20);
- One RCT of ear acupressure plus acupuncture plus conventional analgesic versus conventional analgesic (A17).

Syndromes

One RCT used syndrome differentiation in the inclusion criteria (A17), requiring that participants were diagnosed as Blood stasis due to *qi* stagnation (*qi zhi xue yu* 气滞血瘀) and Blood and *qi* dual deficiency (*xue qi kui xu* 血气亏虚). Another study developed the acupuncture protocol based on *bi* syndrome (*bi zheng* 痹症) in CM theory (A1)

Frequently Used Ear Points in Randomised Controlled Trials of Ear Acupuncture or Ear Acupressure plus Acupuncture

The ear points used most frequently in the five RCTs were TF4 *Shenmen* 神门 (n = 5) and AH6a *Jiaogan* 交感 (n = 4)

Risk of Bias for Ear Acupuncture or Ear Acupressure plus Acupuncture

Four parallel RCTs are included in this risk of bias assessment excluding the single crossover study (A20). One RCT (A1) included comparisons with a sham control and a no acupuncture (waitlist) control group, so there were five comparisons for blinding. For sequence generation, all studies were described as 'randomised' and provided details of sequence generation, so all were judged 'low risk' (Table 7.15). Three studies described a reliable method of allocation concealment and were judged 'low risk', while one study (A17) was judged 'unclear risk' due to the lack of a relevant statement. Two comparisons that used sham acupuncture were judged 'low risk' for blinding of participants and outcome assessors, while the open-label studies as well as the no acupuncture arm in the three-arm study were 'high risk' for blinding of participants. Blinding of study personnel was not described in any study, so all were judged as 'high risk' of bias since it is difficult to blind the people who perform acupuncture. As the measurements for pain are subjective outcomes reported by participants, blinding of outcome assessors was judged as 'high risk'

Table 7.15 Risk of Bias of Randomised Controlled Trials of Ear Acupuncture or Ear Acupressure plus Acupuncture

Risk of Bias Domain	Low Risk *n* (%)	Unclear Risk *n* (%)	High Risk *n* (%)
Sequence generation	4 (100)	0 (0)	0 (0)
Allocation concealment	3 (75)	1 (25)	0 (0)
Blinding of participants*	2 (40)	0 (0)	3 (60)
Blinding of personnel*	0 (0)	0 (0)	5 (100)
Blinding of outcome assessors*	2 (40)	0 (0)	3 (60)
Incomplete outcome data	4 (100)	0 (0)	0 (0)
Selective reporting	1 (25)	3 (75)	0 (0)

*Based on five comparisons.

of bias if participants were not blinded to the treatments. There were no drop-outs or few drop-outs so all were assessed as 'low risk' of bias for incomplete outcome data. One study (A1) reported all outcomes in its protocol, so it was judged 'low risk of bias' for selective outcome reporting. The other studies were judged 'unclear risk' since their protocols were unavailable.

Ear Acupuncture plus Acupuncture versus Sham Controls

Two RCTs (A1.1, A18) compared ear acupuncture plus traditional acupuncture with sham acupuncture controls for AIMSS. All participants had BPI ≥3 for the worst pain item.

In the three-arm RCT (A1), 226 breast cancer participants were randomised into the real acupuncture (n = 110), sham acupuncture (n = 59), or no acupuncture (waitlist) control (n = 57) groups. The real acupuncture and sham acupuncture treatments consisted of twelve 30 to 45-minute sessions administered over a period of six weeks (two per week) followed by one session per week for six weeks. At every treatment visit, the patients assigned to the true interventions group received the traditional acupuncture prescription and the ear acupuncture protocol in one ear, with the alternate ear used at the next visit. The acupuncture points were TE5 *Waiguan* 外关, LI4 *Hegu* 合谷, GB41 *Zulinqi* 足临泣, GB34 *Yanglingquan* 阳陵泉, ST41 *Jiexi* 解溪, and KI3 *Taixi* 太溪. The ear acupuncture points were TF4 *Shenmen* 神门, CO10 *Shen* 肾, CO12 *Gan* 肝 (liver), CO14 *Fei* 肺 (lung), and AH6 *Jiaogan* 交感. A joint-specific protocol allowed additional points for up to three of the patient's most painful joint areas. The sham acupuncture consisted of a core standardised prescription of minimally invasive, shallow needle insertion using thin, short needles at non-acupuncture points. The sham acupuncture protocol also included joint-specific treatments and application of adhesives to non-acupuncture points on the ear. The no acupuncture (waitlist) group received no acupuncture treatments and no other intervention after randomisation. Twenty participants did not have baseline or outcome data and could not be evaluated.

The research group for the above three-arm RCT (A1) also conducted a two-arm RCT (A18) that enrolled 43 AIMSS participants to receive real acupuncture or sham acupuncture (A18) using an identical acupuncture protocol but the treatment was twice a week for six weeks. In this two-arm RCT, five participants did not initiate, or discontinued, the intervention due to loss to follow-up (real acupuncture = 2; sham acupuncture = 1) or scheduling difficulties (real acupuncture = 1; sham acupuncture = 1).

Pain Intensity

Both studies reported pain intensity measures on BPI. In one study (A1.1), there was no significant difference between groups for BPI-worst pain. The other study (A18) reported a significantly greater reduction in the true intervention group compared to the sham acupuncture group for BPI-worst pain. However, the pooled result showed no difference between groups (MD –1.44 [–3.39, 0.51], I^2 = 86%) with considerable heterogeneity (Table 7.16).

Table 7.16 Ear Acupuncture plus Acupuncture versus Sham Controls: Pain Intensity

Outcome	Condition, Pain Intensity (N. Participants)	Effect Size MD [95% CI], I^2	Included Studies
BPI - worst pain	AIMSS, BPI ≥3 for the worst pain item (155)	–0.51 [–1.24, 0.22]	A1.1
BPI - worst pain	AIMSS, BPI ≥3 for the worst pain item (38)	–2.50 [–3.73, –1.27]*	A18
Pooled result	2 studies (193)	–1.44 [–3.39, 0.51] 86%	A1.1, A18

*Statistically significant. Abbreviations: AIMSS, aromatase inhibitor-associated musculoskeletal symptoms; BPI, Brief Pain Inventory; CI, confidence interval; MD, mean difference; N., number.

Quality of Life

The two studies reported data on QOL. One study (A1.1) used the 19 item Functional Assessment of Cancer Therapy-Endocrine Symptoms (FACT-ES)[28] for which higher scores indicate better QOL. There was no significant difference between groups for FACT-ES (MD 1.87 [−2.78, 6.52], n = 155).

The other study (A18) reported QOL measured by FACT-G, which consisted of physical, social/family, emotional, and functional.[24] Five response levels ('not at all' to 'very much') were ranked for each subscale. Higher scores indicate better QOL. The physical subscale showed a significantly greater improvement in the true intervention group compared with the sham control (MD 4.40 [0.58, 8.22], n = 38) but there were no significant differences for the social/family subscale (MD −0.10 [−4.10, 3.90], n = 38), emotional subscale (MD 3.20 [−0.09, 6.49], n = 38), or functional subscale (MD 1.60 [−1.20, 4.40], n = 38).

Ear Acupuncture plus Acupuncture versus No Acupuncture

Three studies (A1.2, A19, A20) were included in this comparison. The previously described three-arm trial on acupuncture for AIMSS (A1) also included a comparison of acupuncture with no acupuncture (A1.2), the results of which are reported in this comparison. The same research group also conducted a randomised, crossover study (A20) of 21 AIMSS participants with BPI ≥3 for the worst pain item. It used the same ear acupuncture plus acupuncture protocol as the three-arm trial (A1), twice weekly for six weeks. It compared the real acupuncture condition with no acupuncture but assessable data were only available for before and after acupuncture treatment, so data were not available for this comparison. Two participants in this study (A20) discontinued treatment due to scheduling difficulties within the first three weeks of treatment.

In another study (A19), 70 cancer patients with chronic pain or dysfunction attributed to neck dissection were randomly assigned to weekly acupuncture versus usual care (e.g. physical therapy, analgesia, and/or anti-inflammatory drugs, per patient preference or physician recommendation) for four weeks. Acupuncture needles were placed at both standard and customised points. Standard distal points (LI4 *Hegu* 合谷, SP6 *Sanyinjiao* 三阴交, GV20 *Baihui* 百会, Extra point *Laozhen* 落枕, auricular TF4 *Shenmen* 神门) were used in all patients. The customised points included (1) scalp acupuncture zones (front, middle and back) on the head chosen according to the primary zone(s) of the pain (these were considered to be customised distal points); (2) local tender points (*ashiyue* 阿是穴) on the body which had the greatest sensitivity to palpation pressure; and (3) the bilateral point LI2 *Erjian* 二间 for patients with dry mouth. The total number of acupuncture points (needles) used ranged from eight points (14 needles) to 26 points (39 needles). Needles were inserted using traditional acupuncture technique to a depth of 0.25 to 0.5 inches and retained for 30 minutes. Needles were stimulated manually, but because the sensitivity of acupuncture points may vary, especially after surgery, no specific *de qi* 得气 response was elicited. Twelve people dropped out, six in the acupuncture group and six in the control group. In each group, three withdrew and three were lost to follow-up.

Pain Intensity

All the studies reported data on pain intensity. Two studies used BPI scores (A1.2, A20) and one study used NRS scores (A19). In each of the RCTs, there were significant reductions within the acupuncture groups but only two studies could be pooled. The pooled result showed a significantly greater reduction in the ear acupuncture plus acupuncture groups compared to the controls that received no acupuncture (MD −1.88 [−2.50, −1.25] $I^2 = 0\%$) without heterogeneity (Table 7.17).

In the pilot crossover RCT (A20), the mean BPI-SF worst pain scores declined after acupuncture treatment (MD 5.3 to 3.3), as did scores for pain severity (3.7 to 2.5), and pain-related interference (3.1 to 1.7) but there were insufficient data for us to conduct significance tests.

Table 7.17 Ear Acupuncture plus Acupuncture versus No Acupuncture: Pain Intensity

Outcome	Condition, Pain Intensity (N. Participants)	Effect Size MD [95% CI]	Included Studies
BPI - worst pain	AIMSS, BPI ≥3 for the worst pain item (152)	−1.76 [−2.49, −1.03]*	A1.2
NRS	Malignant tumour, moderate or severe pain (58)	−2.20 [−3.41, −0.99]*	A19
Pooled result	2 studies (210)	−1.88 [−2.50, −1.25]* 0%	A1.2, A19

*Statistically significant. Abbreviations: AIMSS, aromatase inhibitor-associated musculoskeletal symptoms; BPI, Brief Pain Inventory; CI, confidence interval; MD, mean difference; N., number; NRS, Numeric Rating Scale.

Quality of Life

One study (A1.2) reported on QOL using FACT-ES. There was no significant difference between groups for FACT-ES (MD 4.72 [−0.18, 9.61], $n = 152$) at the end of the treatment.

Ear Acupressure plus Acupuncture plus Conventional Analgesic versus Conventional Analgesic

One RCT (A17) enrolled 60 participants with cancer pain (cancer type unspecified) to receive a combination of ear acupressure plus acupuncture plus conventional analgesics based on the WHO three-step analgesic ladder or conventional analgesics alone. The acupuncture points consisted of a standardised group including the ear points TF4 *Shenmen* 神门, AH6a *Jiaogan* 交感, AT4 *Pizhixia* 皮质下 for acupressure and the traditional points LI4 *Hegu* 合谷 and LR3 *Taichong* 太冲 for acupuncture. In addition, there was an individualised group of two ear points based on the location of tumour invasion and Chinese medicine theory as follows: CO13 *Pi* 脾 and CO4 *Wei* 胃 for gastric cancer, and CO14 *Fei* 肺 and HX2 *Zhichang* 直肠 for rectal cancer. Acupuncture was administered every other day for three sessions followed by a rest of two days as a treatment course, and there were eight courses of treatment. Ear acupressure was done twice a week, using each ear alternately, for a total of 16 times. Both therapies were used simultaneously and the treatment duration was eight weeks. There was no drop-out.

Pain Intensity and Duration of pain

There was a significantly greater reduction in the integrative therapy group for BPI-pain severity at the end of the treatment (MD −1.77 [−2.64, −0.90] n = 60) but the between-group difference was not statistically significant for BPI-pain interference (MD 0.32 [−0.69, 1.33], n = 60).

The average duration of pain was significantly shorter in the integrative group (MD −2.12 [−2.57, −1.67] hours per day, n = 60) than in the conventional analgesic group.

GRADE for Ear Acupuncture plus Acupuncture

Assessments of ear acupuncture plus acupuncture versus sham acupuncture for pain intensity were conducted using the GRADE approach. Two RCTs (A1.1, A18) were included. The pooled result of a mean −1.44 points reduction in BPI- worst pain was not significant, but the heterogeneity (I^2 = 86%) was considerable. The certainty of the evidence was reduced by two categories to 'low' due to the statistical heterogeneity and small sample size (Table 7.18)

Non-controlled Clinical Trial of Ear Acupuncture plus Acupuncture

In a pragmatic pilot study (A26), participants with moderate or severe cancer pain (NRS ≥4) received a maximum of 10 acupuncture treatments on traditional points according to pain location and on four ear points, TF4 *Shenmen* 神门 and three points based on the French system Cingulate gyrus, Point zero, and Subcortex. Of the 115 patients screened, 52 (45%) were eligible and agreed to participate.

Table 7.18 GRADE for Pain Intensity: Ear Acupuncture plus Acupuncture versus Sham Controls

Outcome	Absolute Effect: With Acupuncture	Absolute Effect: With Sham Acupuncture	Relative Effect (95% CI) N. Studies (Participants	Certainty of the Evidence (GRADE)
BPI - worst pain	**3.72 points** Average difference: 1.44 points lower (95% CI: 3.39 points lower to 0.51 points higher	**5.16 points**	**MD −1.44** (−3.39 to 0.51 points) 2 (193)	⊕⊕◯◯ LOW[1,2]

Note: 1) Statistical heterogeneity was considerable; 2) Both randomised controlled trials had small sample sizes. Abbreviations: BPI, Brief Pain Inventory; CI, confidence interval; GRADE, Grading of Recommendations Assessment, Development and Evaluation; MD, mean difference N., number. See Table 7.16 for included studies

Eleven (21%) were lost to follow-up, leaving 41 who completed all study procedures.

Mean BPI-pain severity was 6.0±1.3 at baseline and 3.8±2.0 at the end of treatment. Prescribed pain medications decreased across the course of the study. Patient satisfaction was high: 87% reported that their expectations were met 'very well' or 'extremely well'; 90% said they were likely to participate again; 95% said they were likely to recommend acupuncture to others; and 90% reported they found the service to be 'useful' or 'very useful.' It was concluded that acupuncture was feasible, safe, and a helpful treatment adjunct for the cancer patients experiencing uncontrolled pain in this study.

Safety of Ear Acupuncture or Ear Acupressure plus Acupuncture

All the RCTs reported on AEs. Three RCTs indicated there were no AEs associated with acupuncture therapy (A17, A18, A20). The three-arm study (A1) reported bruising was the most common AEs related to acupuncture therapy. More patients in the real acupuncture group experienced grade 1 bruising (47%) than that in the sham control group (25%). There was one episode of grade 2 presyncope in the real acupuncture group and one episode in the sham control group, and no grade 3 or higher AEs. One study (A19) reported no serious AEs were attributed to acupuncture therapy. Twenty-seven minor events were noted in the study. The most common included temporary increase in pain, minor bruising or bleeding, and constitutional symptoms. The single non-controlled study (A26) mentioned there were no AEs associated with the acupuncture therapy.

Studies of Moxibustion

Two RCTs, no CCTs and no non-controlled studies of moxibustion were identified. One study (A10) compared moxibustion with sham moxibustion while another study (A6) investigated the effects of moxibustion plus conventional analgesic versus conventional analgesic alone. The two RCTs enrolled 324 participants with ages ranging from 26 to 89 years. Following dropouts, 322 participants completed the studies. Neither study used syndrome differentiation. The abdominal points CV4 *Guanyuan* 关元 and CV12 *Zhongwan* 中脘 were used in both studies.

Risk of Bias for Moxibustion

One study (A10) used a secure, computerised database to generate the random sequence, so it was judged 'low' risk for this aspect and 'low' for allocation concealment, as the database ensured full allocation concealment (Table 7.19). The other study (A6) did not report sufficient details on methodological aspects, so it was judged 'unclear' risk for sequence generation and allocation concealment. The study that used a sham control (A10) was judged 'low' risk for blinding of participants and outcome assessors, while the other study was judged 'high' risk. Since blinding of personnel is challenging in moxibustion therapy, both studies were judged 'high' risk. There were no dropouts or few dropouts, so both were assessed as 'low' risk of bias for incomplete outcome data. No protocols could be located, so both were judged 'unclear' risk for selective outcome reporting.

Table 7.19 Risk of Bias of Randomised Controlled Trials of Moxibustion

Risk of Bias Domain	Low Risk *n* (%)	Unclear Risk *n* (%)	High Risk *n* (%)
Sequence generation	1 (50)	1 (50)	0 (0)
Allocation concealment	1 (50)	1 (50)	0 (0)
Blinding of participants	1 (50)	0 (0)	1 (50)
Blinding of personnel[1]	0 (0)	0 (0)	2 (100)
Blinding of outcome assessors	1 (50)	0 (0)	1 (50)
Incomplete outcome data	2 (100)	0 (0)	0 (0)
Selective reporting	0	2 (100)	0 (0)

Note: 1) Blinding of personnel (acupuncturists) is challenging in moxibustion.

Real Moxibustion versus Sham Moxibustion

The sham-controlled two-arm RCT (A10; *n* = 16) investigated the efficacy and safety of moxibustion for relieving cancer pain in patients with metastatic cancer and moderate or severe pain (NRS ≥4). All participants received moxibustion at CV4 *Guanyuan* 关元 and CV12 *Zhongwan* 中脘 plus three *ashi* points 阿是穴, using a moxa cone (1.4 cm diameter, 1.5 cm height, and 150 mg) placed directly on the skin surface. For the real moxibustion group, the moxa cone was removed just before the skin was burnt (when less than 0.5 cm of unburned moxa remained). After one cone was burnt, it was removed and another one was placed on the same point repeatedly for 10 minutes at each session, once daily for seven consecutive days. The sham therapy involved removing the moxa cone earlier so as not to deliver complete heat stimulation to the treatment points (when more than 1 cm of unburned moxa remained). The blinding of the sham moxibustion was credible according to a blinding credibility test. Two participants dropped out during the study period (group not specified); one failed to attend at day 3 due to aggravation of ascites, and the other patient failed to attend at day 2 due to aggravation of pancreatic cancer.

Pain Intensity

The results showed there was a significantly greater reduction in BPI total scores (MD –1.32 [–2.22, –0.42], *n* = 14), BPI-pain intensity (MD –1.28 [–2.22, –0.34], *n* = 14), and BPI pain interference (MD –1.36 [–2.44, –0.28], *n* = 14) in favour of the real moxibustion group at the end of treatment.

Analgesic Dose

For analgesic dose, as morphine equivalent, there was no significant difference between groups for total dose (MD –44.71 [–121.97, 32.55] mg/d, *n* = 14) or change in dose (MD 1.14 [–10.87, 13.15] mg/d, *n* = 14). The authors noted that change in opioid dose was mainly associated with incidents of breakthrough pain.

Quality of Life

At the end of treatment, there was no significant difference between groups for QOL on FACT-G (MD 6.72 [–7.06, 20.50], *n* = 14).

Moxibustion plus Conventional Analgesic versus Conventional Analgesic

An open-label RCT (A6; *n* = 308) compared moxibustion in conjunction with conventional analgesics based on the WHO three-step analgesic ladder compared to conventional analgesics alone for cancer pain. Moxibustion was applied at CV12 *Zhongwan* 中脘, CV8 *Shenque* 神阙 and CV4 *Guanyuan* 关元 using a moxa stick placed 2–3 cm away from the skin over the points to bring a mild warmth to the point location and allow the skin to become slightly red. Treatment was once a day, from one day before until three days after chemotherapy. Each treatment lasted for 20 minutes and two treatments were delivered daily for a total treatment course of four weeks.

All participants received analgesics according to the three-step ladder. The control group did not receive moxibustion.

Pain Intensity

Scores on the NRS at the end of the treatment were significantly lower in the group that also received moxibustion compared to the group that only received conventional therapy (MD −1.45 [−1.75, −1.15], *n* = 308).

Quality of Life

For QOL, on the FACT-G total scores there were significantly greater improvements in the group that received moxibustion in addition to conventional therapy (MD 15.53 [14.66, 16.40], *n* = 308) compared to the no moxibustion group.

Safety of Moxibustion

Only one RCT (A10) reported on AEs, and it indicated there were no AEs associated with moxibustion, although one patient complained about the smell from the moxa as it burned.

Clinical Evidence for Commonly Used Acupuncture Interventions

Due to the diversity in the types of cancer pain and the location of the pain, about 65 traditional acupuncture points and six ear points were included in Chapter 2 based on recommendations in guidelines and contemporary books.

The traditional points used in three or more clinical trials (RCT, CCT and/or non-controlled) were:

- LI4 *Hegu* 合谷 (*n* = 14), PC6 *Neiguan* 内关 (*n* = 6), LI11 *Quchi* 曲池 (*n* = 4), and TE5 *Waiguan* 外关 (*n* = 4) on the arm;

- ST36 *Zusanli* 足三里 (*n* = 11), SP6 *Sanyinjiao* 三阴交 (*n* = 8) and GB34 *Yanglingquan* 阳陵泉 (*n* = 7) on the leg;
- LR3 *taichong* 太冲 (*n* = 7), KI3 *Taixi* 太溪 (*n* = 6), GB41 *Zulinqi* 足临泣 (*n* = 4) and ST41 *Jiexi* 解溪 (*n* = 3) on the foot;
- CV12 *Zhongwan* 中脘 (*n* = 4); and CV4 *Guanyuan* 关元 (*n* = 3) and on the abdomen;
- GV20 *Baihui* 百会 (*n* = 4) on the head.

Of these points, only KI3 *Taixi* 太溪, GB41 *Zulinqi* 足临泣 and ST41 *Jiexi* 解溪 were not mentioned in Chapter 2.

The ear points used in three or more clinical studies (RCT, CCT and/or non-controlled) were TF4 *Shenmen* 神门 (*n* = 9), AH6a *Jiaogan* 交感 (*n* = 8), CO12 *Gan* 肝 (*n* = 5), AT4 *Pizhixia* 皮质下 (n = 4), CO10 *Shen* 肾 (*n* = 4) and CO14 *Fei* 肺 (*n* = 3). Of these, the first three points were recommended in the sources summarised in Chapter 2.

There was a high degree of overlap between the traditional points and ear points included in Chapter 2 and the points used in multiple clinical trials in Chapter 7. This was not surprising since many traditional acupuncture points can be used for pain in the local area or along the course of the meridian. Nevertheless, it does demonstrate that the points tested in the clinical trials were commonly used points for which there was expert consensus regarding their application in cancer pain.

Summary of Clinical Evidence for Acupuncture and Related Therapies

This summary covers the key points of Chapter 7 including a dot-point summary of the main pain-related and QOL results for each category of acupuncture therapy.

Acupuncture and Electroacupuncture

For acupuncture and electroacupuncture, most of the evidence was based on 10 RCTs (574 participants) with supporting data from one CCT, and seven non-controlled studies (three case-series, one retrospective case-series, and three case reports). The results are summarised below.

Acupuncture or Electroacupuncture versus Sham Controls

Sham controls were used in five RCTs. Both groups used the same conventional management.

- Reduction in NRS scores for pain intensity (2 RCTs, n = 87) but heterogeneity was substantial. The GRADE assessment was Low (Table 7.7);
- No improvement on FACT-G (1 RCT, n = 29) or QLQ-C30 (1 RCT, n = 27).

Acupuncture or Electroacupuncture plus Conventional Analgesic versus Conventional Analgesic

Four RCTs did not use a sham control. Both groups used the same conventional analgesic medications.

- Reduction in NRS/VAS scores for pain intensity (3 RCTs, n = 180), but the heterogeneity was substantial. The GRADE assessment was Very Low (Table 7.8);
- Reduction in BPI scores (1 RCT, n = 45);
- Reduction in analgesic onset time, improvement in duration of analgesia, reduction in average frequency of breakthrough pain, reduction in maintenance dose of analgesics (1 RCT, n = 60);
- Improvement on QLQ-C30 (2 RCTs, n = 124) without heterogeneity.

Electroacupuncture plus Conventional Analgesic plus Zolpidem versus Conventional Analgesic plus Zolpidem

In one RCT (A7) the test group received electroacupuncture plus conventional analgesics plus zolpidem while the control group did not receive acupuncture.

- Reduction in NRS scores for pain intensity (1 RCT, n = 100).

Acupuncture plus Kinesiotherapy versus Kinesiotherapy

One RCT (A5) evaluated acupuncture plus kinesiotherapy for rehabilitation of physical and functional disorders in women undergoing breast cancer surgery.

- Reduction in VAS scores for pain intensity (1 RCT, n = 48).

Acupuncture versus Fentanyl Transdermal Patch

One CCT (A22) compared electroacupuncture to fentanyl transdermal patch analgesia and found no significant difference between groups for VAS scores.

- No difference in VAS scores for pain intensity (1 CCT, n = 65).

Non-controlled Studies of Acupuncture or Electroacupuncture

All seven non-controlled studies (n = 95) reported improvements in cancer pain when acupuncture or electroacupuncture were combined with standard medical and supportive care.

Ear Acupuncture and Ear Acupressure

Ear acupuncture or ear acupressure was used in four RCTs (227 participants) and two non-controlled studies. The results for each comparison are summarised below.

Ear Acupuncture versus Sham Ear Acupuncture

Two RCTs used sham controls.

- Reduction in NRS/VAS scores for pain intensity (2 RCTs, n = 80), with substantial heterogeneity. The GRADE assessment was 'low' (Table 7.13);

- Reduction in the maintenance dose of analgesic medication (1 RCT, *n* = 23).

Ear Acupressure plus Conventional Analgesic versus Conventional Analgesic

Two open-label RCTs compared ear acupressure plus conventional analgesics with conventional analgesics alone.

- Reduction in NRS/VAS scores for pain intensity (2 RCTs, *n* = 106), with substantial heterogeneity. The GRADE assessment was 'very low' (Table 7.14);
- Reduction in the maintenance dose of analgesic medication (1 RCT, *n* = 46);
- No difference on KPS (1 RCT, *n* = 60).

Non-controlled Studies of Ear Acupuncture or Ear Acupressure

Both non-controlled studies (*n* = 70) found reductions in pain intensity following ear acupuncture or ear acupressure.

Ear Acupuncture or Ear Acupressure plus Acupuncture

Ear acupuncture or ear acupressure plus traditional acupuncture were used in five RCTs (420 participants) and one non-controlled study. The results for each comparison are summarised below.

Ear Acupuncture plus Acupuncture versus Sham Controls

Two RCTs used sham controls.

- No reduction in BPI - worst pain scores (2 RCTs, *n* = 193), with considerable heterogeneity. The GRADE assessment was 'low' (Table 7.18);

- Improvement in QOL on FACT-G - physical (1 RCT, $n = 38$);
- No difference in QOL on FACT-G - social, FACT-G - emotional, or FACT-G - functional (1 RCT, $n = 38$);
- No difference in QOL on FACT-ES (1 RCT, $n = 155$).

Ear Acupuncture plus Acupuncture versus No Acupuncture

Three RCTs did not use a sham control and the control group received no additional acupuncture.

- Reduction in NRS/BPI scores for pain (2 RCTs, $n = 210$);
- No difference on FACT-ES (1 RCT, $n = 152$).

Ear Acupressure plus Acupuncture plus Conventional Analgesic versus Conventional Analgesic

In one RCT, ear acupressure was combined with manual acupuncture plus conventional analgesics while the control group only received the same conventional analgesics.

- Reduction in BPI pain severity scores, shorter duration of pain (1 RCT, $n = 60$);
- No difference in BPI pain interference scores (1 RCT, $n = 60$).

Non-controlled Study of Ear Acupuncture plus Acupuncture

The single case-series study ($n = 41$) found pain relief following treatment with individualized ear acupuncture plus traditional acupuncture.

Moxibustion

Moxibustion was investigated in 2 RCTs (324 participants). The results for each comparison are summarised below.

Moxibustion versus Sham Moxibustion

One RCT used a sham control.

- Reduction in BPI scores for pain (1 RCT, $n = 14$);
- No reduction in analgesic dose (1 RCT, $n = 14$);
- No difference on QOL using FACT-G (1 RCT, $n = 14$).

Moxibustion plus Conventional Analgesic versus Conventional Analgesic

In one RCT, moxibustion was combined with conventional analgesics while the control group only received the same conventional analgesics.

- Reduction in NRS scores for pain intensity (1 RCT, $n = 308$);
- Improvement in QOL on FACT-G (1 RCT, $n = 308$).

Safety of Acupuncture Therapies

Regarding the safety of the acupuncture interventions, 14 of the 21 RCTs mentioned safety. Local dermal symptoms such as bruising and rash were the most frequently reported adverse events (AEs) for the application of acupuncture. No dropouts were attributed to side effects related to acupuncture treatment. Overall, acupuncture was a relatively safe treatment for cancer pain control. No AEs were reported for moxibustion.

References

1. Chiu HY, Hsieh YJ, Tsai PS. (2017) Systematic review and meta-analysis of acupuncture to reduce cancer-related pain. *Eur J Cancer Care (Engl)* **26(2)**.
2. Li H. (2016) A systematic review of randomized controlled trials of acupuncture treatment for cancer pain [Master's thesis]. Heilongjiang University of Chinese Medicine.

3. Hu C, Zhang H, Wu W, *et al.* (2016) Acupuncture for pain management in cancer: A systematic review and meta-analysis. *Evid Based Complement Alternat Med* **2016:** 1720239.
4. Paley CA, Johnson MI, Tashani OA, Bagnall AM. (2015) Acupuncture for cancer pain in adults. *Cochrane Database Syst Rev* **(10):** CD007753.
5. Zhou J, Liang Y, Chen Q, Fang JQ. (2014) Meta-analysis on randomized controlled clinical trials of auricular acupuncture on cancer pain. *Chinese Archives of Traditional Chinese Medicine* **(10):** 2326–2330.
6. Zheng Y, Yu YH, Fang FF. (2014) Meta-analysis on wrist-ankle acupuncture of cancerous pain. *Journal of Liaoning University of Traditional Chinese Medicine* **(01):** 152–155.
7. Choi TY, Lee MS, Kim TH, *et al.* (2012) Acupuncture for the treatment of cancer pain: A systematic review of randomised clinical trials. *Support Care Cancer* **20(6):** 1147–1158.
8. Peng H, Peng HD, Xu L, Lao LX. (2010) Efficacy of acupuncture in treatment of cancer pain: A systemaitic review. *J Chin Integr Med* **8(6):** 501–509.
9. Lee H, Schmidt K, Ernst E. (2004) Acupuncture for the relief of cancer-related pain: A systematic review. *Eur J Pain* **9(4):** 437–444.
10. Bardia A, Barton DL, Prokop LJ, *et al.* (2006) Efficacy of complementary and alternative medicine therapies in relieving cancer pain: A systematic review. *J Clin Oncol* **24(34):** 5457–5464.
11. Pan Y, Yang K, Shi X, *et al.* (2018) Clinical benefits of acupuncture for the reduction of hormone therapy-related side effects in breast cancer patients: A systematic review. *Integr Cancer Ther* **17(3):** 602–618.
12. Yang GS, Kim HJ, Griffith KA, *et al.* (2017) Interventions for the treatment of aromatase inhibitor-associated arthralgia in breast cancer survivors: A systematic review and meta-analysis. *Cancer Nurs* **40(4):** E26–E41.
13. Chen L, Lin CC, Huang TW, *et al.* (2017) Effect of acupuncture on aromatase inhibitor-induced arthralgia in patients with breast cancer: A meta-analysis of randomized controlled trials. *Breast* **33:** 132–138.
14. Lee PL, Tam KW, Yeh ML, Wu WW. (2016) Acupoint stimulation, massage therapy and expressive writing for breast cancer: A systematic review and meta-analysis of randomized controlled trials. *Complement Ther Med* **27:** 87–101.
15. Chien TJ, Liu CY, Chang YF, *et al.* (2015) Acupuncture for treating aromatase inhibitor-related arthralgia in breast cancer: A systematic review and meta-analysis. *J Altern Complement Med* **21(5):** 251–260.

16. Bae K, Yoo HS, Lamoury G, *et al.* (2015) Acupuncture for aromatase inhibitor-induced arthralgia: A systematic review. *Integr Cancer Ther* **14(6):** 496–502.
17. Dos Santos S, Hill N, Morgan A, *et al.* (2010) Acupuncture for treating common side effects associated with breast cancer treatment: A systematic review. *Med Acupunct* **22(2):** 81–97.
18. Chao LF, Zhang AL, Liu HE, *et al.* (2009) The efficacy of acupoint stimulation for the management of therapy-related adverse events in patients with breast cancer: A systematic review. *Breast Cancer Res Treat* **118(2):** 255–267.
19. Tao WW, Jiang H, Tao XM, *et al.* (2016) Effects of acupuncture, tuina, tai chi, qigong, and traditional Chinese medicine five-element music therapy on symptom management and quality of life for cancer patients: A meta-analysis. *J Pain Symptom Manage* **51(4):** 728–747.
20. Lau CH, Wu X, Chung VC, *et al.* (2016) Acupuncture and related therapies for symptom management in palliative cancer care: Systematic review and meta-analysis. *Medicine (Baltimore)* **95(9):** e2901.
21. Lian WL, Pan MQ, Zhou DH, Zhang ZJ. (2013) Effectiveness of acupuncture for palliative care in cancer patients: A systematic review. *Chin J Integr Med* **20(2):** 136–147.
22. Garcia MK, McQuade J, Haddad R, *et al.* (2013) Systematic review of acupuncture in cancer care: A synthesis of the evidence. *J Clin Oncol* **31(7):** 952–960.
23. Pan CX, Morrison RS, Ness J, *et al.* (2000) Complementary and alternative medicine in the management of pain, dyspnea, and nausea and vomiting near the end of life: A systematic review. *J Pain Symptom Manage* **20(5):** 374–387.
24. Cella DF, Tulsky DS, Gray G, Sarafian B, Linn E, Bonomi A, Silberman M, Yellen SB, Winicour P, Brannon J, *et al.* (1993) The Functional Assessment of Cancer Therapy scale: development and validation of the general measure. *J Clin Oncol.* **11(3):** 570–579. doi: 10.1200/JCO.1993.11.3.570.
25. Cheung YB, Thumboo J, Goh C, Khoo KS, Che W, Wee J. (2004) The equivalence and difference between the English and Chinese versions of two major, cancer-specific, health-related quality-of-life questionnaires. *Cancer.* **101(12):** 2874–2880. doi: 10.1002/cncr.20681. PMID: 15529310.
26. Aaronson NK, Ahmedzai S, Bergman B, Bullinger M, Cull A, Duez NJ, Filiberti A, Flechtner H, Fleishman SB, de Haes JC, *et al.* (1993) The

European Organization for Research and Treatment of Cancer QLQ-C30: a quality-of-life instrument for use in international clinical trials in oncology. *J Natl Cancer Inst.* **85(5):** 365–376. doi: 10.1093/jnci/85.5.365. PMID: 8433390.

27. Bruera E, Kuehn N, Miller MJ, Selmser P, Macmillan K. (1991) The Edmonton Symptom Assessment System (ESAS): a simple method for the assessment of palliative care patients. *J Palliat Care.* **7(2):** 6–9. PMID: 1714502.
28. Fallowfield LJ, Leaity SK, Howell A, Benson S, Cella D. (1999) Assessment of quality of life in women undergoing hormonal therapy for breast cancer: validation of an endocrine symptom subscale for the FACT-B. *Breast Cancer Res Treat.* **55(2):** 189–199. doi: 10.1023/a:1006263818115. PMID: 10481946.

References to Included Studies

Study Number	Reference
A1	Hershman DL, Unger JM, Greenlee H, *et al.* (2018) Effect of acupuncture vs sham acupuncture or waitlist control on joint pain related to aromatase inhibitors among women with early-stage breast cancer. *JAMA* **320(2):** 167.
A2	Kim K, Lee S. (2018) Intradermal acupuncture along with analgesics for pain control in advanced cancer cases: A pilot, randomized, patient-assessor-blinded, controlled trial. *Integr Cancer Ther* **17(4):** 1137–1143.
A3	Ruela LO, Iunes DH, Nogueira DA, *et al.* (2018) Effectiveness of auricular acupuncture in the treatment of cancer pain: Randomized clinical trial. *Rev Esc Enferm USP* **52:** e03402.
A4a	王颖. (2016) 电针联合羟考酮缓释片治疗晚期非小细胞肺癌癌痛的临床研究. 学位论文. 浙江中医药大学 2–14.
A4b	王颖, 王晓艳, 王辉, 张亚萍, 方红明 (2017) 电针联合羟考酮缓释片治疗晚期非小细胞肺癌癌痛30例. 浙江中医杂志 **52(9):** 684–685.
A5	Giron PS, Haddad CA, Lopes de Almeida Rizzi SK, *et al.* (2016). Effectiveness of acupuncture in rehabilitation of physical and functional disorders of women undergoing breast cancer surgery. *Support Care Cancer* **24(6):** 2491–2496.

(*Continued*)

(*Continued*)

Study Number	Reference
A6	李玲, 高翠霞, 何炜, 马桂霞, 王炜炜, 司慧彬, 孟雨姗. (2016) 温阳艾灸法联合三阶梯止痛法对癌痛患者止痛效果和生活质量的影响. 中医研究 **29(9):** 48–50.
A7	沈陆斐, 陈文宇, 吕晓东, 刘加良, 杨新妹, 姚明, 倪华栋. (2016) 电针对改善肺癌疼痛患者睡眠质量的疗效观察. 医学研究杂志 **45(6):** 87–90.
A8	郭宗兵, 郭广红, 杨际平, 邵颖. (2015) 针刺治疗对胃癌晚期患者疼痛和生活质量的影响. 国际中医中药杂志 **37(4):** 371–373.
A9	王敬, 芦殿荣, 毕然, 舒晓宁. (2015) 耳穴埋豆干预骨转移中重度癌性疼痛临床观察 30 例. 云南中医中药杂志 **36(2):** 43–45.
A10	Lee J, Yoon SW. (2014) Efficacy and safety of moxibustion for relieving pain in patients with metastatic cancer: A pilot, randomized, single-blind, sham-controlled trial. *Integr Cancer Ther* **13(3):** 211–216.
A11	Mao JJ, Xie SX, Farrar JT, *et al.* (2014) A randomised trial of electro-acupuncture for arthralgia related to aromatase inhibitor use. *Eur J Cancer* **50(2):** 267–276.
A12	Bao T, Cai L, Giles JT, *et al.* (2013) A dual-center randomized controlled double blind trial assessing the effect of acupuncture in reducing musculoskeletal symptoms in breast cancer patients taking aromatase inhibitors. *Breast Cancer Res Treat* **138(1):** 167–174.
A13	Chen H, Liu TY, Kuai L, *et al.* (2013) Electroacupuncture treatment for pancreatic cancer pain: A randomized controlled trial. *Pancreatology* **13(6):** 594–597.
A14	Oh B, Kimble B, Costa DS, *et al.* (2013) Acupuncture for treatment of arthralgia secondary to aromatase inhibitor therapy in women with early breast cancer: Pilot study. *Acupunct Med* **31(3):** 264–271.
A15	沈健美, 张文涛, 吴倩影, 王东升. (2013) 电针经穴治疗晚期肝癌患者癌性疼痛临床研究. 辽宁中医药大学学报 **15(9):** 189–191.
A16	朱利楠, 王瑞林, 宗红, 樊青霞. (2013) 磁珠耳穴贴压联合奥施康定治疗癌症神经病理性疼痛的疗效观察. 中华物理医学与康复杂志 **35(7):** 579–581.
A17	蒋坤融. (2011) 针刺四关穴结合耳压治疗癌性疼痛的临床研究. 学位论文. 广州中医药大学.

Study Number	Reference
A18	Crew KD, Capodice JL, Greenlee H, *et al.* (2010) Randomized, blinded, sham-controlled trial of acupuncture for the management of aromatase inhibitor-associated joint symptoms in women with early-stage breast cancer. *J Clin Oncol* **28(7):** 1154–1160.
A19	Pfister DG, Cassileth BR, Deng GE, *et al.* (2010) Acupuncture for pain and dysfunction after neck dissection: Results of a randomized controlled trial. *J Clin Oncol* **28(15):** 2565–2570.
A20	Crew KD, Capodice JL, Greenlee H, *et al.* (2007) Pilot study of acupuncture for the treatment of joint symptoms related to adjuvant aromatase inhibitor therapy in postmenopausal breast cancer patients. *J Cancer Surviv* **1(4):** 283–291.
A21	Alimi D, Rubino C, Pichard-Leandri CE, *et al.* (2003) Analgesic effect of auricular acupuncture for cancer pain: A randomized, blinded, controlled trial. *J Clin Oncol* **21(22):** 4120–4126.
A22	Xu LL, Wan YX, Huang J and Xu F. (2018) Clinical analysis of electroacupuncture and multiple acupoint stimulation in relieving cancer pain in patients with advanced hepatocellular carcinoma. *J Cancer Res Ther* **14(1):** 99–102.
A23	Miller KR, Patel JN, Symanowski JT, *et al.* (2019) Acupuncture for cancer pain and symptom management in a palliative medicine clinic. *Am J Hosp Palliat Care* **36(4):** 326–332.
A24	Su CF. (2018) Home care with acupuncture increased the quality of life in a patient with advanced cancer with neuropathic pain induced by bone metastasis: A case report. *J Integr Med* **16(3):** 208–210.
A25	Yeh CH, Chien LC, Chiang YC, *et al.* (2015) Auricular point acupressure as an adjunct analgesic treatment for cancer patients: A feasibility study. *Pain Manag Nurs* **16(3):** 285–293.
A26	Garcia MK, Driver L, Haddad R, *et al.* (2014) Acupuncture for treatment of uncontrolled pain in cancer patients: A pragmatic pilot study. *Integr Cancer Ther* **13(2):** 133–140.
A27	Vinjamury SP, Li JT, Hsiao E, *et al.* (2013) Effects of acupuncture for cancer pain and quality of life: A case series. *Chin Med* **8(1):** 15.
A28	Paley CA, Johnson MI. (2011) Acupuncture for cancer-induced bone pain: A pilot study. *Acupunct Med* **29(1):** 71–73.

(*Continued*)

(*Continued*)

Study Number	Reference
A29	Tuck CM. (2010) A 54-year-old woman with degenerative back pain. *Acupunct Med* **28(1):** 46–48.
A30	Mao JJ, Bruner DW, Stricker C, *et al.* (2009) Feasibility trial of electroacupuncture for aromatase inhibitor-related arthralgia in breast cancer survivors. *Integr Cancer Ther* **8(2):** 123–129.
A31	Jenner C, Filshie J. (2002) Galactorrhoea following acupuncture. *Acupunct Med* **20(2–3):** 107–108.
A32	Alimi D, Rubino C, Leandri EP, Brule SF. (2000) Analgesic effects of auricular acupuncture for cancer pain. *J Pain Symptom Manage* **19(2):** 81–82.

8

Clinical Evidence for Other Chinese Medicine Therapies

OVERVIEW

In addition to Chinese herbal medicine and acupuncture, other therapies are used in Chinese medicine. These include forms of remedial massage, cupping, exercise therapies and special dietary interventions for specific diseases and/or symptoms. This chapter reviews and assesses the evidence for these other therapies for cancer pain and includes studies of remedial massage.

Introduction

Besides Chinese herbal medicine (CHM), acupuncture and moxibustion, Chinese medicine (CM) includes a range of other CM therapies for managing diseases and maintaining health. These include but are not limited to:

- Remedial massage therapies, such as the *tui na* 推拿 and *an mo* 按摩 forms of remedial massage;
- Exercise therapies such as the various styles of *tai chi* (*tai ji quan* 太极拳), various forms of *dao yin yang sheng gong* 导引养生功 and various types of *qi gong* 气功;
- Cupping therapy; and
- Dietary therapies based on CM theory.

Previous Systematic Reviews

Systematic reviews of various types of complementary therapies,[1,2] integrative therapy,[3] massage therapy,[4–10] *tai chi/qi gong*[11–13] and cupping therapy[14] for relief of pain and other symptoms in cancer patients were identified. However, only a few studies were of Chinese massage therapy for cancer pain, and none of the studies of *tai chi/qi gong* were cancer pain-specific. No systematic review of Chinese dietary therapy for cancer pain was located.

Identification of Clinical Studies

The search and selection process identified one randomised controlled trial (RCT), zero non-randomised controlled clinical trials (CCT) and one non-controlled study of other Chinese medicine therapies for cancer pain as eligible for inclusion (Fig. 8.1).

One RCT and one non-controlled study were of Chinese massage therapy (O1, O2). Studies of other types of massage therapy including reflexology were excluded. A single-group study from Korea tested hand massage using an aromatic oil composed of bergamot, lavender and frankincense for hospice patients with terminal cancer. It reported a reduction in pain score but the paper was written in Korean and only the abstract was available in English so it was not possible to determine if the massage style was a form of *tui na* 推拿, *an mo* 按摩 or another method.[15] Two RCTs of Chinese dietary therapy were excluded since not all participants had pain due to cancer at baseline.[16,17] One Chinese study of cupping for cancer pain was identified but the control group used the drug dextropropoxyphene which has been discontinued so this study was excluded.[18] All the studies of *tai chi/qi gong* were of quality of life measures and did not require pain to be present at baseline, so these were excluded.

Summary of Clinical Evidence for Other Chinese Medicine Therapies

Clinical evidence was available for one RCT and one non-controlled study of Chinese remedial massage.

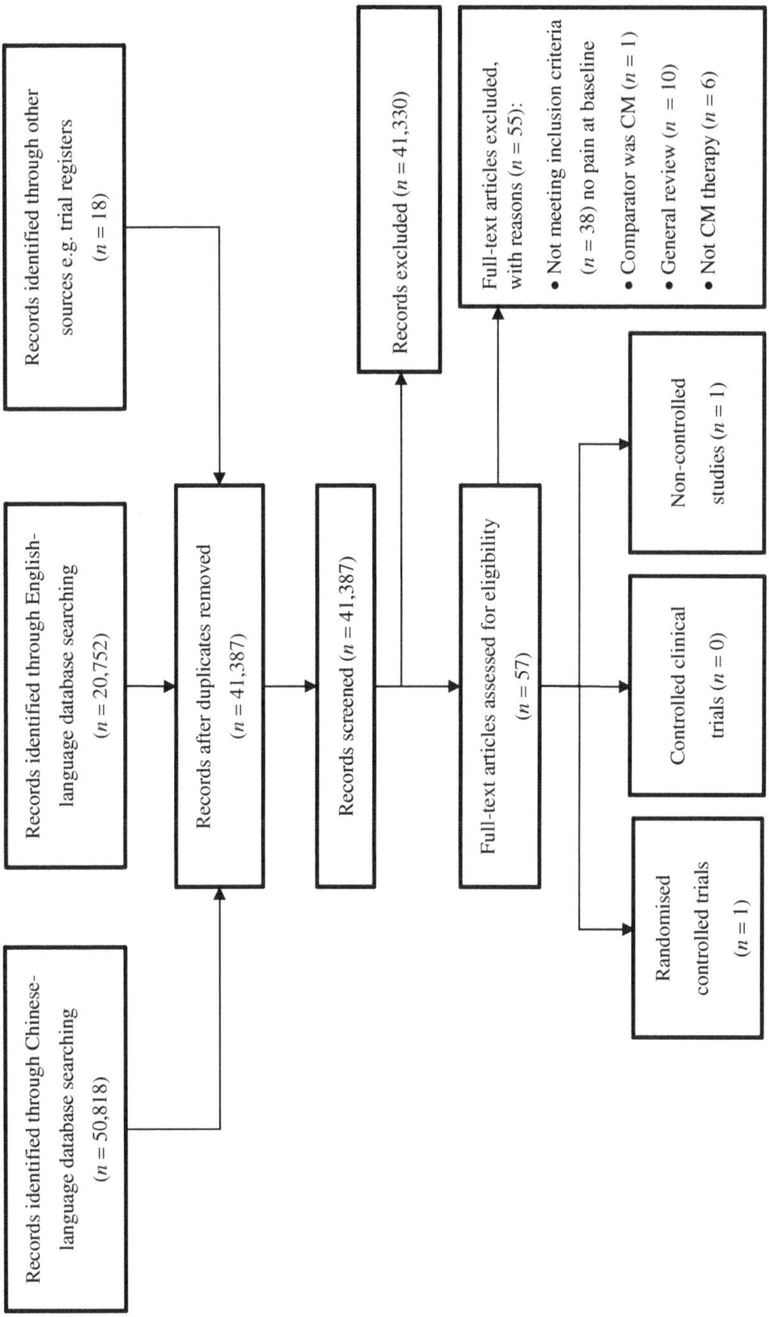

Fig. 8.1 Flowchart of study selection process: Other therapies

Chinese Remedial Massage

Of the potential studies of massage, most did not use a form of Chinese massage therapy, were of foot massage or hand massage, and/or were for a range of symptoms including pain but did not require pain at baseline. Only one RCT (O1) and one non-controlled study (O2) were included. No CCTs were identified.

Randomised Controlled Trials

One multi-centre RCT (five centres) conducted in Taiwan was of an unnamed remedial massage intervention that appeared to be a form of *an mo* 按摩 that only included participants who had cancer pain associated with bone metastases and had a pain intensity of VAS ≥ 4 on a ten-point scale (O1). It compared a full-body massage that was adapted to the person and the location of the bone metastases. The duration of a massage session was about 45 minutes and this was compared to a 45-minute session of social attention as an inactive control. Each group included 36 in-patient participants who received three sessions delivered by trained nurses over three to four days.

Risk of Bias

The risk of bias was judged to be low for sequence allocation which was conducted using computer-based minimisation to minimise variance between groups due to differences in pain intensity, analgesic use and other variables. Due to the obvious differences in interventions, we judged the risk of bias to be high for blinding of participants, and investigators, and unclear risk for outcome assessors. There were two drop-outs in the massage group and three in the social attention group after session one. These were documented as 'having physical distress' (T = 1, C = 2); 'progress of disease' (T = 1, C = 0); and 'feeling stressed' (T = 0, C = 1); and intent-to-treat (ITT) analysis was conducted, so the study was judged as 'low risk' for incomplete data. All data appear to have been reported but there was no reference to a trial protocol, so the study was judged 'unclear risk' for selective outcome reporting.

Results

The outcome measure for pain was a visual analogue scale (VAS) for present pain intensity. This was presented in a vertical form since Chinese patients are accustomed to reading from top the bottom. It comprised a 100-mm line with 'pain as bad as it could be' (10 points) at the top and 'no pain' (0 points) at the bottom. The VAS was assessed immediately prior to each session and 20 minutes after each session. Results were presented for differences within and between groups for each of the three sessions. The authors reported that the intention-to-treat (ITT) analysis found greater pain reductions in the massage group after each session. Our analysis of the mean data based on as-treated numbers found no baseline imbalances and similar between-groups results for session 1: MD −1.60 [−2.65, −0.55], $n = 72$; session 2: MD −1.40 [−2.36, −0.44], $n = 67$; and session 3: MD −1.60 [−2.70, −0.50] $n = 67$; indicating significantly greater improvements in the massage therapy group compared to the social attention control group. The authors reported that a reduction of one point or more was considered clinically significant.

In addition, the authors reported significant improvements in VAS for mood in the first two sessions but not the third session, in VAS for relaxation after each session, but no significant differences for a sleep VAS. The authors reported there were no adverse events associated with the massage.

Non-controlled Studies

The single non-controlled study (O2) was the pilot for the above RCT. It tested the same massage intervention in 30 in-patients with bone metastases and pain using the same VAS for pain at various time points after the massage. In addition, a questionnaire based on the Short-Form McGill Pain Questionnaire and the brief pain inventory was used to assess pain at 16–18 hours post-intervention.

The results for the pain VAS showed significant reductions in pain compared to before the intervention at all time-points from immediately after massage to 16–18 hours after massage. The pain questionnaire showed a reduction in total scores and in the sub-scores for number of pain locations, present pain and worst pain. In addition, there were significant reductions in VAS for anxiety. No patient reported any adverse effect of the massage. In the recruitment phase, some patients refused participation due to allodynia and concern over the safety of massage and whether it could provoke bone pain.

Summary of Clinical Evidence for Other Chinese Medicine Therapies

Only two studies were included in this section. The non-controlled pilot study and the subsequent RCT suggest that a massage intervention in Chinese patients with metastatic bone pain produced clinically significant pain relief following the intervention. Although the non-controlled study suggested that pain relief was still present at 16–18 hours post-intervention, the RCT only provided assessable data at 20 minutes post-intervention, so it was not possible to determine how long the pain relief persisted. Three massage sessions were delivered; each produced a similar result, so there appeared to be no tolerance. Despite the presence of bone metastases, there were no adverse effects. However, the authors noted that the massage was adapted to the patient, areas of metastasis and tumours were avoided, and people with allodynia were excluded. These aspects suggest that massage may only be applicable to certain cancer pain patients and it is unclear how long the effects persist or how many sessions could be tolerated. Both these studies were limited by lack of blinding and the studies may not have provided complete data for all outcome measures. Consequently, it was not possible to draw any conclusions regarding the effectiveness of these therapies in cancer pain.

A Cochrane review found low-quality evidence for massage therapy (any type) versus no massage therapy for improving cancer pain in the short term[4] and another review found a similar result.[8] A recent clinical guideline for integrative therapies in breast cancer included massage therapy interventions for depression/mood disturbances (B grade evidence), anxiety and stress reduction (C grade evidence), but did not include an assessment of massage therapy for cancer pain,[19] while a wide-ranging review of non-pharmacologic therapies for pain noted that massage therapy was a low-risk intervention that has shown effects in various types of chronic pain but did not make mention of cancer pain.[20]

Overall, the evidence for Chinese remedial massage for treating people with cancer pain is promising but not sufficient for a conclusion to be made regarding its efficacy and safety. However, it is important to note that massage therapy should avoid pressure on lesion areas and be adapted to the needs of the individual person. For dietary therapies, exercise therapies and cupping, there is very little assessable evidence of direct relevance to people with pain due to cancer.

References

1. Bardia A, Barton DL, Prokop LJ, *et al.* (2006) Efficacy of complementary and alternative medicine therapies in relieving cancer pain: A systematic review. *J Clin Oncol* **24(34):** 5457–5464.
2. Cassileth B, Trevisan C, Gubili J. (2007) Complementary therapies for cancer pain. *Curr Pain Headache Rep* **11(4):** 265–269.
3. Running A, Seright T. (2012) Integrative oncology: Managing cancer pain with complementary and alternative therapies. *Curr Pain Headache Rep* **16(4):** 325–331.
4. Shin ES, Seo KH, Lee SH, *et al.* (2016) Massage with or without aromatherapy for symptom relief in people with cancer. *Cochrane Database Syst Rev* **(6):** CD009873.
5. Calenda E. (2006) Massage therapy for cancer pain. *Curr Pain Headache Rep* **10(4):** 270–274.
6. Liu Y, Fawcett TN. (2008) The role of massage therapy in the relief of cancer pain. *Nurs Stand* **22(21):** 35–40.
7. Somani S, Merchant S, Lalani S. (2013) A literature review about effectiveness of massage therapy for cancer pain. *JPMA* **63(11):** 1418–1421.
8. Lee SH, Kim JY, Yeo S, *et al.* (2015) Meta-analysis of massage therapy on cancer pain. *Integr Cancer Ther* **14(4):** 297–304.
9. Jane SW, Wilkie DJ, Gallucci BB, Beaton RD. (2008) Systematic review of massage intervention for adult patients with cancer: A methodological perspective. *Cancer Nurs* **31(6):** E24–E35.

10. Boyd C, Crawford C, Paat CF, *et al.* (2016) The impact of massage therapy on function in pain populations: A systematic review and meta-analysis of randomized controlled trials: Part ii, cancer pain populations. *Pain Med* **17(8):** 1553–1568.
11. Tao WW, Jiang H, Tao XM, *et al.* (2016) Effects of acupuncture, tuina, tai chi, qigong, and traditional Chinese medicine five-element music therapy on symptom management and quality of life for cancer patients: A meta-analysis. *J Pain Symptom Manage* **51(4):** 728–747.
12. Klein PJ, Schneider R, Rhoads CJ. (2016) Qigong in cancer care: A systematic review and construct analysis of effective qigong therapy. *Support Care Cancer* **24(7):** 3209–3222.
13. Zeng Y, Luo T, Xie H, *et al.* (2014) Health benefits of qigong or tai chi for cancer patients: A systematic review and meta-analyses. *Complement Ther Med* **22(1):** 173–186.
14. Kim JI, Lee MS, Lee DH, *et al.* (2011) Cupping for treating pain: A systematic review. *Evid Based Complement Alternat Med* **2011:** 467014.
15. Chang SY. (2008) Effects of aroma hand massage on pain, state anxiety and depression in hospice patients with terminal cancer. *Taehan Kanho Hakhoe Chi* **38(4):** 493–502.
16. Wu TH, Chiu TY, Tsai JS, *et al.* (2008) Effectiveness of Taiwanese traditional herbal diet for pain management in terminal cancer patients. *Asia Pac J Clin Nutr* **17(1):** 17–22.
17. Wu TH, Chiu TY, Chen CY, Yang LL. (2006) Evaluation of herb drug rice milk for palliation of terminal cancer pain 藥膳米漿緩解癌末疼痛之評估. 安寧療護雜誌 **11(2):** 137–149.
18. Huang ZF, Li HZ, Zhang ZJ, *et al.* (2006) Observations on the efficacy of cupping for treating 30 patients with cancer pain. *Shanghai Journal of Acupuncture and Moxibustion* **25(8):** 14–15.
19. Greenlee H, DuPont-Reyes MJ, Balneaves LG, *et al.* (2017) Clinical practice guidelines on the evidence-based use of integrative therapies during and after breast cancer treatment. *CA Cancer J Clin* **67(3):** 195–232.
20. Tick H, Nielsen A, Pelletier KR, *et al.* (2018) Evidence-based nonpharmacologic strategies for comprehensive pain care: The consortium pain task force white paper. *Explore (NY)* **14(3):** 177–211.

References to Included Studies

Study Number	Reference
O1	Jane SW, Chen SL, Wilkie DJ, *et al.* (2011). Effects of massage on pain, mood status, relaxation, and sleep in Taiwanese patients with metastatic bone pain: A randomized clinical trial. *Pain* **152(10):** 2432–2442.
O2	Jane SW, Wilkie DJ, Gallucci BB, *et al.* (2009). Effects of a full-body massage on pain intensity, anxiety, and physiological relaxation in Taiwanese patients with metastatic bone pain: A pilot study. *J Pain Symptom Manage* **37(4):** 754–763.

9

Clinical Evidence for Combination Therapies

OVERVIEW

The searches identified one randomised controlled trial, one non-randomised controlled clinical trial and no non-controlled studies. The randomised controlled trial used an oral Chinese herbal medicine combined with transcutaneous electrical nerve stimulation on acupuncture points. The controlled clinical trial combined a topical Chinese herbal medicine with *an mo* 按摩 remedial massage. Both studies assessed the effects of the combination therapies on pain and adverse effects associated with pain medications.

Introduction

Combination therapies are defined as two or more Chinese medicine (CM) interventions administered together, for example Chinese herbal medicine (CHM) plus acupuncture. No previous systematic review of CHM combined with acupuncture or other combinations of CM therapies for cancer pain could be located.

Identification of Clinical Studies

The searches identified one randomised controlled trial (RCT) (C1) that tested the combination of an oral CHM plus transcutaneous electrical nerve stimulation (TENS) on acupuncture points (acu-TENS), and one non-randomised controlled clinical trial (CCT) that tested the combination of a topical CHM and *an mo* 按摩 (C2) (Fig. 9.1). No non-controlled study satisfied the inclusion criteria.

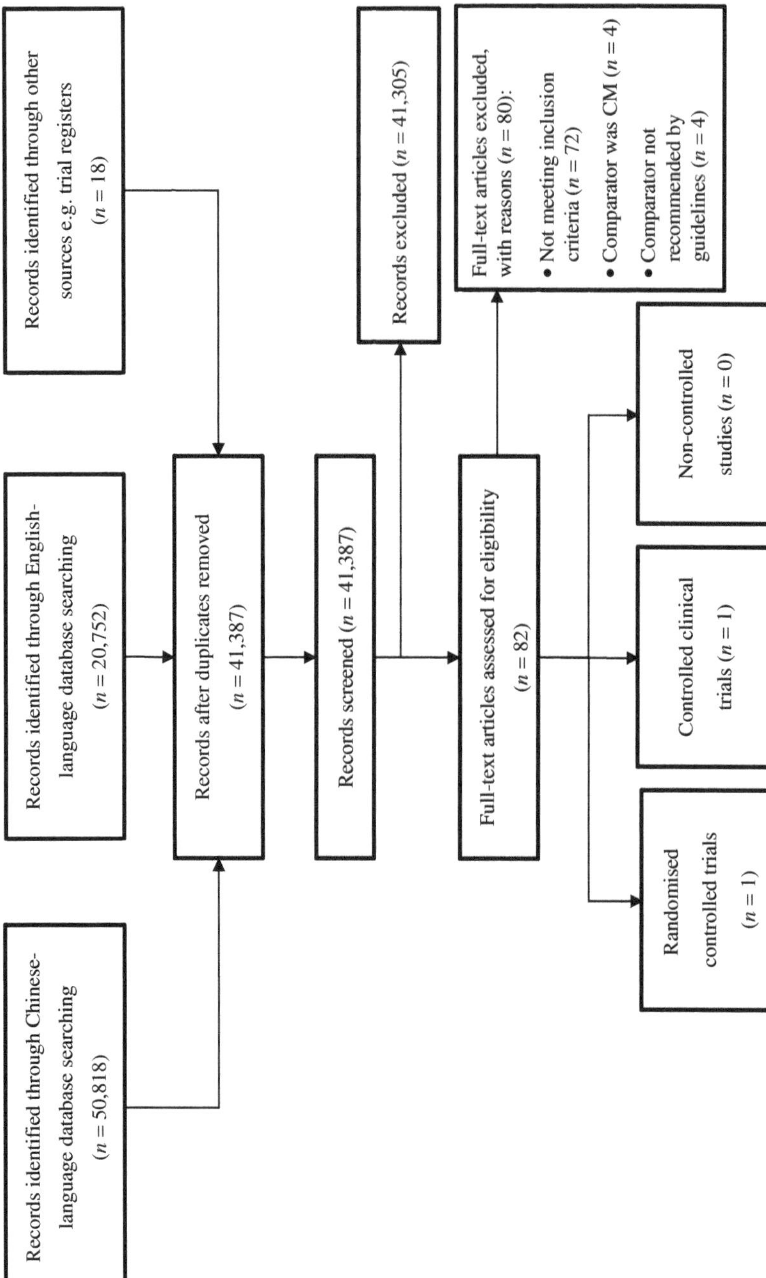

Fig. 9.1 Flowchart of study selection process: Combination therapies

Randomised Controlled Trials of Combination Therapies

Only one RCT (C1) of oral CHM plus acu-TENs was included in this section. This study was conducted in mainland China and enrolled 165 participants whose ages ranged from 18 to 70 years. There were no drop-outs. The study did not mention Chinese medicine syndrome differentiation.

In this study, all participants had various malignancies with moderate or severe pain (NRS ≥ 4). All were treated with morphine sulfate sustained-release tablets (4 ≤ NRS ≤ 6, started with 10 mg; 7 ≤ NRS ≤ 10, started with 20 mg), taken once every 12 hours, with the dose adjusted according to the patient's pain relief for four weeks. In the CM group, the people (*n* = 84) also received an oral formula designed by the authors called *Xiao ji zhi tong fang* 消积止痛方 (*chuan xiong* 川芎, *tao ren* 桃仁, *hong hua* 红花, *yan hu suo* 延胡索, *ru xiang* 乳香, *mo yao* 没药, *wu ling zhi* 五灵脂, *huai niu xi* 怀牛膝, *huang qi* 黄芪, *gan cao* 甘草, etc.) one packet per day in two doses for four weeks, plus TENs was applied at LI4 *Hegu* 合谷, ST36 *Zusanli* 足三里, EX-B2 *Jiajixue* 夹脊穴 and *ashi* points 阿是穴 for four weeks.

For sequence generation the risk of bias was judged 'low risk' due to the description of the details of a proper method of randomisation. There was no mention of a method of allocation concealment, so the risk of bias was judged as 'unclear risk'. There was no mention of blinding of participants, personnel or outcome assessors so these domains were all judged as 'high risk' for blinding of participants and personnel and 'unclear risk' for blinding of outcome assessors. Since there were no drop-outs, the study was judged 'low risk' for incomplete outcome data. No protocol could be located but all the outcomes appear to have been reported, so the study was judged 'unclear risk' for selective outcome reporting.

There was a significantly greater reduction in the integrative medicine group for NRS scores (MD –0.36 [–0.42, –0.30], *n* = 165) and analgesic onset time (MD –16.09 [–22.09, –10.09] minutes, *n* = 165), and there was a significantly greater increase in duration of

Table 9.1 Oral CHM plus Acu-TENs plus Conventional Analgesic versus Conventional Analgesic: Adverse Reactions (Criteria Not Specified)

Adverse Reaction	Effect Size RR [95% CI]	Included Studies (*n* Participants)
Nausea and vomiting	0.14 [0.06, 0.34]*	C1 (165)
Constipation	0.51 [0.32, 0.81]*	
Dizziness	0.75 [0.29, 1.92]	
Drowsiness	0.85 [0.52, 1.38]	

*Statistically significant.
Abbreviations: CI, confidence interval; *n*, number; RR, relative risk.

analgesia (MD 1.67 [0.51, 2.83] hours, *n* = 165) compared to the control that received morphine sulfate sustained-release tablets alone.

This study also reported on adverse reactions but did not specify which criteria were used. There were significant reductions in the incidence of people experiencing nausea and vomiting (RR 0.14 [0.06, 0.34]) and constipation (RR 0.51 [0.32, 0.81]) in the integrative group, but no significant difference between groups in the incidence of dizziness and drowsiness (Table 9.1).

Controlled Clinical Trials of Combination Therapies

One CCT was identified (C2). This study specifically recruited 50 people (34–83 years old) with various malignancies and bone metastases. All had moderate or severe pain (NRS ≥ 4). Thirty people in the CM group received *Mo tong gao* 摩痛膏 (*fu zi* 附子, *wu tou* 乌头, *nan xing* 南星, *san qi* 三七, *bing pian* 冰片, *ding xiang* 丁香, etc.) which was a formula designed by the hospital. This was made into pills, and then mixed with 10 ml of ginger juice, heated and stirred to make a paste which was applied to the local pain area. Then *an mo* 按摩 remedial massage was applied on this pain area until the paste turned dry. A gauze dressing was used to cover the paste. This was repeated every 48 hours for six days. Twenty people in the control group were treated with fentanyl transdermal system (4.2 mg every 72 hours) for six days. This study was conducted in mainland China, did not mention syndrome differentiation in the selection criteria and there were no drop-outs.

Table 9.2 Topical CHM plus *An Mo* 按摩 versus Fentanyl Transdermal System: Adverse Reactions (Criteria Not Specified)

Adverse Reaction	Effect Size RR [95% CI]	Included Studies (*n* Participants)
Nausea and vomiting	0.04 [0.002, 0.65]*	C2 (50)
Constipation	0.06 [0.004, 1.06]	
Dizziness	0.10 [0.005, 1.78]	
Skin rash	3.39 [0.17, 67.05]	

*Statistically significant.
Abbreviations: CI, confidence interval; *n*, number; RR, relative risk.

The results showed no difference for NRS scores between groups (MD 0.49 [–0.95, 1.93], *n* = 50). The analgesic onset time was 10–20 minutes in the CM group and 10–20 hours in the control group, since it takes 12–24 hours for the fentanyl to reach a stable plasma concentration, and 24–72 hours to reach the peak plasma concentration.

For adverse reactions, the study did not specify which criteria were used. There was a significant reduction in the incidence of nausea and vomiting (RR 0.04 [0.002, 0.65]) in the CHM plus *an mo* 按摩 group (Table 9.2) but no significant differences between groups for constipation (RR 0.06 [0.004, 1.06]), dizziness (RR 0.10 [0.005, 1.78]) and skin rash (RR 3.39 [0.17, 67.05]).

Safety of Combination Therapies

The RCT (C1) did not mention the safety of the CHM or acu-TENS. The CCT (C2) mentioned two cases of rash in the CHM plus *an mo* 按摩 group. The rash disappeared after the CM therapies were stopped.

Summary of Clinical Evidence for Combination Therapies

The single RCT used an oral CHM that included ingredients identified as effective for pain in Chapter 6 (i.e. *yan hu suo* 延胡索, *ru xiang*

乳香, *mo yao* 没药) combined with acu-TENS on acupuncture points that are recommended for pain relief in cancer (see Chapter 2).

With regard to the effects of TENS (all types), a Cochrane review of three RCTs of TENS for cancer pain reported the results were inconclusive.[1] A review of 38 RCTs of TENS for various types of pain found that variation in methodological quality and the way TENs was applied may account for the inconclusive results of reviews.[2] More recently, in a series of eight case reports of patients with cancer pain due to sarcoma who received individualised TENS for two months, seven patients experienced pain reduction and in three patients the reduction was clinically significant.[3] A retrospective cohort study (n = 87) at a major US cancer centre found that 69.7% of patients reported a benefit but a proportion were not responsive.[4] These reviews and studies did not identify any safety issues with TENs.

The topical CHM used in the CCT included a number of the ingredients identified in Chapter 6 (i.e. *fu zi* 附子, *wu tou* 乌头, *bing pian* 冰片, *ding xiang* 丁香) as having antinociceptive effects, and a few studies have indicated that *an mo*-style remedial massage may improve cancer pain (see Chapter 8).

Overall, the evidence for combination CM therapies for people with pain due to cancer is very limited. This area appears to have received little attention from clinical researchers and it presents study design challenges since multiple control groups would be needed to determine if any of the observed benefits were due the combination of the therapies compared to the therapies separately.

References

1. Hurlow A, Bennett MI, Robb KA, *et al.* (2012) Transcutaneous electric nerve stimulation (tens) for cancer pain in adults. *Cochrane Database Syst Rev* **(3):** CD006276.
2. Bennett MI, Hughes N, Johnson MI. (2011) Methodological quality in randomised controlled trials of transcutaneous electric nerve stimulation for pain: Low fidelity may explain negative findings. *Pain* **152(6):** 1226–1232.

3. Loh J, Gulati A. (2013) Transcutaneous electrical nerve stimulation for treatment of sarcoma cancer pain. *Pain Manag* **3(3):** 189–199.
4. Loh J, Gulati A. (2015) The use of transcutaneous electrical nerve stimulation (tens) in a major cancer center for the treatment of severe cancer-related pain and associated disability. *Pain Med* **16(6):** 1204–1210.

References to Included Studies

Study Number	Reference
C1	吴文通, 王芳, 钱尤. (2017) 中西医结合治疗中重度癌痛的临床疗效观察. 中华中医药学刊 **35(2):** 492–494.
C2	徐中伟, 東家和, 邹菁, 周荣耀. (2001) 摩痛膏治疗转移性骨癌疼痛的疗效观察. 辽宁中医杂志 **28(3):** 146–147.

10

Summary and Conclusions

OVERVIEW

The main findings of the previous chapters are summarised in this chapter. Cross-references between chapters are provided for syndrome differentiation, herbal formulas, acupuncture and related therapies, acupuncture points and other Chinese medicine therapies. The main results of the clinical trials and the associated meta-analyses are summarised and discussed as well as the quality of the evidence and its limitations. The implications of the findings of the chapters for the clinical management of cancer pain using Chinese medicine are discussed and future directions for clinical and experimental research are proposed.

Introduction

The mainstay in the management of pain due to cancers is the application of analgesic medications based on the World Health Organisation (WHO) analgesic ladder and modified according to the needs of the patient to achieve optimal pain relief. Within this framework, various Chinese medicine (CM) therapies are used mainly to enhance pain relief and reduce analgesic use, improve quality of life (QOL) outcomes and relieve some of the adverse reactions associated with analgesic use.

Using the 'whole-evidence' approach which is applied throughout this series, the main contemporary clinical recommendations for the use of CM in cancer pain were identified and summarised in Chapter 2 to provide a reference point for the classical medical literature (in Chapter 3) and the evidence derived from the clinical trials that were assessed (in Chapters 5, 7, 8 and 9). In addition, for the main herbs used in the Chinese herbal medicine (CHM) formulas that were tested in Chapter 5, the experimental evidence for their effects on pain is reviewed in Chapter 6.

Contemporary CM textbooks and clinical guidelines provide a range of different CM therapies that may be applicable in the management of cancer pain (Chapter 2). These include CHMs administered as oral formulas, as topical preparations or as enemas; various types of acupuncture therapies including manual acupuncture, electro-acupuncture, moxibustion, ear acupuncture or acupressure and scalp acupuncture; as well as other CM therapies including exercise therapies such as *dao yin* 导引 and *qi gong* 气功, psychological therapy and music therapy.

These CM therapies may be used singly or in combination, but their use is generally adjunctive to conventional treatment, monitoring, and assessment within an integrative approach to cancer pain management.

In this chapter, the main results of the clinical trials are summarised, and the recommendations derived from contemporary CM textbooks and guidelines (Chapter 2) are cross-referenced to the findings of Chapters 3, 5, 7, 8 and 9 to identify points of similarity and difference.

Chinese Medicine Syndrome Differentiation

In Chapter 2, six main syndromes were identified for cancer pain based on the *Guideline of Diagnosis and Treatment of Tumours in TCM* (肿瘤中医诊疗指南)[1] which also provided one or more guiding CHM formulas for each syndrome (Table 2.1). Since there was no national standard for syndrome differentiation available at the time of writing, additional syndromes and formulas were identified from major textbooks, and these are summarised in Table 2.2.

A number of the syndrome names are similar, and some contain multiple concepts leading to overlap between the concepts expressed in the names. Therefore, to facilitate comparison between chapters, the principal components of the syndromes from Chapter 2 were

Table 10.1 Summary of Chinese Syndromes Included in Chapters 2, 3, 5 and 7

Syndrome Names[1]	Chapter 2 (Included)	Chapter 3 (Included)	Chapter 5 (No. of Studies)[2]		Chapter 7 (No. of Studies)[3]
			RCT	Non-controlled	RCT
Blood stasis: *xue yu* 血瘀/*yu xue* 瘀血	Yes	No	6 (5 o, 1 t)	2 (o, o +t)	1
Qi stagnation/Liver depression: *qi zhi* 气滞/肝郁	Yes	Yes	3 (2 o, 1 t)	1 (o + t)	1
Phlegm dampness: *tan shi* 痰湿	Yes	Yes	0	0	0
Deficient cold: *xu han* 虚寒	Yes	Yes[4]	1 (t)	0	0
Heat: *re* 热	Yes	Yes	2 (o)	0	0
Toxin: *du* 毒	Yes	Yes	0	0	0
Qi deficiency: *qi xu* 气虚	Yes	No	1 (o)	0	2
Blood deficiency: *xue xu* 血虚	Yes	No	0	0	1
Yin deficiency: *yin xu* 阴虚	Yes	No	3 (2 o, 1 t)	1 (o)	0
Yang deficiency: *yang xu* 阳虚	Yes	No	0	0	0
Kidney deficiency: *shen xu* 肾虚	No	No	3 (o)	0	0

[1]Some studies included more than one syndrome.
[2]There were no CCTs in Chapter 5.
[3]The studies in Chapter 8 and Chapter 9 did not mention any specific syndromes.
[4]This was *han* 寒 (cold) due to external pathogens, so it is different to *xu han* 虚寒, but similar herbs were used.
Abbreviations: o, oral CHM; RCT, randomised controlled trial; t, topical CHM.

identified and listed along with any syndromes that appeared two or more times in the clinical chapters (Table 10.1). Most of the data on syndromes used in the clinical trials were from the studies of orally or topically administered CHMs (Chapter 5) but some were available for the acupuncture studies (Chapter 7). In all the CHM studies that used syndrome differentiation, the syndrome was an inclusion criterion and one formula was used, but one acupuncture study (A16) varied treatment according to syndrome differentiation. None of the studies in Chapter 8 or Chapter 9 made mention of syndrome differentiation. In the classical literature (Chapter 3) the citations did not use syndrome differentiation in the same manner as contemporary CM, but some citations provided explanations of aetiology that were consistent with particular syndromes, so when these were present in one or more citations, 'Yes' was marked in Table 10.1.

The most frequently mentioned of the concepts in the syndrome names was Blood stasis (*xue yu* 血瘀/*yu xue* 瘀血) which appeared in six of the randomised controlled trials (RCTs) of CHM (five oral, one topical) and in two of the non-controlled CHM studies in Chapter 5. It also appeared in one acupuncture RCT. The next most frequent was *qi* stagnation (*qi zhi* 气滞) including Liver *qi* depression (*gan yu* 肝郁), which appeared in three RCTs of CHM (two oral, one topical), one non-controlled study of CHM and one acupuncture RCT. The next most frequent were the deficiency syndromes. *Yin* deficiency (*yin xu* 阴虚) was mentioned in three RCTs of CHM (two oral, one topical) and one non-controlled study of CHM. Kidney deficiency (*shen xu* 肾虚) was equally frequent with three RCTs of oral CHM and one non-controlled study of CHM, but it was not mentioned in the syndromes included in Chapter 2. *Qi* deficiency (*qi xu* 气虚) was mentioned only once in Chapter 5 (one oral RCT) but twice in the acupuncture RCTs, while Blood deficiency (*xue xu* 血虚) did not appear in Chapter 5 and was mentioned once in one of the acupuncture RCTs. Deficient cold (*xu han* 虚寒) appeared in one RCT of oral CHM. Of the pathogens, heat (*re* 热) appeared in two RCTs of oral CHM but phlegm/damp (*tan shi* 痰湿) and toxins (*du* 毒) did not appear in the syndromes mentioned in any of the clinical studies.

In the classical literature, the main pathogens described were external cold (*han* 寒) or cold *qi* (*han qi* 寒气), heat (*re* 热), phlegm (*tan* 痰) and toxins (*du* 毒). In the citations relating to 'breast rock' (*ru yan* 乳岩), *qi* stagnation (*yu* 郁, *yu zhi* 郁滞), especially in relation to the emotions and the Liver, was the most frequently mentioned factor.

Overall, the syndromes that appeared frequently in the clinical studies were included Chapter 2. In the case of Kidney deficiency (*shen xu* 肾虚), this syndrome can be included within the scope of *yin* deficiency (*yin xu* 阴虚) and *yang* deficiency (*yang xu* 阳虚), so this difference is mainly related to terminology. Although there were more clinical studies of topical CHM than oral CHM in Chapter 5, syndromes were more likely to be mentioned in studies of oral CHM.

Chinese Herbal Medicine

In contemporary China, conventional medications are combined with CHMs in the management of cancer pain and the adverse effects of cancer therapies. This integrative approach is usually under the oversight of a multidisciplinary team which monitors the patient's responses and adjusts medications accordingly. Chapter 2 provides lists of oral CHM formulas according to the presenting syndromes. These are a guide and are usually modified according to the circumstances and needs of the particular patients, their symptoms and signs, and the conventional medications they receive. Topical CHM preparations are listed without syndromes in Chapter 2 but topical CHMs may also be prescribed according to the presenting syndromes. It should be noted that due to the diversity in the types of cancers and the locations of pain, Chapter 2 can only provide an overview of the CHM formulas used in cancer pain and is not comprehensive.

In the classical literature (Chapter 3), oral and topical CHMs were used in the management of painful conditions that were at least broadly consistent with cancer pain. However, it is not possible to be certain that these conditions would now be diagnosed as cancer. This is particularly the case in the conditions categorised as *ji ju* 积聚 or *zheng jia* 症/癥瘕 which could refer to a diverse range of palpable masses. In the case of *ru yan* 乳岩, which referred to hard lumps in the breast, the descriptions were generally consistent with breast cancer, but other conditions were also possible. Except in a few case studies, we do not know if the CHMs produced any beneficial effects. We can only assume that the authors included them because they believed they were effective.

The studies included in Chapter 5 were all required to only include people who had a clear diagnosis of cancer and had pain that was related to the cancer at the beginning of the study. Only validated outcome measures were used. Therefore, we can be reasonably confident that the clinical studies were measuring changes in pain due to cancer, rather than pain due to mixed aetiologies. The results of the analyses in Chapter 5 are summarised in detail at the end of the chapter, so only brief summaries of the main results of the RCTs are provided here.

For the effects of the oral CHMs on pain relief, one RCT showed pain reduction that was less than that of ibuprofen (H1). When CHMs were combined with conventional analgesic medications, there was no additional improvement in pain intensity based on two placebo-controlled RCTs (Table 5.3), but the pool of five open-label RCTs showed a significant benefit for combining CHM with conventional analgesic medications (Table 5.5). The GRADE assessment for the placebo-controlled studies was 'moderate' (Table 5.10) but it was 'very low' for the open-label studies (Table 5.11). For pain due to use of aromatase inhibitors, the pool of two RCTs (H10, H11) found a significant reduction when compared to calcium carbonate and vitamin D3 tablets.

For frequency of breakthrough pain, when an oral CHM was combined with conventional analgesic medication, one placebo-controlled RCT (H3) found no significant difference between groups, while one open-label RCT (H5) found a significant reduction in the CHM plus conventional analgesic medication group. For medication dosage, one placebo-controlled RCT (H2) found a significant reduction in average dose and the other (H3) found a reduction in total dose. In the open-label RCTs, there was a reduction in the pooled maintenance dose (H6, H8). For total analgesic dose, in one RCT (H5) this was reduced in people with moderate pain but not in people with severe pain. For analgesic onset time, the CHM had less effect than ibuprofen (H1) and when a CHM was combined with a conventional analgesic (H6), there was no difference in analgesic onset time.

Overall, for the oral CHMs the results were mixed for effects on pain intensity and frequency of breakthrough pain, but reductions in the dosage of conventional analgesics required for pain relief were found in multiple studies. Considering that most studies would have based the conventional treatments on the analgesic ladder, it is likely that conventional medication dosages would have been varied in response to the pain relief requirements of the patients, so the addition of a CHM was less likely to provide any detectable increase in pain relief. Similarly, for breakthrough pain, this would have been treated with additional analgesia as it occurred. Where an effect of the CHMs could be detected was in changes in the dosages of analgesic medications required over time. This was evident but only five studies reported this outcome and there was variation in how this was reported. Very little data on analgesic onset time were available and the available data suggested that the oral CHMs did not have any significant effect. This could be expected, since there is no apparent way in which the addition of an oral CHM could increase onset time compared to the various conventional analgesics.

In the studies of topical CHMs, there was a greater reduction in pain intensity in a comparison with placebo (H13) and no difference between groups for topical CHM versus tramadol (H14). This suggested that the topical CHM did produce an independent analgesic effect. When the topical CHMs were combined with conventional analgesic medications, there was an additional reduction in pain intensity in the pool of three placebo-controlled RCTs (Table 5.16) and in the 11 open-label studies (Table 5.18). The GRADE assessment for the placebo-controlled studies was 'moderate' (Table 5.26) but it was 'low' for the open-label studies (Table 5.27). There was no significant reduction in pain intensity in the single RCT of oral plus topical CHM combined with analgesic medication (H30).

For frequency of breakthrough pain, in one placebo-controlled RCT of topical CHM plus conventional analgesic medication (H15) there was a reduction in average frequency per person; in one open-label RCT (H28) there was a significant reduction in average frequency per person per week; while another open-label RCT (H23) found no reduction in average frequency per person per day. For dosage of conventional analgesic medications, two of the placebo-controlled RCTs (H15, H17) reported reductions. In the open-label RCTs, a pool of three studies (Table 5.21) found a reduction in the analgesic maintenance dose; one (H28) found a reduction in average dose per day while another (H23) found no difference in total dose. The single RCT of oral plus topical CHM combined with analgesic medication (H30) found a reduction in analgesic maintenance dose.

Analgesic onset time was reduced in the topical CHM group compared with oral tramadol (H14). When topical CHMs were used in combination with conventional analgesic medications, there was no reduction in analgesic onset time in one placebo-controlled RCT (H16), but there was a reduction in the pool of two open-label RCTs (Table 5.19). Duration of analgesia was not different in the comparison with tramadol (H14) but the pooled effect for two open-label RCTs of CHM plus conventional analgesic medication showed a significant increase (Table 5.20).

Overall, for the topical CHMs more studies were available (17 RCTs) than for the oral CHMs (12 RCTs). Significant reductions in pain intensity were found when topical CHMs were combined with conventional analgesic medications in both the placebo-controlled and open RCTs. For breakthrough pain, the results were mixed and based on only three studies. As with the oral CHMs, the addition of topical CHMs appeared to result in reductions in analgesic medication dose in most studies. Again, the results for analgesic onset time were mixed, as were the results for duration of analgesia. In the case of the topical CHMs, the reduction in pain intensity may have been due to an additional analgesic effect from direct absorption through the skin but the magnitude of the reduction was small (less than 1 point on NRS). As with the oral CHMs, reduction in analgesic dosage may be a more meaningful outcome.

Five different measures relating to QOL were reported, but relatively few studies reported on QOL. For the open-label studies of oral CHMs combined with conventional analgesic medications, there were improvements on the Chinese QOL scale[2] in one study (H4) and in the pooled result of four studies for KPS (Table 5.6). There was no difference on the brief pain inventory (BPI) in one study (H8). For topical CHMs combined with conventional analgesic medications, in the placebo-controlled studies there was an improvement in one study (H15) on the National Comprehensive Cancer Network

(NCCN) impact of pain measurement but no difference in the pooled result of two RCTs for Karnofsky Performance Status (KPS) (H15, H17). In the open-label RCTs, there were improvements in the pooled results of three RCTs for QLQ-C30 (Table 5.22), and seven RCTs for KPS (Table 5.24) but no significant differences in the pooled result of four RCTs on the Chinese QOL scale (Table 5.23) and in one study that used the NCCN impact of pain measurement (H23). The pooled results tended to show heterogeneity, so there was considerable variation in the results for QOL. The study of oral plus topical CHM (H30) also used the NCCN impact of pain measurement and found no significant difference between groups.

It could be expected that QOL was related to pain outcomes but variability in outcome reporting prevented any assessment of such a relationship. It is also likely that the durations of some studies were too short for the assessment of change in QOL to be feasible.

A few studies reported on symptoms related to the adverse effects of analgesic medications. For the orally administered CHMs, there were fewer gastrointestinal reactions in the CHM group compared to ibuprofen (H1) but in the placebo-controlled studies of CHM plus conventional analgesic medications the pooled results showed no differences in the incidences of adverse reactions (Table 5.4). In the open-label studies, one found significant reductions (Table 5.8) but the other found no differences between groups (Table 5.9). In one study that focused on opioid-induced constipation (H12), there was a significant reduction in Cleveland Clinic Constipation Score (CCS).

In the placebo-controlled studies of topical CHMs combined with analgesic medications, one study found no difference in opioid-related symptoms but there was an increased incidence of allergies in the group that used the topical CHM (Table 5.17), while in another RCT (H17) there was no difference in nausea and vomiting but the incidence of constipation decreased. In the open-label studies the pooled results showed reductions in nausea and vomiting, and constipation, but not in other symptoms (Table 5.25).

With regard to the safety of the CHMs, skin reactions were reported in six of the RCTs of topical CHMs and in one study skin allergies led to five drop-outs (Table 5.30). In the RCTs of oral CHMs there were three deaths in one RCT (H2), of which two were in the CHM group, but the authors reported that all the deaths were unrelated to the interventions. In another RCT of oral CHM there was one case of diarrhoea. However, only eight RCTs reported details on adverse events (AEs) while ten simply stated that there were no AEs related to the CHMs. The other RCTs did not mention AEs, so the reporting of safety data was too incomplete for an accurate safety assessment. It is possible that there were interactions between the CHMs and the conventional medications, but none were reported. Considering the complexity of the clinical condition in advanced cancers and the relatively short durations of the studies, it is likely that only severe interactions could have been identified. Based on the available data, the topical CHMs appeared to increase the incidence of skin allergies. For incidence of opioid-related adverse reactions, there were either no differences or reductions, mainly in constipation. It seems probable that these reductions were due to reductions in opioid dose, but it was not possible to test such an association.

Chinese Herbal Medicine Formulas in Key Clinical Guidelines and Textbooks, Classical Literature and Clinical Studies

This section provides an overview of the CHM formulas that appeared in multiple chapters. In Chapter 2, 31 different orally administered formulas, seven different topical formulas and one enema preparation were listed. In Table 10.2 only the CHM formulas from Chapter 2 that appeared in other chapters are listed, plus any formulas that appeared in two or more clinical studies in Chapters 5 and 9, including modified versions of the same formula.

There was very little overlap between the oral formulas listed in Chapter 2 and those used in the classical literature (Chapter 3). In Chapter 2, *Er chen tang* 二陈汤 plus *Yi yi ren tang* with modifications 薏苡仁汤等加减 was suggested for phlegm-dampness pain (*tan shi teng tong* 痰湿疼痛), while in the classical literature *Er chen tang* 二陈汤 plus another formula or additional ingredients appeared in two citations for breast masses (*ru yan* 乳岩) with pain. In none of these cases was it clear whether the *Er chen tang* 二陈汤 was being

Table 10.2 Summary of Oral Chinese Herbal Medicine Formulas Included in Chapters 2, 3, 5 and 9

Formula Names[1,2]	Chapter 2 (Included)	Chapter 3 (No. of Citations)	Chapter 5 (No. of Studies)[3] RCT	Chapter 5 (No. of Studies)[3] Non-controlled	Chapter 9 (No. of Studies)[2] RCT/CCT
Oral formulas					
Chai hu shu gan san, jia wei 柴胡疏肝散,加減	Yes	0	2	0	0
Yuan hu zhi tong ke li/ jiao nang 元胡止痛颗粒/胶囊	Yes	0	1	0	0
Er chen tang plus *Yi yi ren tang jia wei* 二陈汤合薏苡仁汤加减	Yes	2 (*Er chen tang* 二陈汤 plus other ingredients)	0	0	0
Other oral formulas in Chapter 2	Yes	0	0	0	0
Xi lu wan 晞露丸	No	6	0	0	0
Da huang wan 大黄丸 no. 1.	No	2	0	0	0
Topical formulas					
Chan su gao 蟾酥膏	Yes	2 (*chan chu* 蟾蜍 only)[4]	0	1 (*Chan su xiao zhong gao* 蟾酥消肿膏)	0
Other topical formulas in Chapter 2	Yes	0	0	0	0

[1]Some formula combinations were used. The list of formulas in Chapter 2 is too long to show here, so only those that appeared in other chapters are included.
[2]The studies in Chapter 9 (one RCT, one CCT) did not mention any of these formulas.
[3]There were no CCTs in Chapter 5.
[4]*Chan chu* 蟾蜍 is the whole toad which provides *chan su* 蟾酥, which is the main ingredient in *Chan su gao* 蟾酥膏 and *Chan su xiao zhong gao* 蟾酥消肿膏.
Abbreviations: CCT, non-randomised controlled clinical trial; RCT, randomised controlled trial.

used for the pain but it is likely that this was not the case, and it had a supporting role for removing phlegm. It should be noted that *Er chen tang* 二陈汤 is common throughout the classical literature and has many applications.

None of the topical CHMs from Chapter 2 appeared in the classical citations but toad (*chan chu* 蟾蜍) was used topically in three classical citations while toad venom (*chan su* 蟾酥) was a major component in the manufactured cataplasm *Chan su gao* 蟾酥膏 which was listed for pain relief in Chapter 2.

The formulas in Chapter 5 were mostly different from those listed in Chapter 2. One oral formula that was listed in the textbooks and also tested in two RCTs was *Chai hu shu gan san* 柴胡疏肝散. This appeared in a modified form in Chapter 2 as *Chai hu shu gan san jia jian* 柴胡疏肝散加减. Its main actions were to soothe the Liver, regulate *qi* and relieve pain. *Chai hu shu gan san* 柴胡疏肝散 was used without modifications in one RCT (H2) for 21 days and was used with slightly different modifications to the version in Chapter 2 in another RCT as *Chai hu shu gan san jia wei* 柴胡疏肝散加味 (H8) for five days. In both RCTs it was used in liver cancer together with opioids.

In the first study ($n = 45$), which was placebo-controlled, *Chai hu shu gan san* 柴胡疏肝散 was combined with fentanyl transdermal system and compared to a placebo for the CHM plus fentanyl transdermal system in people with advanced liver cancer. After 21 days there was no significant additional reduction in pain scores on the numerical rating scale (NRS) in the test group but there was a significant reduction in the dose of fentanyl transdermal system (Table 5.12). It should be noted that patients could adjust their dose of this medication to achieve a desired degree of pain relief, so medication dose was an important outcome. There were no differences between groups in adverse reactions. In an open RCT ($n = 46$) in liver cancer *Chai hu shu gan san jia wei* 柴胡疏肝散加味 was combined with morphine sustained-release tablets. After five days, there were no significant differences between groups for NRS, maintenance dose of the morphine, or scores on BPI. The results for these two studies are summarised in Table 5.31.

The other formula listed in Chapter 2 was *Yuan hu zhi tong ke li* 元胡止痛颗粒. The encapsulated form, *Yuan hu zhi tong jiao nang* 元胡止痛胶囊, was tested in one open RCT (H7) in combination with morphine sulfate sustained-release tablets for seven days in people with advanced malignant tumours ($n = 60$). There was no significant difference between groups for NRS scores but there was improvement in KPS and on some measures of immune function. For adverse reactions to analgesic medications, there were reductions in nausea and vomiting, and constipation, in the combined therapy group (Table 5.32).

In the case of topical formulas, none of those from Chapter 2 directly appeared in the clinical trials in Chapter 5. However, a topical formula closely related to *Chan su gao* 蟾酥膏 was used in a case study of a woman with bone metastases (H33) which reported that *Chan su xiao zhong gao* 蟾酥消肿膏 provided rapid pain relief. None of the clinical studies employed a CHM enema. None of the formulas in Chapter 9 appeared in Chapter 2 or Chapter 5.

Although there was very little overlap in the formulas used in Chapters 2, 5 and 3 in terms of their names, at the level of ingredients there was greater similarity. Of the herbs in Chapter 6 (i.e. *bing pian* 冰片, *xi xin* 细辛, *yan hu suo* 延胡索, *chuan wu* 川乌 or *wu tou* 乌头, *cao wu* 草乌, *da huang* 大黄, *mo yao* 没药, *ru xiang* 乳香, *ding xiang* 丁香, *quan xie* 全蝎 and *xue jie* 血竭), which were based on the herbs most frequently used in the topical formulas in Chapter 5, all except for *da huang* 大黄 were components of a least one of the formulas, topical or oral, listed in Chapter 2. When compared to the ingredients of the formulas in the classical literature, which were mainly oral (Chapter 3), only *bing pian* 冰片, *xi xin* 细辛 and *cao wu* 草乌 did not appear. Chapter 9 only included two formulas which included five of the herbs from Chapter 6: *bing pian* 冰片, *yan hu suo* 延胡索, *wu tou* 乌头, *mo yao* 没药, *ru xiang* 乳香 and *ding xiang* 丁香. Notably, each of the herbs included in Chapter 6 has received research attention for effects on pain.

Acupuncture and Related Therapies

The acupuncture interventions derived from the textbooks that were included in Chapter 2 involved manual acupuncture or electroacupuncture or moxibustion on traditional points and *ashi* points 阿是穴, and ear acupuncture. In the classical literature (Chapter 3), there were only 33 citations that mentioned the use of acupuncture

Table 10.3 Summary of Acupuncture Therapies Included in Chapters 2, 3, 7 and 9

Acupuncture Therapy[1]	Chapter 2 (Included)	Chapter 3 (No. of Citations)	Chapter 7 (No. of Studies)[2]			Chapter 9 (No. of Studies)[2]
			RCT	CCT	Non-controlled	RCT/CCT
Acupuncture/electro-acupuncture	Yes	33	15	1	8	0
Moxibustion	Yes	15	2	0	0	0
Ear acupuncture/ear acupressure	Yes	0	9	0	3	0
Scalp acupuncture	No	0	1[3]	0	0	0

[1]Some studies used more than one intervention e.g. acupuncture plus moxibustion, traditional acupuncture plus ear acupressure. These are counted separately in this table.
[2]There were no non-controlled studies in Chapter 9.
[3]The main interventions were at traditional points and ear points, plus scalp zones corresponding to the pain location which varied according to the participant.
Abbreviations: CCT, non-randomised controlled clinical trial; RCT, randomised controlled trial.

points for conditions that could have been cancer pain. Of these, nine made specific mention of needling and 15 mentioned moxibustion, but many did not make mention of the point stimulation method. Since acupuncture was not contra-indicated, we expect the use acupuncture was implied in all 33 citations (Table 10.3). In Chapter 7, 32 clinical trials were included and there were none in Chapter 9. Of the studies in Chapter 7, the majority (24 studies) used acupuncture at traditional points with only two studies (both RCTs) using moxibustion alone. Ear acupuncture or ear acupressure was used in 12 studies but this included six studies that combined traditional and ear acupuncture points. Two RCTs and one non-controlled study used ear acupressure alone and the same number used ear acupuncture alone. In one RCT (A19) that included a standard protocol of traditional acupuncture and ear acupuncture, scalp acupuncture zones were added as a customised component, but the names of the zones were not provided.

Of the specific types of cancer pain, aromatase inhibitor-associated musculoskeletal symptoms (AIMSS) was the most commonly researched, with six RCTs (A1, A11, A12, A14, A18, A20) and one non-controlled study (A30). The next most common type was metastatic disease, with three RCTs (A9, A10, A16) and three non-controlled studies (A24, A28, A29).

In the RCTs of acupuncture at traditional points, comparisons with sham acupuncture showed significantly greater reductions in pain intensity (two RCTs, GRADE: Low, Table 7.7) but no improvements in QOL (two RCTs). In the open label studies of acupuncture combined with conventional analgesics there were significantly greater reductions in pain intensity in the integrative medicine groups (three RCTs, GRADE: Very Low, Table 7.8) and improvements in QOL (two RCTs, Table 7.5).

For ear acupuncture versus sham controls, there were significantly greater reductions in pain intensity (two RCTs, GRADE: Low, Table 7.13). In the open label studies of ear acupressure combined with conventional analgesics, pain intensity was reduced (two RCTs, GRADE: Very Low, Table 7.14) but there was no significant difference in KPS scores (one RCT).

For ear acupuncture plus acupuncture versus sham controls, there was no significant difference for BPI-worst pain (two RCTs, Table 7.16; GRADE: Low, Table 7.18). Of the QOL measures, only FACT-G physical showed a significant improvement (one RCT). In a comparison between ear acupuncture plus acupuncture versus no acupuncture, there was a significant reduction in pain intensity (two RCTs, Table 7.17) but no significant difference in QOL on FACT-ES (one RCT). In an open-label study of ear acupressure plus acupuncture plus conventional analgesics, there was a significant reduction in BPI-pain severity and duration of pain (one RCT).

When real moxibustion was compared to sham moxibustion (one RCT), there were significant reductions in BPI total scores and BPI-pain severity but no significant difference for analgesic dose. For moxibustion combined with conventional analgesics (one RCT) there was a significant reduction in pain intensity and improvement in QOL on FACT-G.

For each of the types of acupuncture and combinations of acupuncture therapies, there tended to be reductions in pain on various measures (NRS, VAS, BPI) and improvements in measures of QOL.

However, due to the differences in the acupuncture therapies, the study designs, the outcome measures and the types of cancer pain, there were few opportunities for pooling data and most meta-analysis pools only included two RCTs. Therefore, there were insufficient data to determine which acupuncture therapies were more effective and whether combining acupuncture therapies (e.g. use of traditional points plus ear points) provided any additional effect. The small numbers of studies in each comparison and the heterogeneity in the pooled results led to the downgrading of the quality of evidence in GRADE to 'low' or 'very low'.

Acupuncture Points Used in Key Clinical Guidelines and Textbooks, Classical Literature and Clinical Studies

In Chapter 2, about 65 differently named traditional points including *ashi* points 阿是穴 plus six ear points were recommended for cancer pain associated with different cancers and pain at different locations (Table 2.3). For the purposes of comparison, the traditional points listed in Table 10.4 include all points in the classical literature (Chapter 3), and points used in two or more clinical studies in Chapters 7 and 9. Chapter 9 is included in this section since the study that included acu-TENS (C1) specified traditional points. All ear acupoints used in Chapter 2 and Chapters 7 and 9 are listed in Table 10.5.

Of the traditional points, 17 points included in Chapter 2 were included in Table 10.4. Of these, the two points CV3 *Zhongji* 中极 and BL23 *Shenshu* 肾俞 were also included in the classical literature (Chapter 3) and these points were each used in one clinical study. CV6 *Qihai* 气海 was included in Chapter 3 and was used in two clinical studies but it was not in Chapter 2. However, the points that were the most frequent inclusions in Chapter 3 (KI17 *Shangqu* 商曲, SP12 *Chongmen* 冲门, BL18 *Ganshu* 肝俞) did not appear in Chapter 2 and were not used in any of the included clinical trials.

In the clinical studies, LI4 *Hegu* 合谷 was the most popular point, being used in 15 studies, followed by ST36 *Zusanli* 足三里

Table 10.4 Summary of Traditional Acupuncture Points Included in Chapters 2, 3, 7 and 9

Points[1]	Chapter 2 (Included)	Chapter 3 (No. of Citations)	Chapter 7 (No. of Studies)			Chapter 9 (No. of Studies)[2]
			RCT	CCT	Non-controlled	RCT
Acupuncture/Electro-acupuncture/Moxibustion						
LI4 *Hegu* 合谷	Yes	0	12	0	2	1
ST36 *Zusanli* 足三里	Yes	0	7	1	3	1
SP6 *Sanyinjiao* 三阴交	Yes	0	5	1	2	0
PC6 *Neiguan* 内关	Yes	0	5	1	0	0
LR3 *Taichong* 太冲	Yes	0	6	0	1	0
GB34 *Yanglingquan* 阳陵泉	Yes	0	6	0	1	0
LI11 *Quchi* 曲池	Yes	0	3	1	0	0
GV20 *Baihui* 百会	Yes	0	3	1	0	0
KI3 *Taixi* 太溪	No	0	5	0	1	0
CV12 *Zhongwan* 中脘	Yes	0	4	0	0	0
TE5 *Waiguan* 外关	Yes	0	4	0	0	0
CV4 *Guanyuan* 关元	Yes	0	3	0	0	0
GB41 *Zulinqi* 足临泣	No	0	4	0	0	0
CV6 *Qihai* 气海	No	1	2	0	0	0
EX-B2 *Jiaji* 夹脊	Yes	0	1	0	1	1
ST41 *Jiexi* 解溪	No	0	3	0	0	0
GB21 *Jianjing* 肩井	No	0	2	0	0	0
EX-HN3 *Sishencong* 四神聪	Yes	0	2	0	0	0
BL60 *Kunlun* 昆仑	Yes	0	1	0	1	0
Ashi points 阿是穴	Yes	0	2	0	1	1
CV3 *Zhongji* 中极	Yes	2	1	0	0	0

(*Continued*)

Table 10.4 (*Continued*)

Points[1]	Chapter 2 (Included)	Chapter 3 (No. of Citations)	Chapter 7 (No. of Studies)			Chapter 9 (No. of Studies)[2]
			RCT	CCT	Non-controlled	RCT
BL23 *Shenshu* 肾俞	Yes	1	0	0	1	0
KI17 *Shangqu* 商曲	No	11	0	0	0	0
SP12 *Chongmen* 冲门	No	9	0	0	0	0
BL18 *Ganshu* 肝俞	No	6	0	0	0	0
LR13 *Zhangmen* 章门	No	2	0	0	0	0
BL17 *Geshu* 膈俞	No	1	0	0	0	0
KI10 *Yingu* 阴谷	No	1	0	0	0	0

[1]Since there are 65 traditional points in Chapter 2, only points used in two or more clinical studies, or points in Chapter 3 are included in this table.
[2]There was one RCT of acu-TENS and no CCTs or non-controlled studies of acupuncture in Chapter 9.
Abbreviations: CCT, non-randomised controlled clinical trial; RCT, randomised controlled trial.

(12 studies), SP6 *Sanyinjiao* 三阴交 (eight studies), and GB34 *Yanglingquan* 阳陵泉 and LR3 *Taichong* 太冲 (seven studies). Two points were used in six studies each: PC6 *Neiguan* 内关, and KI3 *Taixi* 太溪. All except for KI3 *Taixi* 太溪 were included in Chapter 2. Of the other points used in two or more clinical studies, most were included in Chapter 2, the exceptions being GB41 *Zulinqi* 足临泣 (four studies), CV6 *Qihai* 气海 (two studies), ST41 *Jiexi* 解溪 (three studies) and GB21 *Jianjing* 肩井 (two studies). Overall, the points used in the clinical studies tended to be included in Chapter 2.

One notable difference between the points mentioned in the clinical studies and those in the classical literature is the clinical studies mainly mentioned points located on the limbs and head, with relatively fewer on the trunk. In contrast, the points used in the classical literature were mainly on the trunk, except for KI10 *Yingu* 阴谷

Table 10.5 Summary of Ear Acupuncture Points Included in Chapters 2, 7 and 9

Points[1]	Chapter 2 (Included)	Chapter 7 (No. of Studies)			Chapter 9 (No. of Studies)[2]
		RCT	CCT	Non-controlled	RCT/CCT
Ear Acupuncture/Ear Acupressure					
TF4 Shenmen 神门	Y	8	0	1	0
AH6a Jiaogan 交感	Y	7	0	1	0
CO12 Gan 肝	Y	5	0	0	0
AT4 Pizhixia 皮质下	Y	3	0	1	0
CO14 Fei 肺	N	3	0	0	0
CO10 Shen 肾	N	4	0	0	0
CO13 Pi 脾	N	2	0	0	0
CO4 Wei 胃	N	2	0	0	0
CO15 Xin 心	Y	0	0	0	0
HX6,7i Erjian 耳尖	Y	0	0	0	0

[1]Ear points are a modern innovation, so Chapter 3 was not included in the comparisons. In some studies, ear points were combined with traditional acupuncture points.
[2]There were no studies that used ear-acupuncture points in Chapter 9.

near the knee. One reason for this difference is both Chapter 2 and the clinical studies mentioned the use of local painful points (*ashi* points), which can vary according to the individual, whereas Chapter 3 only included specific point names. It is likely that many of the points used in the classical literature were located near to the pain, which was mainly on the trunk.

Of the abdominal points in Chapter 2 that were used in multiple clinical studies, only CV12 *Zhongwan* 中脘 (four studies) is located in the upper abdomen on the midline, while the classical literature included the lateral points KI17 *Shangqu* 商曲 and LR13 *Zhangmen* 章门 instead. On the lower abdomen, Chapter 2 and the clinical studies included CV6 *Qihai* 气海 (two studies), CV4 *Guanyuan* 关元 (three studies) and CV3 *Zhongji* 中极 (one study), all on the midline. Chapter 3 included two of these points, CV6 *Qihai* 气海 and CV3

Zhongji 中极, plus one lateral point SP12 *Chongmen* 冲门. All these points are still used for abdominal pain.

Also included in Chapter 2 and in the clinical studies were EX-B2 *Jiaji* 夹脊 points which are located on the back lateral to the spine and are used according to the pain location. Of the points in the classical literature, three are located lateral to the spine — BL17 *Geshu* 膈俞, BL18 *Ganshu* 肝俞 and BL23 *Shenshu* 肾俞 — and these points can be used for relief of local pain in a similar manner to the nearby EX-B2 *Jiaji* 夹脊 points. Considering the diversity of local points that could be used, it is not surprising that the classical literature and Chapter 2 differed in the points included. However, it remains apparent that distal points on the arm and legs were not typically used in the classical literature for pain associated with masses located in the trunk.

Ear points did not appear in the classical literature. In the clinical studies the most popular points were TF4 *Shenmen* 神门 (nine studies), AH6a *Jiaogan* 交感 (eight studies), CO12 *Gan* 肝 (five studies), and AT4 *Pizhixia* 皮质下 (four studies) all of which were included in Chapter 2. Of the other five ear points included in one or more clinical studies, none was included in Chapter 2. Considering that many ear points could be used according to the pain location, it was not feasible for Chapter 2 to list all possibilities. Nevertheless, the clinical studies and Chapter 2 were in agreement regarding most of the principal ear points.

Other Chinese Medicine Therapies

This section summarises the results from Chapters 2, 3, 8 and 9 for the use of other CM therapies (see Table 10.6).

The books and guidelines reviewed in Chapter 2 mentioned the use of therapeutic exercises, *qi gong* 气功, music therapy and psychological support in the management of pain due to cancers. In the classical literature in Chapter 3, a number of authors mentioned the importance of regulating the emotions in the management of breast cancers and one suggested quiet forms of *qi gong* 气功, but no details of the method were given.

Table 10.6 Summary of Other Chinese Medicine Therapies Included in Chapters 2, 3, 8 and 9

Other Therapy	Chapter 2	Chapter 3 (No. of Citations)	Chapter 8 (No. of Studies)[1]		Chapter 9 (No. of Studies)[2]	
			RCT	Non-controlled	RCT	CCT
Exercises including *dao yin* 导引 and *qi gong* 气功	Yes	1	0	0	0	0
Therapeutic massage including *tui na* 推拿 and *an mo* 按摩	No	0	1	1	0	1
Acu-TENS[3]	No	0	0	0	1	0
Dietary interventions	Yes	0	0	0	0	0
Psychological support	Yes	1	0	0	0	0
Music therapy	Yes	0	0	0	0	0

[1]There were no CCTs in Chapter 8.
[2]There were no non-controlled studies in Chapter 9.
[3]Acu-TENS is transcutaneous electrical nerve stimulation (TENS) on acupuncture points.
Abbreviations: CCT, non-randomised controlled clinical trial; RCT, randomised controlled trial.

The clinical trials in Chapter 8 included one unblinded RCT of *an mo* 按摩 remedial massage in hospital in-patients with cancer pain associated with bone metastases, and a single non-controlled study that was the pilot for the RCT. Both studies reported reductions in pain following the remedial massage sessions. There were also improvements in mood and relaxation but not in sleep. There was no assessment in the RCT of how long the pain relief persisted. No safety issues were identified but the people delivering the intervention took particular care to adjust the remedial massage to the particular patient and avoided lesions and metastatic sites.

One of the studies of combination therapies in Chapter 9 included *an mo* 按摩 applied to the pain region in conjunction with a topical herbal paste. In this case it appeared that one function of the *an mo* 按摩 was to rub in the analgesic paste. The area was then covered with a dressing. In comparison with the fentanyl transdermal system, there was no significant difference in pain scores after six days of treatment, suggesting that the topical treatment was effective, and there was a reduction in nausea and vomiting (Table 9.2), but the study was not blind.

The only RCT in Chapter 9 tested the combination of acu-TENS, an oral CHM formula and morphine sulfate sustained-release tablets. The combination group had significantly greater reductions in pain intensity and analgesic onset time plus some reductions in adverse reactions to opioids (Table 9.1). However, the study was open-label and it is not possible to determine whether the acu-TENS provided an additional benefit.

No clinical studies of *qi gong* 气功, *tai chi* 太极, other exercise therapies, food therapies, music therapy or a CM-style of psychological support were included. One reason was all participants in a study were required to have pain due to the cancer or cancer therapy at baseline in order for the study to be included in the chapter. In addition, most cancer pain patients were in hospital and receiving multiple treatments, so delivering these kinds of therapies may have been the impractical.

Limitations of the Evidence

In each chapter we aimed to provide overviews of the current state of the evidence at the time of writing; however, there are limitations to the scope and depth of their coverage and in how the data can be interpreted.

The contemporary management of pain in cancer is a complex topic so Chapter 1 could only hope to be an overview of the main points. It was based mainly on the available guidelines supplemented with other resources and aimed to be an introduction to the topic. Due to these limitations, it should not be considered comprehensive and the most up-to-date guidelines should be consulted for detailed information.

The overview of CM for cancer pain in Chapter 2 was based on a Chinese guideline and supplemented with information drawn from textbooks. At the time of writing, no official guideline for CM in cancer pain was available and the guideline used was focused on oral

CHM. Hence the chapter focused on the use of oral CHM based on syndrome differentiation. However, much of contemporary CM practice involves the integrative application of oral and topical CHMs as adjuncts to conventional analgesic medications. This aspect was not considered in detail in the guideline and textbooks, and is a major limitation of the chapter. Also, information on the application of acupuncture in cancer pain was limited and was not linked to syndrome differentiation. There was also very little information on other CM therapies, so these were only mentioned briefly.

The information provided in Chapter 3 was based on searches of the *Zhong Hua Yi Dian*. This is a large digital collection of classical and pre-modern Chinese medicine books, but it does not include every available book, so it should be considered a representative sample of the literature. Since cancer pain was not a unitary concept in classical Chinese medicine, the search approach was to combine terms relevant to masses and cancers with terms specific to pain. This approach produced a sample of citations that combined both criteria, but it is likely that some relevant citations were missed. Also, due to the nature of descriptions in the pre-modern literature, we could not be certain that the conditions described were 'cancer pain' in the modern sense. In order to provide an overview of the topic, we included citations that we judged as relevant and possible instances of cancer pain. Some of the included citations were likely examples while others were less likely. Representative passages were translated. It is important to note that the treatments used have been superseded and we do not know whether any were effective.

The clinical studies included in Chapters 5, 7, 8 and 9 were limited to those that enrolled participants who had pain due to the cancer or the cancer treatment at the beginning of the study. Studies were excluded if some patients did not have pain at baseline; the pain was due to the surgery since post-surgical pain can occur in many diseases; or the pain was due to non-cancer causes. Nevertheless, the exact cause of pain can be difficult to determine so it is possible that some of the people included in the studies may have had pain that appeared due to the cancer but may have had a mixed aetiology.

In Chapter 5, the application of these criteria resulted in the exclusion of many studies of pain in cancer in which pain was one aspect of the patient experience, but it was unclear whether all patients had pain due to the cancer at baseline. Consequently, many of the included studies were of advanced cancers in which the pain was moderate to severe.

Established pain scales, mainly NRS and VAS, were used as outcome measures and we included incident data for breakthough pain. However, most studies tested combinations of CHM plus conventional analgesic medications (mainly opioids) so the results mainly assessed any additional changes in the integrative therapy groups. Considering that opioids are known to effectively control pain and it is standard practice to adjust opioid dosage according to pain intensity and to respond in a timely manner to breakthrough pain, there was little scope for the CHMs to produce additional pain relief, even when they produced analgesic effects. As the results demonstrated, in the studies of oral CHMs there were few reductions in pain intensity and when there were reductions in pooled results, there was heterogeneity and the magnitude of the effect was small (less than 1 point of NRS). For the topical CHMs there was more evidence of reductions in pain intensity, but the magnitudes were still small. This difference may have been due to a greater analgesic effect of topically applied CHMs or it may have simply been due to the larger number of studies of topical CHM providing more power to detect an effect. Whichever the case, the meta-analysis pools tended to be small in terms of numbers of studies and participants. Heterogeneity also limited confidence in the findings. These limitations were reflected in the GRADE assessments.

Another main category of outcome measure was analgesic dose. This was reported in multiple studies but the methods of reporting were variable, leading to few opportunities for data pooling. In general, there were reductions or no differences in both the oral and topical CHM studies, blinded and open-label, and there were no examples of increases. This suggests that the analgesic effects of the CHMs allowed reductions in conventional medication use but the data were based mainly on single studies and due to the variations in the way analgesic dose was measured and the units used, the magnitudes of the effects were not comparable between studies. Therefore, it was not possible to use this outcome to determine which CHMs showed the greatest analgesic effects.

Quality of life was assessed for the included studies. Very few data were available for the oral CHMs with the only poolable data showing an improvement in KPS. For the topical CHMs more poolable data were available. These indicated an improvement on QLQ-C30 and on KPS but no significant change on the Chinese scale. However, all these pools were marred by heterogeneity, so we can only conclude that the effects were variable from study to study. In retrospect, the main way the CHMs could have improved QOL in people with advanced cancers and pain, would be via pain relief. As the results showed, the magnitude of additional pain relief was small and did not reach statistical significance in a substantial proportion of studies. Another avenue would have been reduction of the adverse effects of the analgesic medications, presumably by allowing dose reductions. However, unlike pain, we do not know the proportion of people who experienced such adverse effects at baseline, and what little data we have on this outcome are mixed. In fact, only one study (H12) focused directly on relieving constipation. So, the positive impact of reductions in the adverse effects of analgesics on QOL may have been small. On the other hand, some topical CHMs produced allergic reactions which would have had negative effects on QOL in those who experienced them. Nevertheless, none of the studies showed significant reductions in QOL.

Another limitation to the evidence for CHM was lack of blinding in most studies. Placebo controls were used in only two out of 12 RCTs of oral CHMs and only four out of 17 RCTs of topical CHMs. This lack of blinding likely led to overestimation of effect sizes in favour of the CHM groups. Also, protocols were not available for any of the studies, so we could only assess selective outcome reporting based on correspondence between the methods and the results sections of the published papers.

The quality of the CHMs was poorly reported. The studies generally provided ingredient lists in Chinese but species names were omitted and quality control data were not included. When calculating the frequencies of ingredients, the Chinese names were converted to scientific names based on the main species used, so there may have be regularisation errors.

Safety data were also inadequate. Even in the studies that reported on adverse events, these tended to be for the CHM group only and it was not always clear whether the frequencies of events, or the number of patients who experienced the event, were reported. Also, causal information was limited to the authors' judgement. Therefore, we could not determine how many adverse events were due to the CHM or the interaction between the CHM and the analgesics or other concomitant medications, and which were unlikely to have been caused by the interventions.

In Chapter 7, of the 32 clinical trials of acupuncture and moxibustion, 21 were RCTs. Ten were sham-controlled RCTs while 11 RCTs were open-label. However, opportunities for meta-analysis of data from blinded studies were greatly reduced due to variations in the acupuncture therapies used (traditional acupuncture, ear acupuncture, combined traditional and ear acupuncture, moxibustion), the pain outcome measures (NRS, VAS, BPI scales) and the different measures of QOL. Consequently, pooled results for blinded studies were few and these were only derived from two studies and based on fewer than 200 participants. Also, most of the blinded studies were of AIMSS and there were little poolable data for other types of cancer pain. Therefore, despite a general tendency for the groups that received acupuncture therapies to improve, the evidence was not strong.

Although 16 of the 21 RCTs mentioned safety, variations in the ways adverse events (AEs) were reported made statistical analysis difficult. Nevertheless, the acupuncture interventions appear to have been relatively safe and it is unlikely there were interactions with the conventional therapies.

Clinical studies for other CM therapies (Chapter 8) were limited to two studies of remedial massage by the same research group so very little data were available in this area. Similarly, data for combinations of CM therapies (Chapter 9) were limited to two studies, one of which included an oral CHM and the other included a topical CHM, each combined with other CM therapies. In these studies, it was not possible to determine whether one of the CM interventions provided a greater contribution to the reported effects.

Implications for Practice

The majority of the clinical studies of CHM in Chapter 5 were on its integrative medicine (IM) use in combination with conventional analgesic medications but there were some direct comparisons with placebo and conventional medications. A major difficulty in interpreting the data was the lack of multiple studies of the same CHM intervention using the same comparison.

In most studies the participants had advanced cancers but there were two studies of AIMSS and one of temporomandibular joint (TMJ) disorder.

Both the studies of oral CHMs for AIMSS (H10, H11) found reductions in pain compared to calcium carbonate plus vitamin D3 tablets. Although calcium combined with vitamin D supplementation is commonly prescribed for AIMSS, one recent clinical trial reported no effect[3] while another clinical trial found a benefit but only in the post-hoc analysis.[4] The results for the CHMs were promising but the studies had small sample sizes, were not blinded and were of short duration with the longest (H10) being three months, and the CHMs were different. Consequently, no conclusion could be made.

For TMJ disorder there was one direct comparison between an oral CHM and ibuprofen. The CHM was less effective, but it was not ineffective. It also produced fewer adverse reactions. However, this was based on one open-label study.

In the studies of pain directly due to cancer, most of the assessable data were for pain intensity, analgesic dosage and measures of QOL. As mentioned earlier, it may be unrealistic to expect substantial changes in pain intensity when conventional analgesic medications are used to keep pain tolerable in both groups, so reduction in analgesic medication dose as a proxy measure of analgesic effect can also be considered. In order to short-list the CHMs that showed promise of effectiveness, we have tabulated IM studies that showed significant reductions in pain intensity (on NRS or VAS) plus significant reductions in the dosages of the conventional analgesics (based on at least one measure). We also included one comparison with placebo (Table 10.7).

In the two IM studies of oral CHMs that were placebo-controlled, there were reductions in the dosages of the analgesic medications in both studies (H2, H3) but only one (H3) produced a significant reduction in pain intensity (Table 5.3). In the open-label studies, only H6 satisfied both criteria.

Table 10.7 Chinese Herbal Interventions that Showed Promising Effects[1] on Pain

Study (o/t)	Comparison	CHM	Analgesic	Duration
H3 (o)	IM (placebo)	*Yi shen gu kang fang* 益肾骨康方	OxyContin®	14 days
H6 (o)	IM	*Bu shen huo xue fang* 补肾活血方	OxyContin®	14 days[4]
H13 (t)	Placebo	*Shuang bai san* 双柏散	None[2]	7 days
H15 (t)	IM (placebo)	*Bing chong zhi tong gao* 冰虫止痛膏	Morphine sulfate sustained-release tablets	10 days[3,4,5]
H17 (t)	IM (placebo)	*Xiao pi zhen tong gao* 消痞镇痛膏	OxyContin®	7 days
H19 (t)	IM	*Xiao zheng zhi tong gao* 消症止痛膏	OxyContin®	7 days[4]
H28 (t)	IM	Cataplasm designed by the authors	Intrathecal injections of morphine	4 weeks[3,4]

[1]Includes studies that showed significant reductions in pain intensity (NRS or VAS) plus reduction in dosage of conventional analgesic (any measure), where relevant.
[2]This was a comparison with placebo in mild pain, so no analgesics were used.
[3]Also reduced frequency of breakthrough pain.
[4]Also improved QOL.
[5]One case of skin rash.
Abbreviations: IM, integrative medicine (CHM + conventional analgesic); o, oral CHM; t, topical CHM.

One of the topical CHMs was compared with placebo in mild pain (H13) and produced relief, at least in the short term, but it was unclear whether it would have produced a similar effect in the IM context in moderate to severe pain. In the IM studies of topical CHMs, two placebo-controlled studies showed effects on pain intensity and analgesic dose. One of these (H15) was reported to have also reduced frequency of breakthrough pain and improved QOL on the NCCN scale although there was no difference in KPS. The other study (H19) also produced no significant change in KPS but both studies were of short duration (seven to ten days) so significant changes in KPS may be unrealistic. Two open-label IM studies of topical CHMs were also included. Of these, one (H28) was notable due to its longer duration (four weeks), reduction in breakthrough pain and improved QOL on QLQ-C30.

The CHMs in Table 10.7 did not appear to have produced adverse events other than one case of skin rash (H15) but as mentioned earlier, safety data were inadequate in many studies. Therefore, while this shortlist of CHMs provides a summary of the best available clinical evidence in cancer pain, it is not possible to recommend particular CHMs.

For acupuncture, the clinical studies suggest that acupuncture therapies can improve cancer pain outcomes but the results from the blinded studies were based mainly on single studies, and relatively small meta-analysis pools (Tables 7.3 and 7.11) with heterogeneity. For AIMSS, there were six RCTs but poolable data were limited and results were sometimes conflicting (Tables 7.16 and 7.17). For QOL, a diversity of measures was used and data pooling was generally not feasible. While there were some significant improvements (Table 7.5) some other results showed no significant changes. Both studies of moxibustion (one blinded, one open-label) reported reductions in pain intensity. The open-label study also found an improvement in QOL. Based on the available data it was not possible to determine whether acupuncture, ear acupuncture, moxibustion or any combination of these was more effective. However, the acupuncture interventions appeared not to have produced any serious AEs so the benefits, even if small, may outweigh the risks. In terms of point selection, the frequency analyses of the acupuncture points used (Tables 10.4 and 10.5) showed that certain points were much more frequent inclusions in clinical studies than other points, so these could be considered for clinical practice.

With regard to other CM therapies (Chapter 8), the only evidence was for remedial massage (*an mo* 按摩) delivered in a hospital context. This improved pain on VAS measured 20 minutes after each 45-minute massage session and improved relaxation when compared to a group who received social attention for an equivalent duration. Unfortunately, the RCT did not provide any longer-term data, although the pilot study suggested an effect may continue for 16–18 hours. The intervention appeared safe provided the practitioner was well trained and avoided strong pressure and lesions.

Implications for Research

Only a small proportion of the clinical studies was adequately blinded. This made it difficult to interpret the results. Future studies should implement adequate blinding. In the studies of orally administered CHM decoctions a suitable control intervention may be difficult to design due the distinctive smell and taste of such decoctions but when manufactured medicines are used, placebo controls are feasible, and these are also feasible when topical cataplasms are used. The use of placebo to facilitate blinding of participants and personnel is an important aspect of trial design to prevent the overestimation of effect sizes and increase confidence that the effects were likely due to the intervention and not just non-specific effects of receiving treatment.[5] Although some included studies did use placebo controls, none reported on the effectiveness of the blinding and it was unclear who, other than the participants, were blinded.

Similarly, acupuncture 'sham' devices have been developed to facilitate blinding,[6,7] some of which were used in the clinical studies in Chapter 7. Unlike orally administered placebo interventions, it is controversial whether 'sham' acupuncture is a type of inert placebo or a type of acupuncture therapy.[8] This is especially problematic in pain, since many named and unnamed local painful points are used for pain and traditional acupuncture did not necessarily require skin penetration. Therefore, it can be difficult to select an acupuncture-like intervention that can achieve blinding and employ an intervention that could not be effective in reducing pain.

In general, the reporting of trial methodology was not adequate in the included studies. The methods used for the generation of the randomisation sequence and the concealment of allocation, and the statistical methods all should be described. The reasons for drop-outs need to be detailed and the analysis should be based on intention to treat (ITT). Only a few of the included studies had trial registration and/or an available protocol. Hence it was difficult to determine whether all outcomes were reported and not just those that favoured the test intervention.[9]

Other inadequacies in the studies of CHMs related to herbal nomenclature and quality control. The ingredients of the CHMs should be described unambiguously using scientific names plus the part used, and any processing. The methods for ensuring the quality of the CHM in terms of its ingredients, the manufacture or preparation of the intervention and an analysis of the chemical constituents should be provided.[10,11]

The information required when reporting on clinical trials is detailed in the Consolidated Standards of Reporting Trials (CONSORT)[12] and the extensions for herbal medicine[13] and acupuncture.[14,15] Lack of endorsement of CONSORT by most Chinese journals has been a contributing factor to the lack of detail in reports of Chinese medicine clinical trials.[16] By improving reporting standards, researchers can make their work more relevant to an international audience and improve the impact of their research.

As Table 10.2 illustrated, few of the CHM interventions listed in the guideline and textbooks (Chapter 2) have been investigated in clinical trials of cancer pain (Chapters 5 and 9). A likely reason is many trials were investigator-initiated and motivated by discovery of novel formulations. Nevertheless, the efficacy of established CHM formulas needs to be tested. One approach could be three-arm studies which include an established CHM and a novel CHM. It is also important to test the effects of syndrome differentiation. Although some of the included CHM studies applied syndrome differentiation, we do not know whether this improved the outcomes compared to the general application of the same formula.

Another disjunction between research and practice was between the clinical and experimental research into CHMs. Whereas the clinical studies mainly used multi-ingredient formulas, the experimental studies (Chapter 6) focused on extracts of single herbs or single compounds. All of the herbs included in Chapter 6 showed evidence of pain-relieving effects in animal models but we cannot simply conclude that these accounted for the effects reported in the clinical studies. While it is important to take a drug discovery approach to the isolation of promising compounds, it is also important to consider how combinations of herbs may act in concert to improve analgesia. Another field for experimental research is the investigation of the herbs used in combination with opioids and other analgesic medications to determine if there are any interactions, both detrimental and beneficial. This is of particular importance since CHMs are typically used in an integrative setting.

In addition, the majority of the CHM formulas were used topically whereas in most, but not all, of the experimental studies, the herbs were administered orally or by intraperitoneal (i.p.) injection. Considering the possible advantages of the topical route, the use of novel methods of topical delivery may be a promising field for further research.

For acupuncture, the findings of the available clinical studies suggest that at least some acupuncture interventions reduced pain associated with various cancers but most of the higher-quality studies were for AIMSS. While there have been multiple studies on metastatic cancer pain, only single RCTs were included for pain due to pancreatic cancer, non-small cell lung cancer, gastric cancer and malignant neuropathic pain. These are all areas that require further clinical research. There is also scope for comparing different types and/or combinations of acupuncture therapies in three-arm studies to determine which is more effective.

References

1. 中华中医药学会. (2008) 肿瘤中医诊疗指南. 北京: 中国中医药出版社.
2. 孙燕. (2001) 内科肿瘤学. 北京: 人民卫生出版, pp. 996–997.
3. Shapiro AC, Adlis SA, Robien K, *et al.* (2016) Randomized, blinded trial of vitamin D3 for treating aromatase inhibitor-associated musculoskeletal symptoms (AIMSS). *Breast Cancer Res Treat* **155(3):** 501–512.
4. Khan QJ, Kimler BF, Reddy PS, *et al.* (2017) Randomized trial of vitamin D3 to prevent worsening of musculoskeletal symptoms in women with breast cancer receiving adjuvant letrozole: The vital trial. *Breast Cancer Res Treat* **166(2):** 491–500.
5. Bian ZX, Moher D, Dagenais S, *et al.* (2006) Improving the quality of randomized controlled trials in Chinese herbal medicine, part ii: Control group design. *Zhong Xi Yi Jie He Xue Bao* **4(2):** 130–136.
6. Zhang CS, Yang AW, Zhang AL, *et al.* (2014) Sham control methods used in ear-acupuncture/ear-acupressure randomized controlled trials: A systematic review. *J Altern Complement Med* **20(3):** 147–161.
7. Zhang CS, Tan HY, Zhang GS, *et al.* (2015) Placebo devices as effective control methods in acupuncture clinical trials: A systematic review. *PloS One* **10(11):** e0140825.
8. Zhang GS, Zhang CS, Tan HY, *et al.* (2018) Systematic review of acupuncture placebo devices with a focus on the credibility of blinding of healthy participants and/or acupuncturists. *Acupunct Med* **36(4):** 204–214.
9. Ellenberg SS. (2012) Protecting clinical trial participants and protecting data integrity: Are we meeting the challenges? *PloS Med* **9(6):** e1001234.
10. Wolsko PM, Solondz DK, Phillips RS, *et al.* (2005) Lack of herbal supplement characterization in published randomized controlled trials. *Am J Med* **118(10):** 1087–1093.
11. Leung KS, Bian ZX, Moher D, *et al.* (2006) Improving the quality of randomized controlled trials in Chinese herbal medicine, part iii: Quality control of Chinese herbal medicine used in randomized controlled trials. *Zhong Xi Yi Jie He Xue Bao* **4(3):** 225–232.
12. Schulz KF, Altman DG, Moher D, Group C. (2010) Consort 2010 statement: Updated guidelines for reporting parallel group randomised trials. *Trials* **11:** 32.
13. Gagnier JJ, Boon H, Rochon P, *et al.* (2006) Reporting randomized, controlled trials of herbal interventions: An elaborated consort statement. *Ann Intern Med* **144(5):** 364–367.

14. MacPherson H, White A, Cummings M, *et al.* (2002) Standards for reporting interventions in controlled trials of acupuncture: The STRICTA recommendations. *J Altern Complement Med* **8(1):** 85–89.
15. MacPherson H, Altman DG, Hammerschlag R, *et al.* (2010) Revised standards for reporting interventions in clinical trials of acupuncture (STRICTA): Extending the CONSORT statement. *J Evid Based Med* **3(3):** 140–155.
16. Chen M, Cui J, Zhang AL, *et al.* (2018) Adherence to CONSORT items in randomized controlled trials of integrative medicine for colorectal cancer published in Chinese journals. *J Altern Complement Med* **24(2):** 115–124.

References to Included Studies

Study Number	Reference
H1	陈琦, 吴芸. (2015) 肿痛安治疗癌症放射治疗后颞下颌关节疼痛的疗效评价. 国际口腔医学杂志 **42(1):** 24–27.
H2	吴敏华, 周月芬, 陈旭烽, 朱月娇, 谢艳茹, 涂建飞. (2013) 柴胡疏肝散辅助芬太尼透皮贴治疗肝癌疼痛. 中西医结合肝病杂志 **23(2):** 83–85.
H3	宋洪丽, 殷玉琨, 周磊, 冯利. (2018) 益肾骨康方联合盐酸羟考酮缓释片治疗中重度癌性躯体痛肾虚血瘀证患者随机对照双盲临床研究. 中医杂志 **59(15):** 1300–1303.
H4	黄敏. (2007) 益气化瘀法配合美施康定治疗中重度癌性疼痛的临床研究. 学位论文. 南京中医药大学 13–21.
H5	李伟锋. (2016) 加减清骨散治疗阴虚内热型骨转移癌痛的临床研究. 学位论文. 广州中医药大学 20–28.
H6	宋程. (2016) 补肾活血方治疗骨转移癌痛临床疗效及镇痛机制研究. 学位论文. 湖南中医药大学 2–10.
H7	王卫华, 周小伟. (2012) 活血行气化瘀法治疗癌性疼痛疗效分析. 山东中医杂志 **31(10):** 725–727.
H8	阿依宝塔·努腊勒木. (2018) 柴胡疏肝散加味治疗肝癌肝郁气滞型癌痛的临床研究. 学位论文. 新疆医科大学 5–13.
H10	赵炜, 关念波, 周蕴明, 张美英. (2018) 强骨止痛方治疗芳香化酶抑制剂所致乳腺癌骨丢失性疼痛. 中国中西医结合外科杂志 **24(1):** 15–20.
H11	钟莹, 郭智涛, 黄映飞, 梁喆盈, 吴玢. (2017) 补肾强筋胶囊治疗乳腺癌芳香化酶抑制剂相关骨关节症状的临床观察. 中医药导报 **23(8):** 38, 39,43.

(*Continued*)

Study Number	Reference
H12	张翔, 李和根, 顾芳红. (2016) 养阴理气汤治疗阿片性便秘的临床研究. 山东中医杂志 **35(2):** 104–107.
H13	冯丽红. (2012) 双柏散外敷为主治疗肝癌轻度癌痛的疗效观察. 学位论文. 广州中医药大学 10–24.
H14	张莹. (2004) 化坚拔毒膜对癌性疼痛的干预作用及其机理研究. 学位论文. 天津中医学院 253–267.
H15	唐倩. (2013) 冰虫止痛膏外用辅助治疗局部癌性疼痛的临床研究. 学位论文. 北京中医药大学 53–70.
H16	王院春, 王希胜, 李仁廷, 惠建荣. (2014) 乌香痛消膏外治癌性疼痛 40 例. 山东中医杂志 **33(3):** 188–189.
H17	宋琳, 蒋益兰, 王容容. (2017) 消痞镇痛膏外敷联合奥施康定片治疗肺癌重度疼痛 30 例临床观察. 中医杂志 **58(21):** 1846–1849.
H19	黄逸姣. (2013) 消症止痛膏联合羟考酮控释片对中重度癌性疼痛的临床研究. 学位论文. 南京中医药大学 16–30.
H23	田娇. (2015) 骨痛贴外用治疗阴寒凝滞型癌性躯体痛的临床观察. 学位论文. 北京中医药大学 31–49.
H28	车瑾, 徐洋, 曹蔚, 洪帆, 秦婷婷. (2018) 鞘内注射阿片类药物联合自拟中药穴位贴敷对中重度癌性疼痛、睡眠和生活质量的影响. 现代中西医结合杂志 **27(18):** 1949–1953.
H30	苏新平, 邓天好, 谭达全. (2016) 中医内外兼治气虚血瘀型骨转移癌痛 56 例临床观察. 中医药导报 **22(1):** 33–35.
H33	刘嘉湘, 郁诗玲, 徐振晔, 施志明. (1985) 蟾酥消肿膏治疗晚期恶性肿瘤疼痛 187 例疗效观察. 辽宁中医杂志 **4:** 30–31.
A1	Hershman DL, Unger JM, Greenlee H, *et al.* (2018) Effect of acupuncture vs sham acupuncture or waitlist control on joint pain related to aromatase inhibitors among women with early-stage breast cancer. *JAMA* **320(2):** 167.
A9	王敬, 芦殿荣, 毕然, 舒晓宁. (2015) 耳穴埋豆干预骨转移中重度癌性疼痛临床观察 30 例. 云南中医中药杂志 **36(2):** 43–45.
A10	Lee J, Yoon SW. (2014) Efficacy and safety of moxibustion for relieving pain in patients with metastatic cancer: A pilot, randomized, single-blind, sham-controlled trial. *Integr Cancer Ther* **13(3):** 211–216.

(*Continued*)

(*Continued*)

Study Number	Reference
A11	Mao JJ, Xie SX, Farrar JT, *et al.* (2014) A randomised trial of electro-acupuncture for arthralgia related to aromatase inhibitor use. *Eur J Cancer* **50(2):** 267–276.
A12	Bao T, Cai L, Giles JT, *et al.* (2013) A dual-center randomized controlled double blind trial assessing the effect of acupuncture in reducing musculoskeletal symptoms in breast cancer patients taking aromatase inhibitors. *Breast Cancer Res Treat* **138(1):** 167–174.
A14	Oh B, Kimble B, Costa DS, *et al.* (2013) Acupuncture for treatment of arthralgia secondary to aromatase inhibitor therapy in women with early breast cancer: Pilot study. *Acupunct Med* **31(3):** 264–271.
A16	朱利楠, 王瑞林, 宗红, 樊青霞. (2013) 磁珠耳穴贴压联合奥施康定治疗癌症神经病理性疼痛的疗效观察. 中华物理医学与康复杂志 **35(7):** 579–581.
A18	Crew KD, Capodice JL, Greenlee H, *et al.* (2010) Randomized, blinded, sham-controlled trial of acupuncture for the management of aromatase inhibitor-associated joint symptoms in women with early-stage breast cancer. *J Clin Oncol* **28(7):** 1154–1160.
A19	Pfister DG, Cassileth BR, Deng GE, *et al.* (2010) Acupuncture for pain and dysfunction after neck dissection: Results of a randomized controlled trial. *J Clin Oncol* **28(15):** 2565–2570.
A20	Crew KD, Capodice JL, Greenlee H, *et al.* (2007) Pilot study of acupuncture for the treatment of joint symptoms related to adjuvant aromatase inhibitor therapy in postmenopausal breast cancer patients. *J Cancer Surviv* **1(4):** 283–291.
A24	Su CF. (2018) Home care with acupuncture increased the quality of life in a patient with advanced cancer with neuropathic pain induced by bone metastasis: A case report. *J Integr Med* **16(3):** 208–210.
A28	Paley CA, Johnson MI. (2011) Acupuncture for cancer-induced bone pain: A pilot study. *Acupunct Med* **29(1):** 71–73.
A29	Tuck CM. (2010) A 54-year-old woman with degenerative back pain. *Acupunct Med* **28(1):** 46–48.
A30	Mao JJ, D. Bruner DW, Stricker C, *et al.* (2009) Feasibility trial of electroacupuncture for aromatase inhibitor-related arthralgia in breast cancer survivors. *Integr Cancer Ther* **8(2):** 123–129.
C1	吴文通, 王芳, 钱尤. (2017) 中西医结合治疗中重度癌痛的临床疗效观察. 中华中医药学刊 **35(2):** 492–494.

Glossary

Term	Acronym	Definition	Reference
95% confidence interval	95% CI	A measure of the uncertainty around the main finding of a statistical analysis. Estimates of unknown quantities, such as the odds ratio comparing an experimental intervention with a control, are usually presented as a point estimate and a 95% confidence interval. This means that if someone were to keep repeating a study in other samples from the same population, 95% of the confidence intervals from those studies would contain the truc value of the unknown quantity. Alternatives to 95%, such as 90% and 99% confidence intervals, are sometimes used. Wider intervals indicate lower precision; narrow intervals, greater precision.	http://handbook.cochrane.org/Version 5.1
Acupressure	—	Application of pressure on acupuncture points.	—

(*Continued*)

(*Continued*)

Term	Acronym	Definition	Reference
Acupuncture	—	The insertion of needles into humans or animals for remedial purposes.	World Health Organisation. (2007) WHO International Standard Terminologies of Traditional Medicine in the Western Pacific Region.
Allied and Complementary Medicine Database	AMED	Alternative medicine bibliographic database.	https://www.ebsco.com/products/research-databases/allied-and-complementary-medicine-database-amed
Aromatase inhibitor-associated musculoskeletal symptoms	AIMSS	Musculoskeletal symptoms such as pain and/or inflammation mainly in the joints, as a side effect of the use of aromatase inhibitors (such as anastrozole) to reduce the risk of breast cancer recurrence.	—
Australian New Zealand Clinical Trial Registry	ANZCTR	Clinical trial registry based in Australia.	http://www.anzctr.org.au/
China National Knowledge Infrastructure	CNKI	Chinese-language bibliographic database.	www.cnki.net
Chinese Biomedical Literature Database	CBM	Chinese-language bibliographic database.	https://cbmwww.imicams.ac.cn
Chinese Clinical Trial Registry	ChiCTR	Chinese clinical trial registry.	http://www.chictr.org
Chinese herbal medicine	CHM	System of herbal medicine used in China and other countries in eastern Asia.	—
Chinese medicine	CM	Traditional system of medicine native to China.	—

(*Continued*)

Term	Acronym	Definition	Reference
Chongqing VIP Information Company	CQVIP	Chinese-language bibliographic database.	www.cqvip
ClinicalTrials.gov	—	Clinical trial registry based in the United States.	https://clinicaltrials.gov/
Cochrane Central Register of Controlled Trials	CENTRAL	Bibliographic database that provides a highly concentrated source of reports of controlled trials.	https://community.cochrane.org/editorial-and-publishing-policy-resource/overview-cochrane-library-and-related-content/databases-included-cochrane-library/cochrane-central-register-controlled-trials-central
Combination therapies	—	Two or more Chinese medicines from different therapy groups (e.g. Chinese herbal medicine, acupuncture therapies or other Chinese medicine therapies) administered together.	—
Convention on International Trade in Endangered Species of Wild Fauna and Flora	CITES	International convention aimed at preventing or regulating trade in threatened and endangered species of plants and animals.	https://www.cites.org/eng/disc/text.php
Controlled clinical trial	CCT	A study in which people are allocated to different intervention groups using methods that are not random.	http://handbook.cochrane.org/

(*Continued*)

(*Continued*)

Term	Acronym	Definition	Reference
Cumulative Index of Nursing and Allied Health Literature	CINAHL	Bibliographic database.	https://www.ebscohost.com/nursing/products/cinahl-databases
Cupping therapy	—	Suction by using a vaccumised cup or jar.	World Health Organisation. (2007) WHO International Standard Terminologies of Traditional Medicine in the Western Pacific Region.
Effect size	—	A generic term for the estimate of the effect of a treatment in a study.	http://handbook.cochrane.org/
Effective rate	—	A measure of the proportion of participants who achieved an improvement.	—
Electroacupuncture	EA	Electric stimulation of the acupuncture needle following insertion.	World Health Organisation. (2007) WHO International Standard Terminologies of Traditional Medicine in the Western Pacific Region.
EU Clinical Trials Register	EU-CTR	European union clinical trial registry.	https://www.clinicaltrialsregister.eu
Excerpta Medica database	Embase	Bibliographic database.	http://www.elsevier.com/solutions/embase
Grading of Recommendations Assessment, Development and Evaluation	GRADE	Approach used to grade quality of evidence and strength of recommendations.	http://www.gradeworkinggroup.org/

(*Continued*)

Term	Acronym	Definition	Reference
Health-related quality of life	HR-QOL	A conceptual or operational measurement that is commonly used in a health care setting as a means to assess the impact of disease on the person.	Brooker C. Mosby. (2010) *Mosby's Dictionary of Medicine, Nursing and Health Professions*. Elsevier, United Kingdom.
Heterogeneity	—	Used in a general sense to describe the variation in, or diversity of, participants, interventions and measurement of outcomes across a set of studies, or the variation in the internal validity of those studies. Used specifically, as statistical heterogeneity, to describe the degree of variation in the effect estimates from a set of studies. Also used to indicate the presence of variability among studies beyond the amount expected due solely to the play of chance.	https://training.cochrane.org/handbook Version 5.1
I^2	—	A measure of study heterogeneity that indicates the percentage of variance in a meta-analysis.	https://training.cochrane.org/handbook Version 5.1
Integrative medicine	IM	Chinese medicine combined with pharmacotherapy or other conventional therapy.	—

(*Continued*)

(*Continued*)

Term	Acronym	Definition	Reference
Karnofsky Performance Status	KPS	A descriptive scale used to determine the ability of a patient to tolerate chemotherapy. Relates to ability to carry out activities of daily living.	Yates JW, Chalmer B, Mckegney FP. (1980) Evaluation of patients with advanced cancer using the Karnofsky performance status. *Cancer* **45(8):** 2220–2224.
Mean difference	MD	In meta-analysis, a method used to combine measures on continuous scales, where the mean, standard deviation and sample size in each group are known.	https://training.cochrane.org/handbook Version 5.1
Meta-analysis	—	The use of statistical techniques in a systematic review to integrate the results of included studies. Sometimes misused as a synonym for systematic reviews, where the review includes a meta-analysis.	—
Moxibustion	—	A therapeutic procedure involving ignited material (usually moxa) to apply heat to certain points or areas of the body surface for managing disease.	World Health Organisation. (2007) WHO International Standard Terminologies of Traditional Medicine in the Western Pacific Region.
National Comprehensive Cancer Network	NCCN	Alliance of leading cancer centres that issues guidelines for CRC and other cancers.	https://www.nccn.org/

(*Continued*)

Term	Acronym	Definition	Reference
National Institutes of Health and National Cancer Institute Common Terminology Criteria for Adverse Events	NCI-CTCAE criteria	Series of criteria for evaluating adverse events associated with cancer therapy.	National Institutes of Health and National Cancer Institute. (2008) Common terminology criteria for adverse events (CTCAE), version 4. National Institutes of Health, MD.
Non-controlled studies	—	Observations made on individuals, usually receiving the same intervention, before and after the intervention but with no control group.	http://handbook.cochrane.org/
Non-steroidal anti-inflammatory drug	NSAID	Non-steroidal anti-inflammatory drugs include commonly used analgesics such as aspirin, paracetamol (acetaminophen) and ibuprofen.	—
Numerical rating scale	NRS	Numerical rating scale for rating pain intensity	See NCCN guidelines at https://www.nccn.org/
Opioid-induced constipation	OIC	A side effect of the use of opioids such as morphine.	—
Other Chinese medicine therapies	—	Other Chinese medicine therapies include all traditional therapies except Chinese herbal medicine and acupuncture/moxibustion, such as *tai chi, qi gong, tui na* and cupping.	—
Oxycodone hydrochloride extended-release tablets	Oxycodone HCl extended-release tablets	Generic name for tablets containing oxycodone hydrochloride that are known by the trade name OxyContin®	—

(*Continued*)

(*Continued*)

Term	Acronym	Definition	Reference
PubMed	PubMed	Bibliographic database.	http://www.ncbi.nlm.nih.gov/pubmed
Qi gong 气功	—	A type of other Chinese medicine therapy that typically involves physical exercises and breathing techniques.	—
Randomised controlled trial	RCT	Clinical trial that uses a random method to allocate participants to treatment and control groups.	—
Risk of bias	—	Assessment of clinical trials to indicate if results may overestimate or underestimate the true effect because of bias in study design or reporting.	https://training.cochrane.org/handbook Version 5.1
Risk ratio (relative risk)	RR	The ratio of risks in two groups. In intervention studies, it is the ratio of the risk in the intervention group to the risk in the control group. A risk ratio of 1 indicates no difference between comparison groups. For undesirable outcomes, a risk ratio that is less than 1 indicates that the intervention was effective in reducing the risk of that outcome.	https://training.cochrane.org/handbook version 5.1
Skeletal-related event	SRE	SREs are complications of cancer that affect the bones including: pathological fracture, the need for radiotherapy to bone (to relieve pain), the need for surgery to bone (to relieve pain), spinal cord compression and hypercalcaemia.	—

(*Continued*)

Term	Acronym	Definition	Reference
Summary of findings	SoF	Presentation of results and rating the quality of evidence based on the GRADE approach.	http://www.gradeworkinggroup.org/
Standardised mean difference	SMD	Similar to mean difference (MD). Used when different instruments are used to measure the same construct. The SMD expresses the intervention effect in standard units rather than the original units of measurement. As a rule of thumb, an SMD of 0.2 represents a small effect, 0.5 a moderate effect and 0.8 a large effect.	https://training.cochrane.org/handbook Version 5.1
Tai chi 太极 (*tai ji* 太极)	—	A Chinese martial art with health benefits.	—
Transcutaneous electrical nerve stimulation	TENS	Application of transdermal electrical current to acupuncture points via conducting pads.	—
Tui na 推拿	—	Chinese massage: rubbing, kneading or percussion of the soft tissues and joints of the body with the hands, usually performed by one person on another, especially to relieve tension or pain.	World Health Organisation. (2007) WHO International Standard Terminologies of Traditional Medicine in the Western Pacific Region.
Visual analogue scale	VAS	Measurement system used for many symptoms but in this book the VAS is for rating pain severity/intensity.	See NCCN guidelines at https://www.nccn.org/
Wangfang database	Wanfang	Chinese-language bibliographic database.	www.wanfangdata.com

(*Continued*)

(*Continued*)

Term	Acronym	Definition	Reference
World Health Organisation	WHO	WHO is the directing and coordinating authority for health within the United Nations system. It is responsible for providing leadership on global health matters, shaping the health research agenda, setting norms and standards, articulating evidence-based policy options, providing technical support to countries, and monitoring and assessing health trends. It has issued a range of criteria for assessing outcomes in cancer.	http://www.who.int/about/en/
Zhong Hua Yi Dian 中华医典	ZHYD	The ZHYD [*Encyclopaedia of Traditional Chinese Medicine*] is a comprehensive series of electronic books on compact disk. The collection was put together by the Hunan electronic and audio-visual publishing house. It is the largest collection of Chinese electronic books and includes the major Chinese ancient works, many of which are from rare manuscripts and are the only existing copies. These books cover the period from ancient times up to the period of the Republic of China (1911–1948).	Hu R, ed. (2014) *Zhong Hua Yi Dian* [*Encyclopaedia of Traditional Chinese Medicine*], 5th ed. Hunan Electronic and Audio-Visual Publishing House, Chengsha.

(*Continued*)

Term	Acronym	Definition	Reference
Zhong Yi Fang Ji Da Ci Dian 中医方剂大辞典	ZYFJDCD	Compendium of Chinese herbal formulas with over 96,592 entries derived from classical Chinese books. The Nanjing Chinese Medicine Institute compiled the ZYFJDCD and first published it in 1993.	Peng HR, ed. (1994) *Zhong Yi Fang Ji Da Ci Dian* [*Great Compendium of Chinese Medical Formulae*]. People's Medical Publishing House, Beijing.

Index

Evidence-based Clinical Chinese Medicine

(*Continued from page ii*)

Vol. 12 *Post-Stroke Shoulder Complications*
Lead Authors: Claire Shuiqing Zhang and Shaonan Liu

Vol. 13 *Post-Stroke Spasticity*
Lead Authors: Claire Shuiqing Zhang and Shaonan Liu

Vol. 14 *Unipolar Depression*
Lead Authors: Yuan Ming Di and Lingling Yang

Vol. 15 *Chronic Heart Failure*
Lead Authors: Claire Shuiqing Zhang and Liuling Ma

Vol. 16 *Atopic Dermatitis*
Lead Authors: Meaghan Coyle and Junfeng Liu

Vol. 17 *Colorectal Cancer*
Lead Authors: Brian H May and Yihong Liu

Vol. 18 *Cancer Pain*
Lead Authors: Brian H May and Yihong Liu

Vol. 20 *Chronic Cough*
Lead Authors: Johannah Shergis and Yuanbin Chen

Vol. 22 *Urinary Tract Infection*
Lead Authors: Meaghan Coyle and Xindong Qin

Vol. 23 *Episodic Migraine*
Lead Authors: Claire Shuiqing Zhang and Shaohua Lyu

Vol. 24 *Menopause*
Lead Authors: Meaghan Coyle and Jian Liu

Vol. 29 *Cervical Radiculopathy*
Lead Authors: Claire Shuiqing Zhang and Dihui Zhang

Forthcoming

Vol. 25 *Rhinosinusitis*
Lead Authors: Brian H May and Wenmin Lin

Vol. 28 *Endometriosis*
Lead Authors: Meaghan Coyle and Yongxia Wang

Lightning Source UK Ltd.
Milton Keynes UK
UKHW020624191021
392457UK00001B/50